Contents

KU-319-996

Contents

Introduction vii

1000 MCQs for
DAVIDSON'S
Principles and Practice of
Medicine

M.J. Ford MD FRCPE

Consultant Physician, Eastern General Hospital, Edinburgh
Honorary Senior Lecturer, Edinburgh University, Edinburgh

A.T. Elder MB ChB FRCPE

Consultant Physician, Eastern General Hospital, Edinburgh
Honorary Senior Lecturer, Edinburgh University, Edinburgh

BRITISH SCHOOL OF OSTEOPATHY
4 SUFFOLK ST., LONDON. SW1Y 4HG
TEL. 01-930 9254-8

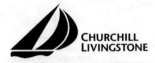
CHURCHILL LIVINGSTONE

NEW YORK EDINBURGH LONDON MADRID MELBOURNE SAN FRANCISCO AND TOKYO 1997

CHURCHILL LIVINGSTONE
Medical Division of Pearson Professional Limited

Distributed in the United States of America by Churhcill
Livingstone Inc., 650 Avenue of the Americas, New York,
N.Y. 10011, and by associated companies, branches and
representatives throughout the world.

This edition published 1997
Previously published as 1200 MCQs in Medicine
Standard edition ISBN 0 443 05462 2

International Student Edition first published 1997
International Student Edition ISBN 0 443 05556 4

British Library Cataloguing in Publication Data
A catalogue record for this book is available from the British
Library

Library of Congress Cataloging in Publication Data
A catalog record for this book is available from the Library of
Congress

Medical knowledge is constantly changing. As new
information becomes available, changes in treatment,
procedures, equipment and the use of drugs become
necessary. The authors and the publishers have, as far as it
is possible, taken care to ensure that the information given in
th text is accurate and up to date. However, readers are
strongly advised to confirm that the information, especially
with regard to drug usage, complies with current legislation
and standards of practice.

The
publisher's
policy is to use
**paper manufactured
from sustainable forests**

Printed by Thomson Press (India) Ltd.

Introduction

Since the book of multiple choice questions supplementing *Davidson's Principles and Practice of Medicine* by Dr P.R. Fleming was first published, medical knowledge has continued to grow at an exponential rate. MCQ companion books to medical textbooks remain both popular and useful methods of self-assessment for medical undergraduates and postgraduates. The aim of this book, like that of its predecessor, is to help students increase the efficiency with which they acquire the factual knowledge necessary for good medical practice. The questions have been arranged to correspond with the chapters of *Davidson's Principles and Practice of Medicine* 17th Edition, and are largely based on the contents of these chapters. In addition, annotated answers have been compiled to enhance the educational value of the book. Most of the answers can be found within the text of *Davidson's*, those that cannot will be found in other popular textbooks of clinical medicine.

The principles and technique

Multiple choice questions are widely used for examination purposes as a reliable and discriminatory test of factual knowledge. Lack of familiarity with the MCQ format may result in unexpected failure, though more usually failure is attributable to a lack of adequate reading and understanding of clinical medicine and the basic sciences. Familiarity with the technique of MCQ examinations is no substitute for the systematic study required to achieve a thorough understanding of medicine.

- Read each stem question and the five items carefully. The questions have been carefully worded to avoid ambiguity and have not been designed to trick the unwary.
- Identify the items which you can answer with confidence and record the answer 'TRUE' or 'FALSE' as appropriate.
- Identify those items to which you do not know the answers. Do not guess the answer if you know nothing about the subject matter. Record the answer 'DO NOT KNOW' and move to the next item.
- There will be items with answers which you may feel you know but lack confidence. After due consideration, record your answer providing this is not a blind guess but informed and intuitive reasoning.
- Concentrate on each stem and item in turn rather than passing quickly from question to question. It is easier to concentrate on the problem in hand than to juggle with several unrelated questions simultaneously.

How to use this book

Students preparing themselves for examinations are recommended to read the appropriate chapters of the textbooks and then to assess themselves using the MCQ technique described.

Record your answers and your reasoning before checking the correct answer. Then return to the appropriate section of a medical textbook and read the relevant text for a more detailed explanation.

SECTION 1
QUESTIONS

1 GENETIC FACTORS IN DISEASE

ANSWERS BEGIN ON P. 142

1.

In humans

Ⓐ somatic cell nuclei contain 22 pairs of homologous autosomes

Ⓑ gamete nuclei are haploid with a single X or Y chromosome

Ⓒ the haploid male cell (sperm) contains 22 autosomes and a Y chromosome

Ⓓ pairing of homologous chromosomes occurs during mitosis

Ⓔ both X chromosomes in females are genetically active

2.

In the chromosomal disorders

Ⓐ aneuploidy is the addition or loss of a chromosome

Ⓑ deletions arise from the loss of a segment of a chromosome

Ⓒ the majority of affected conceptions result in miscarriage

Ⓓ identical deletions produce the same effects whether inherited from father or mother

Ⓔ translocation is the exchange of segments between chromosomes

3.

The karyotype of a

Ⓐ human is usually identified using bone marrow cells

Ⓑ female with Down's syndrome is 46,XX,−21

Ⓒ male with Klinefelter's syndrome is 47,XXY

Ⓓ female with Turner's syndrome is 45,X

Ⓔ male with Trisomy 18 (Edwards syndrome) is 47,XX,+18

4.

Which of the following conclusions can be deduced from the pedigree shown below?

Ⓐ the proband was a female in whom the disease was present

Ⓑ the proband's grandparents were consanguineous

Ⓒ one of the proband's parents had died of the disease

Ⓓ the proband was a monozygotic twin

Ⓔ the disease is transmitted in an autosomal recessive pattern

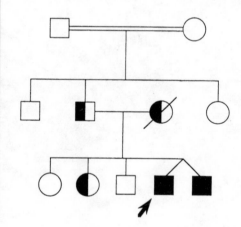

5.

In X-linked dominant inheritance

Ⓐ there is a 50% chance of an affected mother having an affected child

Ⓑ affected children of an affected mother will all be female

Ⓒ affected children of an affected father can be of either sex

Ⓓ male to male transmission occurs frequently

Ⓔ an identical pedigree could be produced by an autosomally transmitted gene

6.

Given the marriage of two heterozygotes carrying the same gene transmitting an autosomal recessive disorder

Ⓐ all of their healthy children will carry the gene

Ⓑ only male children will be affected

Ⓒ each of their children has a 1 in 4 chance of being affected

Ⓓ 75% of families with an only child will have a healthy child

Ⓔ 1 in 16 of their grandchildren will be affected

7.

In autosomal dominant inheritance

Ⓐ affected individuals are usually heterozygotes

Ⓑ affected individuals rarely have an affected parent

Ⓒ male offspring are more likely to be affected than female

Ⓓ unaffected children of an affected parent have a 50% chance of transmitting the condition

Ⓔ clinical disease is always found in genetically affected individuals

8.

In Down's syndrome

Ⓐ non-disjunction of chromosome 21 producing trisomy 21 is the usual cause

Ⓑ translocation accounts for 25% of those affected

Ⓒ translocations often involve chromosomes 21 and 13,14 or 15

Ⓓ the majority of siblings have chromosomal abnormalities

Ⓔ the commonest chromosomal abnormality is polyploidy

9.

Characteristic features of Klinefelter's syndrome include

Ⓐ Fallot's tetralogy

Ⓑ mental retardation

Ⓒ short stature

Ⓓ normal gonadotrophin levels

Ⓔ gynaecomastia

10.

Characteristic features of Turner's syndrome include

Ⓐ primary amenorrhoea

Ⓑ tall stature

Ⓒ webbing of the neck

Ⓓ cubitus valgus

Ⓔ aortic coarctation

11.

Given a husband with haemophilia and his unaffected wife

Ⓐ none of their sons will be affected

Ⓑ all of their daughters will carry the haemophilic gene

Ⓒ a daughter with Turner's syndrome may also have haemophilia

Ⓓ all of his sisters will be carriers

Ⓔ his maternal grandfather could have had haemophilia

12.
The following disorders are transmitted in an autosomal dominant mode
Ⓐ phenylketonuria
Ⓑ polyposis coli
Ⓒ achondroplasia
Ⓓ cystic fibrosis
Ⓔ Marfan's syndrome

13.
The following disorders are transmitted in an X-linked recessive mode
Ⓐ vitamin D resistant rickets
Ⓑ Christmas disease
Ⓒ nephrogenic diabetes insipidus
Ⓓ haemochromatosis
Ⓔ Duchenne muscular dystrophy

14.
The following disorders are transmitted in an autosomal recessive mode
Ⓐ albinism
Ⓑ acute intermittent porphyria
Ⓒ Friedreich's ataxia
Ⓓ Wilson's disease
Ⓔ Gilbert's syndrome

15.
The following disorders are caused by single gene disorders
Ⓐ cleft lip
Ⓑ sickle-cell anaemia
Ⓒ Alzheimer's disease
Ⓓ cystic fibrosis
Ⓔ familial hypercholesterolaemia

16.
In man
Ⓐ each of the 20 amino acids has only one specific DNA triplet codon
Ⓑ during transcription of DNA into RNA, introns are excised
Ⓒ translation of RNA occurs within the cell nucleus
Ⓓ 2–3% of babies have a genetically attributable anomaly
Ⓔ change of a single base pair of DNA can produce clinically detectable disease

17.
The risk of a child developing congenital pyloric stenosis is greater if
Ⓐ the child is female rather than male
Ⓑ the mother rather than the father had the disorder
Ⓒ two siblings rather than one sibling had the disorder
Ⓓ the mother is aged 40 than if she is aged 20
Ⓔ a brother was severely affected rather than mildly affected

18.
In screening for genetic disorders
Ⓐ congenital hypothyroidism is detected by measurement of neonatal thyroxine
Ⓑ asymptomatic carriers of cystic fibrosis can now be identified
Ⓒ the identification of homocystinuria is treated by dietary methionine restriction
Ⓓ haemoglobin electrophoresis is useful in the detection of haemophilia A
Ⓔ ophthalmoscopy is useful in screening the relatives of individuals with familial polyposis coli

19.
Measurement of maternal alpha-fetoprotein is
Ⓐ mandatory in the management of pregnancy
Ⓑ an effective method of diagnosing fetal malformations prenatally
Ⓒ measured at 12 weeks gestation
Ⓓ elevated in neural tube defects of the fetus
Ⓔ elevated in Down's syndrome

20.
The following conditions and genetic markers have been associated with each other
Ⓐ ankylosing spondylitis and HLA B27
Ⓑ peptic ulcer disease and blood group A
Ⓒ atherosclerosis and apolipoprotein A-1
Ⓓ insulin-dependent diabetes mellitus and HLA B8
Ⓔ Reiter's disease and HLA B27

21.

In the laboratory analysis of DNA

Ⓐ restriction endonucleases are used to join small segments of DNA

Ⓑ gene probes must be single stranded to be of use in hybridisation

Ⓒ the polymerase chain reaction is used to amplify small segments of genomic DNA

Ⓓ restriction fragment length polymorphisms are useful in gene tracking

Ⓔ a low recombination fraction suggests that a gene and its marker are closely linked

22.

The following genetic terms are defined as follows

Ⓐ dominant: a trait expressed in a heterozygote

Ⓑ allele: alternative forms of a gene at a given locus

Ⓒ proband: the person who first attracted medical attention to the family

Ⓓ penetrance: frequency of expression of a gene

Ⓔ mosaic: cells of different genotype in a person

23.

Amniocentesis is

Ⓐ usually performed around 16 weeks gestation

Ⓑ best performed with ultrasound guidance

Ⓒ associated with a higher fetal risk than chorionic villus sampling

Ⓓ a useful source of cytological material for genetic analysis

Ⓔ helpful in the diagnosis of Duchenne muscular dystrophy

2 IMMUNOLOGICAL FACTORS IN DISEASE

ANSWERS BEGIN ON P. 145

1.

In the innate immune system

Ⓐ neutrophil leucocytes phagocytose particulate antigens

Ⓑ monocytes develop into tissue macrophages

Ⓒ natural killer cells produce interferons

Ⓓ acute phase proteins bind complement to enhance opsonisation

Ⓔ macrophage-derived interleukin-1 mediates the febrile response

2.

In the adaptive immune system

Ⓐ small granular lymphocytes transform into killer cells

Ⓑ T lymphocytes produce helper, suppressor and cytotoxic cells

Ⓒ helper cells facilitate B cell-mediated killer cell activity

Ⓓ delayed hypersensitivity reactions are mediated by T cells

Ⓔ interleukin-2 is a lymphokine stimulating B cell proliferation

3.

The following statements about immunoglobulins are true

Ⓐ They are secreted by transformed T lymphocytes

Ⓑ IgA is produced by B cells in the lamina propria of the gut

Ⓒ IgG is the only immunoglobulin to cross the placental barrier

Ⓓ IgA comprises 75% of the immunoglobulins in normal serum

Ⓔ IgD is mainly found on the surface of B lymphocytes

4.

Pathophysiological functions of immunoglobulins shown below include

Ⓐ IgG — neutralisation of soluble toxins

Ⓑ IgA — agglutination of bacteria

Ⓒ IgM — complement activation to produce cell lysis

Ⓓ IgD — protection against viruses

Ⓔ IgE — major regulator of B cell functions

5.

The following statements about the complement system are true

Ⓐ Only the classical pathway produces both C3 and C5 convertases

Ⓑ Components of the classical pathway are mainly beta globulins

Ⓒ The classical pathway is triggered by bacterial endotoxin

Ⓓ The alternative pathway is triggered by immune complexes

Ⓔ C1 esterase inhibitor deficiency produces angio-oedema

6.

The following statements about mast cells are true

Ⓐ Mast cells are tissue eosinophils

Ⓑ Mast cells mediate delayed hypersensitivity

Ⓒ Mast cells are activated by the complement components C3 and C5

Ⓓ Mast cells are inactivated by opiate analgesics

Ⓔ Mast cells release leukotrienes, prostaglandins and histamine

7.

In immediate (anaphylactic) hypersensitivity reactions

Ⓐ eosinophils release histaminase to suppress inflammation

Ⓑ the severity depends on the antigen's portal of entry

Ⓒ most manifestations are due to mast cell degranulation

Ⓓ parenteral adrenaline therapy should be given for severe reactions

Ⓔ urticaria is always induced by foreign antigen

8.

In delayed hypersensitivity reactions

Ⓐ T cells recruit macrophages in the development of the response

Ⓑ the provoking infectious agents are typically extracellular

Ⓒ antigen within the macrophage occasionally persists undestroyed

Ⓓ contact eczema is usually caused by haptens such as nickel

Ⓔ Langerhans cells in the dermis present the antigen in eczema

9.

The deposition of immune complexes

Ⓐ produces a vasculitis within vessel walls

Ⓑ in tissues depends upon their size and local haemodynamics

Ⓒ procures an Arthus reaction in the skin 10 days after exposure

Ⓓ in serum sickness results in tissue damage within 12–24 hours

Ⓔ in extrinsic allergic alveolitis is caused by IgA antibodies

10.

Aetiological factors in the development of the spectrum of autoimmune disorders include

Ⓐ loss of suppressor T cell control of helper T cells

Ⓑ immunological exposure to sequestrated antigens

Ⓒ bacterial mimicry of tissue antigen producing a cross-reaction

Ⓓ drug-induced immune complexes activating complement

Ⓔ genetic variations in the major histocompatibility complex

11.

The following statements about the major histocompatibility complex in man are true

Ⓐ The MHC comprises the HLA gene cluster on chromosome 6

Ⓑ The MHC encodes five classes of HLA antigens

Ⓒ Class 1 antigens are located on all nucleated cells but not platelets

Ⓓ Class 2 antigens are on lymphocytes, monocytes and macrophages

Ⓔ Complement components are coded on an adjacent locus

12.

The following diseases are strongly associated with the HLA antigens shown below

Ⓐ narcolepsy — DR2

Ⓑ ankylosing spondylitis — B27

Ⓒ myasthenia gravis — B8

Ⓓ rheumatoid arthritis — A3

Ⓔ haemochromatosis — DR4

13.

The following statements about drug effects on the immune system are true

Ⓐ Chlorpheniramine blocks all histamine receptors

Ⓑ Sodium cromoglycate inhibits the degranulation of mast cells

Ⓒ Adrenaline blocks the T cell release of lymphokines

Ⓓ Corticosteroids inhibit neutrophil adherence to endothelium

Ⓔ Cyclosporin suppresses B cells and T helper cells

14.
In primary hypogammaglobulinaemia
Ⓐ cell mediated immunity is also abnormal
Ⓑ B lymphocytes are usually present
Ⓒ treatment with immunoglobulins each month is effective
Ⓓ isolated IgA deficiency is associated with gluten enteropathy
Ⓔ susceptibility to fungal infections is increased

15.
In primary thymic hypoplasia (Di George syndrome)
Ⓐ fungal and viral infections invariably occur
Ⓑ serum immunoglobulin concentrations are normal
Ⓒ there is severe lymphopenia
Ⓓ hypoparathyroidism may be associated
Ⓔ neonatal death is usual

16.
In acquired immunodeficiency syndrome (AIDS)
Ⓐ the infectious agent is a retrovirus containing DNA
Ⓑ the virus infects helper T lymphocytes
Ⓒ B lymphocytes are activated to produce hypergammaglobulinaemia
Ⓓ monocytes with the T4 surface antigen are also infected
Ⓔ immune-mediated thrombocytopenia is common

17.
In immunisation
Ⓐ passive immunisation provides only temporary protection
Ⓑ tetanus protection is achieved using a live attenuated vaccine
Ⓒ diphtheria protection is achieved using an inactivated toxin
Ⓓ acute demyelinating encephalomyelitis is a complication of passive immunisation
Ⓔ BCG protects against tuberculosis in HIV positive individuals

18.
Plasmapheresis is of proven value in the treatment of
Ⓐ Crohn's disease
Ⓑ Graves' exophthalmos
Ⓒ Waldenstrom's macroglobulinaemia
Ⓓ Post-infective polyneuropathy (Guillain–Barré syndrome)
Ⓔ Haemochromatosis

19.
In transplantation and graft rejection
Ⓐ humorally mediated immune responses are the principal cause of rejection
Ⓑ ABO antigen groups have a major role in rejection pathogenesis
Ⓒ antigen typing is best undertaken on donor blood lymphocytes
Ⓓ the chance of a close HLA match between unrelated people is about 1 in 100
Ⓔ transplanted bone marrow T lymphocytes react against the recipient

20.
The following are important in down-regulating immune responses to specific antigens
Ⓐ reducing the antigen concentrations
Ⓑ increasing specific antibody concentrations
Ⓒ CD8 cells
Ⓓ CD4 cells
Ⓔ anti-idiotype antibodies

21.
The following are autoimmune diseases
Ⓐ Goodpasture's syndrome
Ⓑ atrophic gastritis
Ⓒ myasthenia gravis
Ⓓ Graves' disease
Ⓔ primary biliary cirrhosis

CLIMATE AND ENVIRONMENTAL FACTORS IN DISEASE

3

ANSWERS BEGIN ON P. 148

1.
The following physiological changes characterise heat acclimatisation
- Ⓐ increased circulatory volume
- Ⓑ increased aldosterone production
- Ⓒ increased heart rate
- Ⓓ increased volume of sweating
- Ⓔ decreased cardiac output

2.
In heat exhaustion
- Ⓐ total water losses of 6–8 litres are typical
- Ⓑ headache, nausea and the absence of thirst are characteristic
- Ⓒ the skin is usually hot and dry
- Ⓓ progression to heatstroke is avoidable with effective therapy
- Ⓔ predominant water depletion is more common in the unacclimatised

3.
Typical features of heat hyperpyrexia (heatstroke) include
- Ⓐ absence or impairment of sweat gland function
- Ⓑ body core temperature > 40° Centigrade
- Ⓒ stigmata of salt and water depletion
- Ⓓ cold clammy skin with peripheral circulatory failure
- Ⓔ insidious onset progressing slowly to altered consciousness

4.
Features consistent with a diagnosis of heatstroke include
- Ⓐ onset in a cool temperate climate
- Ⓑ history of exertion while wearing close-fitting garments
- Ⓒ development of acute renal failure
- Ⓓ coma and severe haemorrhage
- Ⓔ recent ingestion of amphetamines

5.
Conditions predisposing to the development of hypothermia include
- Ⓐ Addison's disease
- Ⓑ hypothyroidism
- Ⓒ hepatic cirrhosis
- Ⓓ poor home circumstances, immobility
- Ⓔ drug overdose

6.
The clinical features of hypothermia include
- Ⓐ hyponatraemia due to haemodilution
- Ⓑ body core temperature < 34° Centigrade
- Ⓒ areflexia and absent pupillary responses
- Ⓓ ECG shows tachycardia with pronounced U waves on the ECG
- Ⓔ asymptomatic acute pancreatitis and lactic acidaemia

7.
Characteristic features of acute mountain sickness include
- Ⓐ onset at 1500 metres above sea level
- Ⓑ response to acetazolamide
- Ⓒ headache, nausea and vomiting
- Ⓓ pulmonary and cerebral oedema
- Ⓔ hypocoagulation states

8.
Following an exposure to radiation
- Ⓐ of 20 Gy, the mortality rate is 100%
- Ⓑ granulocytes are the most sensitive cells to low-dose radiation exposure
- Ⓒ of 10 Gy, bone marrow cannot regenerate
- Ⓓ of 2 Gy, pneumonitis and intestinal ulceration develop
- Ⓔ of 2 mSv, the effect is equivalent to one year's background radiation

9.

In environmental exposure to lead

Ⓐ the principal source is from the inhalation of automobile emissions

Ⓑ a predominantly motor neuropathy would suggest toxic levels of exposure

Ⓒ the detection of lead in the blood implies toxicity

Ⓓ a microcytic anaemia is typical of toxicity in children

Ⓔ treatment is confined to symptomatic individuals

10.

The clinical features of chronic mercury poisoning include

Ⓐ sensorineural deafness and optic neuropathy

Ⓑ peripheral paraesthesiae and cerebellar ataxia

Ⓒ erethism with sweating, flushing, excitability and memory loss

Ⓓ acute pulmonary oedema, circulatory failure and renal failure

Ⓔ intestinal mucosal necrosis with gastrointestinal bleeding

11.

The following statements about barotrauma are true

Ⓐ Barometric pressure at sea level is 100 mmHg

Ⓑ Shallow water blackout is due to hyperventilation and hypocarbia

Ⓒ Lung volume doubles on ascending from depth of 10 m to the surface

Ⓓ Hyperinflation with air embolism occurs only in dives > 5 metres

Ⓔ Middle ear 'squeeze' typically ruptures the oval or round window

12.

The following statements about decompression sickness are true

Ⓐ Symptoms are usually apparent within 1 hour of surfacing

Ⓑ Painful lymphoedema is typically due to thoracic duct obstruction

Ⓒ Dissolved nitrogen accumulates particularly in skeletal muscle

Ⓓ Headache, abdominal pain, vertigo and dyspnoea are characteristic

Ⓔ Recompression restores neurological normality even after paraparesis

DISEASES DUE TO INFECTION

ANSWERS BEGIN ON P. 150

4

1.
Diseases typically acquired from animals include
Ⓐ leptospirosis
Ⓑ bartonellosis
Ⓒ Q fever
Ⓓ Lyme disease
Ⓔ hepatitis A

2.
Diseases usually spread via the faecal-oral route include
Ⓐ poliomyelitis
Ⓑ cholera
Ⓒ hepatitis E (non-A, non-B hepatitis)
Ⓓ hepatitis B
Ⓔ salmonellosis

3.
Schedules of immunisation in the UK should include
Ⓐ *Haemophilus influenzae* type B at the age of 3 years
Ⓑ polio vaccine on 3 occasions during the first year of life
Ⓒ mumps, measles and rubella at the age of 6 months
Ⓓ diphtheria, tetanus and pertussis at 2, 3, and 4 months
Ⓔ diphtheria, tetanus and polio vaccination in the first year of school

4.
Contraindications to active immunisation include
Ⓐ atopic disposition
Ⓑ HIV infection if live vaccines are required
Ⓒ pregnancy if live vaccines are required
Ⓓ chronic cardiac or respiratory failure
Ⓔ recent passive immunisation if live vaccines are required

5.
Live viruses are usually used for active immunisation against
Ⓐ poliomyelitis
Ⓑ pertussis
Ⓒ typhoid fever
Ⓓ mumps, measles and rubella
Ⓔ hepatitis B

6.
Indications for passive immunisation with human immunoglobulin include prevention of
Ⓐ hepatitis A and B
Ⓑ tetanus
Ⓒ rabies
Ⓓ meningococcaemia
Ⓔ chickenpox

7.
Notification is a statutory obligation in the following infections
Ⓐ food poisoning
Ⓑ leptospirosis
Ⓒ viral hepatitis
Ⓓ meningococcaemia
Ⓔ measles and rubella

8.
Noteworthy factors in the assessment of pyrexia of unknown origin include
Ⓐ history of travel abroad
Ⓑ occupational history
Ⓒ leisure activities
Ⓓ recent drug therapy
Ⓔ contact with animals and pets

9.

In the classification of HIV infection

Ⓐ group A = acute seroconversion simulating glandular fever

Ⓑ group B = persistent generalised lymphadenopathy

Ⓒ group C = constitutional symptoms and oral candidosis

Ⓓ group A1/B1/C1 all have absolute CD4 count >500/mm^3

Ⓔ asymptomatic infection = group B

10.

Presenting features of HIV infection include

Ⓐ hairy leucoplakia

Ⓑ atypical pneumonia

Ⓒ thrombocytopenic purpura

Ⓓ pulmonary tuberculosis

Ⓔ candidiasis and cryptosporidiosis

11.

HIV infection

Ⓐ is caused by an RNA retrovirus

Ⓑ associated with drug abuse is commoner than sexually acquired HIV in the UK

Ⓒ characteristically does not involve B lymphocytes

Ⓓ principally affects suppressor rather than helper T lymphocytes

Ⓔ has a better prognosis in the presence of Kaposi's sarcoma

12.

In a schoolchild with measles

Ⓐ infection is due to a single-stranded RNA paramyxovirus

Ⓑ rhinorrhoea and conjunctivitis occur at the onset

Ⓒ Koplik's spots appear at the same time as the skin rash

Ⓓ the skin rash typically desquamates as it disappears

Ⓔ infectivity is confined to the prodromal phase

13.

Characteristic complications of measles include

Ⓐ pneumonia

Ⓑ encephalitis

Ⓒ pancreatitis

Ⓓ myocarditis

Ⓔ otitis media

14.

In patients with rubella infection

Ⓐ the RNA virus spreads by the faecal-oral route

Ⓑ the transient polyarthritis is more marked in children than in adults

Ⓒ infectivity is present for 7 days before and after the rash

Ⓓ suboccipital lymphadenopathy with a macular rash behind the ears is typical

Ⓔ the risk of serious fetal damage is < 5% after the 16th week of pregnancy

15.

Typical complications of rubella include

Ⓐ an 80% risk of fetal damage within the first 6 weeks of pregnancy

Ⓑ post-viral encephalitis

Ⓒ gastroenteritis and acute appendicitis

Ⓓ polyarthritis

Ⓔ pericarditis

16.

The characteristic features of mumps include

Ⓐ infection with an RNA paramyxovirus by air-borne spread

Ⓑ high infectivity for 3 weeks after the onset of parotitis

Ⓒ presentation with an acute lymphocytic meningitis

Ⓓ abdominal pain attributable to mesenteric adenitis

Ⓔ orchitis which is usually bilateral and predominantly occurs prepubertally

17.
The features of herpes simplex virus infections include

Ⓐ recurrent genital ulcers
Ⓑ acute gingivostomatitis
Ⓒ encephalitis
Ⓓ shingles
Ⓔ paronychia

18.
The following statements about glandular fever are true

Ⓐ infection is usually attributable to the Epstein–Barr virus
Ⓑ presentation is with fever, headache and abdominal pain
Ⓒ sore throat suggests CMV rather than EBV infection
Ⓓ meningo-encephalitis and hepatitis are recognised complications
Ⓔ severe oro-pharyngeal swelling requires prednisolone therapy

19.
The clinical features of chickenpox include

Ⓐ infection due to varicella zoster virus from air-borne spread
Ⓑ high infectivity until 7 days after the last crop of vesicles
Ⓒ clinical response to acyclovir therapy in the immunocompromised
Ⓓ palatal rash appears before involvement of the trunk then face
Ⓔ constitutional symptoms are particularly severe in children

20.
Recognised complications of chickenpox include

Ⓐ pneumonia particularly in children rather than adults
Ⓑ proliferative glomerulonephritis
Ⓒ acute pancreatitis
Ⓓ encephalitis with cerebellar involvement
Ⓔ myocarditis

21.
The characteristic features of rabies include

Ⓐ a rhabdovirus infection transmitted in animal saliva
Ⓑ an incubation period of 4–8 days
Ⓒ a poor prognosis if symptoms develop
Ⓓ encephalitis or ascending paralysis
Ⓔ active and passive vaccination are useful in prevention and therapy

22.
The clinical features of Lassa fever include

Ⓐ fever, exudative pharyngitis and intercostal myalgia
Ⓑ infection with an arenavirus transmitted in rats' urine
Ⓒ renal, hepatic and circulatory failure
Ⓓ incubation period of 2–3 months
Ⓔ clinical response to tribavirin and immunoglobulin therapy

23.
The clinical features of yellow fever include

Ⓐ a togavirus infection transmitted by mosquitoes
Ⓑ an incubation period of 3–6 weeks
Ⓒ peripheral blood leucocytosis in contrast to viral hepatitis
Ⓓ fever, headache and severe myalgia with bone pains
Ⓔ response to tribavirin drug therapy

24.
Clinical features of dengue include

Ⓐ mosquito-borne infection with an incubation of 5–6 day
Ⓑ continuous or saddleback fever
Ⓒ rigor. headache, photophobia and backache
Ⓓ morbilliform rash and cervical lymphadenopathy
Ⓔ protection by vaccination every 10 years in endemic areas

25.
Diseases attributable to chlamydial infection include
A psittacosis
B epidemic typhus
C trachoma
D lymphogranuloma venereum
E Q fever

26.
In trachoma
A blepharospasm is common presenting feature
B upper eyelid follicular conjunctivitis is typical
C acute ophthalmia neonatorum is a recognised presentation
D tetracycline eye drops are indicated
E blindness is usually due to cataracts

27.
The typical features of psittacosis include
A an incubation period of 2 weeks
B constitutional upset with fever, headache and myalgia
C pulmonary infiltrates on chest X-ray not apparent clinically
D birds surviving the disease are no longer infectious
E prompt resolution with sulphonamide therapy

28.
Diseases attributable to mycoplasmal infection include
A haemolytic anaemia
B pelvic inflammatory disease
C pneumonia
D myocarditis
E urethritis and prostatitis

29.
The typical clinical features of typhus fevers include
A rickettsial infection from arthropods
B parasitisation of the endothelium of small blood vessels
C fever, headache and back pain and cutaneous haemorrhages
D mortality over 90%
E response to chloramphenicol or tetracycline therapy

30.
Features consistent with the diagnosis of Q fever include
A exposure to sheep, cattle and unpasteurised milk
B an incubation period of 1−2 weeks
C pneumonia in the absence of fever, headache or myalgia
D blood culture-negative endocarditis
E prompt clinical response to sulphonamide therapy

31.
The clinical features of Lyme disease include
A infection with the tick-borne spirochaete Borrelia burgdorferi
B an expanding erythematous rash (erythema chronicum migrans)
C cranial nerve palsies
D asymmetrical large joint recurrent oligoarthritis
E response to tetracycline or penicillin therapy

32.
The clinical features of relapsing fevers include
A infection with borrelial spirochaetes
B an incubation period of 1−3 months
C rigors, headache, mental confusion and jaundice
D hepatosplenomegaly and thrombocytopenic purpura
E response to erythromycin or tetracycline therapy

33.
The typical features of leptospirosis include

Ⓐ incubation period of 1–3 months

Ⓑ exposure risk in abattoirs, farms and inland waterways

Ⓒ fever, severe myalgia, headache and conjunctival suffusion

Ⓓ meningitis in *L. icterohaemorrhagica* rather than *L. canicola* infection

Ⓔ myocarditis, hepatitis and acute renal failure

34.
Sexually-transmissible viral diseases include

Ⓐ cytomegalovirus

Ⓑ hepatitis A, B and C

Ⓒ papovavirus

Ⓓ herpes simplex

Ⓔ molluscum contagiosum

35.
The following statements about syphilis are true

Ⓐ Infection is usually caused by *Treponema pertenue*

Ⓑ Untreated, infectivity is restricted to the first 2 months

Ⓒ The distinction between early and late syphilis is made at 2 years

Ⓓ The incubation period for primary syphilis is typically 2–4 weeks

Ⓔ Tertiary and quarternary syphilis usually develop within 5 years

36.
The characteristic features of secondary syphilis include

Ⓐ fever and a macular rash occurring 8 weeks after the chancre

Ⓑ condylomata lata in warm moist areas appearing as flat papules

Ⓒ generalised lymphadenopathy and oro-genital mucous ulceration

Ⓓ CSF pleocytosis is present in 90% indicating meningovascular disease

Ⓔ soft early diastolic murmur on cardiac auscultation

37.
Characteristic features of late (tertiary and quaternary) syphilis include

Ⓐ negative specific treponemal antigen tests

Ⓑ destructive granulomas (gummas) in bones, joints and the liver

Ⓒ sensory ataxia

Ⓓ aneurysms of the ascending aorta

Ⓔ poor response of gummas to antibiotic therapy

38.
The typical clinical features of gonorrhoea include

Ⓐ an incubation period of 2–3 weeks

Ⓑ anterior urethritis and cervicitis

Ⓒ right hypochondrial pain due to perihepatitis

Ⓓ pustular haemorrhagic rash and acute large joint arthritis

Ⓔ good response to ciprofloxacin therapy in penicillin allergy

39.
Features suggestive of non-gonococcal urethritis include

Ⓐ urethral culture of *Chlamydia trachomatis*

Ⓑ urethral culture of *Ureaplasma urealyticum*

Ⓒ keratoderma and peripheral oligoarthritis

Ⓓ painless genital ulceration

Ⓔ good response to penicillin therapy

40.
The typical features of lymphogranuloma venereum include

Ⓐ mononuclear cell exhibiting Donovan bodies within the lesion

Ⓑ transient genital ulceration 1–5 weeks after chlamydial infection

Ⓒ fever, weight loss and inguinal lymphadenopathy

Ⓓ proctitis and rectal stricture

Ⓔ response to tetracycline therapy

41.
Recognised causes of genital ulcers include
Ⓐ herpes zoster
Ⓑ chancroid
Ⓒ primary syphilis
Ⓓ Behçet's syndrome
Ⓔ gonorrhoea

42.
Anogenital herpes simplex is typically associated with
Ⓐ type 1 more often than type 2 herpes simplex infection
Ⓑ primary attacks more severe and prolonged than recurrent attacks
Ⓒ fever with painful genital ulceration and lymphadenopathy
Ⓓ sacral dermatomal pain and urinary retention
Ⓔ absence of clinical response to oral acyclovir

43.
Scarlet fever is typically associated with
Ⓐ rigors, headache and acute pharyngitis or tonsillitis
Ⓑ generalised punctate erythema desquamating on resolution
Ⓒ group B rather than group A streptococcal infection
Ⓓ generalised rather than localised lymphadenopathy
Ⓔ a membranous adherent pharyngeal exudate

44.
The typical features of erysipelas include
Ⓐ group A haemolytic streptococcal skin infection
Ⓑ absence of constitutional symptoms
Ⓒ well-defined area of cutaneous erythema and oedema
Ⓓ commoner in young rather than elderly patients
Ⓔ prompt response within 48 hours to benzyl penicillin

45.
Staphylococcal infection is associated with
Ⓐ resistance to benzyl penicillin therapy
Ⓑ necrotising enterocolitis
Ⓒ bronchopneumonia
Ⓓ toxic shock syndrome
Ⓔ cellulitis

46.
Clinical features suggesting toxic shock syndrome include
Ⓐ onset 24–48 hours after food ingestion
Ⓑ fever, myalgia, vomiting and diarrhoea
Ⓒ hypotension and hypovolaemia
Ⓓ prompt clinical response to benzyl penicillin
Ⓔ generalised erythema desquamating on resolution

47.
In bacteraemic shock
Ⓐ endotoxin initiates disseminated intravascular coagulation
Ⓑ peripheral vascular resistance falls initially
Ⓒ acute circulatory failure is usually due to cardiac failure
Ⓓ leucocytosis and thrombocythaemia indicate a poor prognosis
Ⓔ antibiotic therapy should await bacteriological results

48.
Diphtheria rather than streptococcal tonsillitis is suggested by
Ⓐ tender cervical lymphadenopathy
Ⓑ blood-stained nasal discharge and marked tachycardia
Ⓒ firm, adherent tonsillar exudate extending beyond the tonsils
Ⓓ paralysis of the soft palate, accommodation or ocular muscles
Ⓔ an incubation period of 2–4 days followed by marked fever

49.
In the treatment of diphtheria

Ⓐ antitoxin should be avoided pending bacteriological confirmation

Ⓑ antitoxin-induced anaphylaxis is best treated with prednisolone

Ⓒ antitoxin-induced serum sickness produces intense bronchospasm

Ⓓ isolation is usually unnecessary

Ⓔ myocarditis typically results in permanent cardiac impairment

50.
In whooping cough

Ⓐ the incubation period is 1–2 weeks

Ⓑ onset with rhinitis and conjunctivitis is characteristic

Ⓒ paroxysmal coughing bouts develop 2–3 weeks after exposure

Ⓓ *Bordetella pertussis* is best cultured from anterior nasal swabs

Ⓔ antibiotic therapy rapidly reduces coughing bouts

51.
The typical features of meningococcal infection include

Ⓐ air-borne spread of infection

Ⓑ abrupt onset with headache, vomiting and meningism

Ⓒ acute circulatory failure and purpuric rash

Ⓓ isolation of serogroups A and C more commonly than group B

Ⓔ control of infection in contacts is best achieved by vaccination

52.
Characteristic features of tetanus include

Ⓐ an incubation period of 2–3 days

Ⓑ muscular spasm typically starting in the masseters

Ⓒ convulsions associated with loss of consciousness

Ⓓ abdominal rigidity without pain or tenderness

Ⓔ bacteriological isolation of *Clostridium tetani* from the wound

53.
In the treatment of tetanus

Ⓐ tetanus toxoid should be given intravenously as soon as possible

Ⓑ wound debridement should be undertaken prior to any other therapy

Ⓒ human antitetanus immunoglobulin should be given immediately

Ⓓ diazepam should be avoided because of the hazards of oversedation

Ⓔ penicillin or metronidazole therapy should be administered

54.
The typical features of botulism include

Ⓐ ingestion of infected water 2–4 hours prior to symptom onset

Ⓑ onset with an afebrile gastroenteritis or postural hypotension

Ⓒ autonomic neuropathy induced by the cholinergic neurotoxin

Ⓓ ocular neuropathy and bulbar palsy developing over 3 days

Ⓔ dramatic clinical response to parenteral antitoxin

55.
Clinical features of anthrax include

Ⓐ occupational exposure to animals and animal products

Ⓑ an incubation period of 1–3 weeks

Ⓒ a painless cutaneous papule with regional lymphadenopathy

Ⓓ gastroenteritis, meningitis or bronchopneumonia

Ⓔ multiple antibiotic resistance is common

56.
Recognised features of brucellosis include

Ⓐ an incubation period of 3 months

Ⓑ fever, night sweats and back pain

Ⓒ hepatosplenomegaly and epididymoorchitis

Ⓓ oligoarthritis and spondylitis

Ⓔ peripheral blood neutrophil leucocytosis

57.
The characteristic features of plague include
Ⓐ an incubation period of less than 7 days
Ⓑ transmission of *Yersinia pestis* in infected fish
Ⓒ presentation is predominantly pneumonic rather than bubonic
Ⓓ rigors, severe headache and painful lymphadenopathy
Ⓔ absence of splenomegaly or hepatomegaly

58.
The typical features of typhoid fever include
Ⓐ faecal-oral spread of *Salmonella typhi* by food handlers
Ⓑ an incubation period of 3–7 days
Ⓒ onset with fever, headache, myalgia and septicaemia
Ⓓ 'rose spots' on the trunk and splenomegaly 7–10 days after onset
Ⓔ diarrhoea and abdominal pain and tenderness 10–14 days after onset

59.
Recognised complications of typhoid fever include
Ⓐ cholecystitis
Ⓑ meningitis
Ⓒ endocarditis
Ⓓ osteomyelitis
Ⓔ pneumonia

60.
Paratyphoid fever rather than typhoid fever is suggested by
Ⓐ onset with vomiting and diarrhoea
Ⓑ an incubation period of 5–7 days
Ⓒ absence of an erythematous macular rash
Ⓓ the development of a reactive arthritis
Ⓔ prominence of intestinal complications

61.
In the diagnosis of the enteric fevers
Ⓐ blood cultures are usually positive 2 weeks after onset
Ⓑ stool cultures are usually positive within 7 days of onset
Ⓒ peripheral blood neutrophil leucocytosis is typically marked
Ⓓ the Widal reaction is typically positive within 7 days of onset
Ⓔ persistent fever despite antibiotics indicates resistant organisms

62.
Symptom patterns suggesting specific food poisoning include
Ⓐ bloody diarrhoea after 12–48 hours— *Campylobacter jejuni*
Ⓑ vomiting and abdominal pain after 3–6 hours–staphylococci
Ⓒ vomiting and abdominal pain after 30–90 minutes—food allergy
Ⓓ bloody diarrhoea after 24–48 hours— *Escherichia coli*
Ⓔ vomiting and diarrhoea after 12–48 hours—salmonella

63.
Bacillary dysentery in the UK
Ⓐ is usually caused by *Shigella dysenteriae*
Ⓑ has an incubation period of 1–7 days
Ⓒ usually arises from contaminated water supplies
Ⓓ is characterised by profuse watery diarrhoea
Ⓔ should be treated with sulphonamide or tetracycline therapy

64.
The characteristic features of cholera include
Ⓐ the recent ingestion of contaminated water or shellfish
Ⓑ an incubation period of 5–10 days
Ⓒ sudden onset of profuse watery diarrhoea followed by vomiting
Ⓓ acute circulatory failure developing within 12 hours of onset
Ⓔ rapidly progressive metabolic alkalosis and dehydration

65.
The following statements about penicillins are true
Ⓐ All penicillins are bactericidal
Ⓑ Like the cephalosporins, they contain a beta-lactam ring
Ⓒ Clavulanic acid inhibits bacterial beta-lactamase
Ⓓ They can safely be used in cephalosporin-allergic patients
Ⓔ They are better given intrathecally in bacterial meningitis

66.
Tetracycline therapy
Ⓐ is bactericidal to sensitive bacteria
Ⓑ is contraindicated in pregnancy
Ⓒ doxycycline can safely be used in renal failure
Ⓓ should be given before meals
Ⓔ is active against rickettsiae, mycoplasmas and chlamydiae

67.
Aminoglycoside drug therapy
Ⓐ is ototoxic and nephrotoxic
Ⓑ should be avoided in patients requiring diuretic therapy
Ⓒ must be monitored using plasma drug concentrations
Ⓓ is effective against anaerobes and *Streptococcus faecalis*
Ⓔ is best avoided in renal failure

68.
Erythromycin is active against the following microorganisms
Ⓐ *Campylobacter jejuni*
Ⓑ *Escherichia coli*
Ⓒ *Legionella pneumophila*
Ⓓ *Mycoplasma pneumoniae*
Ⓔ *Clostridium welchii*

69.
Chloramphenicol is active against the following microorganisms
Ⓐ *Haemophilus influenzae*
Ⓑ *Salmonella typhi*
Ⓒ *Klebsiella pneumoniae*
Ⓓ *Pseudomonas aeruginosa*
Ⓔ *Brucella abortus*

70.
Ciprofloxacin is highly active against the following microorganisms
Ⓐ *Escherichia coli*
Ⓑ *Brucella abortus*
Ⓒ *Proteus mirabilis*
Ⓓ *Streptococcus pneumoniae*
Ⓔ *Bacteroides fragilis*

71.
The following statements about antibiotic therapy are true
Ⓐ Chloramphenicol therapy should be avoided in neonates
Ⓑ Metronidazole is effective in giardiasis and amoebiasis
Ⓒ Co-trimoxazole is effective in pneumocystis pneumonia
Ⓓ Sodium fusidate is effective in staphylococcal osteomyelitis
Ⓔ Ciprofloxacin is effective in syphilis

72.
Indications for appropriate chemoprophylaxis include
Ⓐ erythromycin in diphtheria contacts
Ⓑ rifampicin in meningitis contacts
Ⓒ penicillin following previous rheumatic fever
Ⓓ rifampicin in susceptible tuberculosis contacts
Ⓔ amoxycillin before dental surgery in patients with cardiac valve prostheses

73.
Antiviral agents active against the following viruses include
Ⓐ ganciclovir—cytomegalovirus
Ⓑ amantadine—orthomyxovirus
Ⓒ tribavirin—respiratory syncytial virus
Ⓓ zidovudine—retrovirus
Ⓔ famciclovir—herpes simplex and zoster virus

74.

Characteristic features of leprosy include

Ⓐ an incubation period of 2–5 years
Ⓑ growth of the organism on Lowenstein–Jensen medium after 2–3 months
Ⓒ spread of the tuberculoid form on prolonged patient contact
Ⓓ spontaneous healing of the earliest macule
Ⓔ a cell-mediated immune response in the lepromatous form

75.

Typical features of tuberculoid leprosy include

Ⓐ cell-mediated immune response around nerves and hair follicles
Ⓑ absence of infectivity of affected patients
Ⓒ palpable thickening of the peripheral nerves
Ⓓ development of erythema nodosum leprosum
Ⓔ persistently negative lepromin skin test

76.

Typical features of lepromatous leprosy include

Ⓐ absence of infectivity of affected patients
Ⓑ unlike the tuberculoid form, organisms are scanty in number
Ⓒ blood-borne spread from the dermis throughout the body
Ⓓ strongly positive lepromin skin test
Ⓔ anaesthetic hypopigmented skin macules and plaques

77.

In the treatment of multi-bacillary leprosy

Ⓐ the combination of rifampicin, clofazimine and dapsone is advisable
Ⓑ patients should be isolated for the first week of chemotherapy
Ⓒ rifampicin should be given for 2 days every month
Ⓓ clofazimine and dapsone should be administered daily
Ⓔ treatment should be continued for 2 years

78.

The following statements about the Plasmodia life cycle are true

Ⓐ Sporozoites disappear from the blood within minutes of inoculation
Ⓑ Merozoites re-entering RBCs undergo both sexual and asexual development
Ⓒ All plasmodia multiply in the liver then subsequently in RBCs
Ⓓ Dormant hypnozoites remain within the liver cells in all species
Ⓔ Fertilisation of the gametocytes occurs in the human RBCs

79.

All species of Plasmodia producing malaria in humans

Ⓐ are transmitted exclusively by anopheline mosquitoes
Ⓑ have a persistent exo-erythrocytic phase often dormant for years
Ⓒ produce the initial symptoms on the release of RBC sporozoites
Ⓓ parasitise RBCs and normoblasts in all stages of development
Ⓔ parasitise capillary endothelium throughout the body

80.

Typical features of *Plasmodium falciparum* malaria include

Ⓐ febrile response more marked than in other forms of malaria
Ⓑ absence of intravascular haemolysis and splenomegaly
Ⓒ infected RBCs causing capillary occlusion throughout the body
Ⓓ rarity of infection in haemoglobin S or C heterozygotes
Ⓔ longer incubation period of 3–4 weeks in non-immune subjects

81.
Recognised clinical features of malaria include

Ⓐ absence of *P. vivax* infection in subjects lacking the Duffy blood group
Ⓑ asymptomatic *P. malariae* parasitaemia persisting for years
Ⓒ rarity of clinical relapses beyond 2 years
Ⓓ presentation with rigors, herpes simplex and haemolytic anaemia
Ⓔ flu-like symptoms, jaundice and hepatosplenomegaly in *P. falciparum*

82.
Complications of *Plasmodium falciparum* malaria include

Ⓐ delirium and coma
Ⓑ blackwater fever
Ⓒ acute renal failure
Ⓓ acute liver failure
Ⓔ acute cardiac failure

83.
The clinical features of amoebic dysentery typically include

Ⓐ an incubation period of 2–4 weeks
Ⓑ presentation with profuse watery diarrhoea
Ⓒ colonic mucosal involvement most marked in the rectum
Ⓓ characteristic appearances of the mucosa on sigmoidoscopy
Ⓔ *Entamoeba histolytica* cysts in the stool are pathognomonic of the disease

84.
Recognised complications of amoebiasis include

Ⓐ severe intestinal haemorrhage
Ⓑ expectoration of amoebic pus from a liver abscess
Ⓒ cerebral abscess
Ⓓ amoebomas of the caecum, colon and rectum
Ⓔ genital and perianal ulceration from cutaneous amoebiasis

85.
In the diagnosis and therapy of amoebiasis

Ⓐ amoebic liver abscesses usually reveal the presence of cysts
Ⓑ stool trophozoites are unlikely in the presence of blood or mucus
Ⓒ liver abscesses are best identified by ultrasound scanning
Ⓓ metronidazole therapy is effective in both liver and colonic disease
Ⓔ furamide therapy should also be given to eliminate colonic cysts

86.
The characteristic features of giardiasis include

Ⓐ an incubation period of 2–3 days
Ⓑ infection transmitted by air-borne droplet spread
Ⓒ predominant parasitisation of the duodenum and jejunum
Ⓓ presentation with watery diarrhoea and malabsorption
Ⓔ clinical response to a metronidazole

87.
Recognised features of toxoplasmosis include

Ⓐ infection derived from cats, pigs and sheep
Ⓑ asymptomatic infection is common in otherwise healthy subjects
Ⓒ congenital infection produces choroidoretinitis and cerebral palsy
Ⓓ glandular fever-like illness with peripheral blood monocytosis
Ⓔ pyrimethamine and sulphadimidine therapy is useful in AIDS

88.

The typical features of African trypanosomiasis include

🅐 transmission of the parasite by the tsetse cattle fly

🅑 an incubation period of 2–3 weeks

🅒 onset with chancre-like skin lesion with local lymphadenopathy

🅓 generalised lymphadenopathy, hepatosplenomegaly and encephalitis

🅔 good prognosis given prompt pentamidine or suramin therapy

89.

Typical features of South American trypanosomiasis include

🅐 spread of the parasite by the reduviid bug of cats and dogs

🅑 Romana's sign with eye closure due to a conjunctival lesion

🅒 latent period of many years before onset of chronic disease

🅓 colonic and oesophageal dilatation due to neuropathy

🅔 response to nifurtimox therapy achieves cure rates of 90%

90.

Typical features of visceral leishmaniasis (kala-azar) include

🅐 spread of *Leishmania donovani* by sandflies from dogs and rodents

🅑 an incubation period of 1–2 weeks

🅒 rigors with hepatomegaly but no splenomegaly

🅓 diagnosis confirmed on peripheral blood film

🅔 clinical response to pentavalent antimonials e.g. stibogluconate

91.

Typical features of South American leishmaniasis include

🅐 nasal and mouth mucosal ulcers

🅑 painful ulcers in the groins or axillae

🅒 marked splenomegaly and lymphadenopathy

🅓 ulcers which heal without scarring

🅔 negative Leishmanin skin test

92.

All forms of schistosomiasis are associated with

🅐 trematode helminths reproducing in freshwater snails

🅑 the passage of cercariae in the urine and/or stool

🅒 cercarial penetration of the skin or mucous membranes

🅓 progression to portal or pulmonary hypertension

🅔 eradication following praziquantel therapy

93.

Typical features of *Schistosoma haematobium* infection include

🅐 disease confined to the urinary tract

🅑 presentation with painless haematuria

🅒 spontaneous resolution within a year of leaving endemic areas

🅓 involvement of the uterine cervix and seminal vesicles

🅔 an endemic disease in China and the Far East

94.

Typical features of *Schistosoma mansoni* infection include

🅐 an endemic disease in Egypt and East Africa

🅑 abdominal pain with loose, blood-stained stools

🅒 progression to jaundice and chronic liver failure

🅓 paraplegia, cor pulmonale and bowel papillomata

🅔 weight loss and malabsorption due to small bowel disease

95.
Typical features of *Schistosoma japonicum* infection include
Ⓐ parasitisation of rodents, domestic animals and man
Ⓑ infestation follows the ingestion of raw fish and crustacea
Ⓒ abdominal pain and diarrhoea due to ileal and colonic involvement
Ⓓ epilepsy, hemiplegia, paraplegia and blindness
Ⓔ morbidity and mortality rate less than that from the other species

96.
Cestode infestation with *Taenia saginata* is associated with
Ⓐ ingestion of undercooked pork
Ⓑ abdominal pain and diarrhoea
Ⓒ presentation with pruritus ani
Ⓓ weight loss and malabsorption
Ⓔ response to praziquantel therapy

97.
Infestation with *Taenia solium* is typically associated with
Ⓐ ingestion of undercooked fish
Ⓑ liberation of larvae in the ileum from ingested ova
Ⓒ larval penetration into the circulation via the stomach
Ⓓ epilepsy and calcified cysts in skeletal muscle
Ⓔ resistance to praziquantel therapy

98.
***Echinococcus granulosus* infestation is usually associated with**
Ⓐ contact with sheep, cattle and dogs
Ⓑ acquisition of hydatid cysts in childhood
Ⓒ cysts in the liver, brain and lungs
Ⓓ absence of dissemination during liver aspiration
Ⓔ prompt response to albendazole therapy if surgically inoperable

99.
In infestation with the nematode *Enterobius vermicularis*
Ⓐ adult threadworms occur in great numbers in the small bowel
Ⓑ presentation with intense pruritus ani is typical
Ⓒ identifiable ova are found on the perianal skin
Ⓓ malabsorption usually develops following heavy infestations
Ⓔ all family members should take piperazine or mebendazole therapy

100.
In infestation with *Ascaris lumbricoides*
Ⓐ the disease follows ingestion of food contaminated with larvae
Ⓑ larval migration through the lungs produces pulmonary eosinophilia
Ⓒ obstruction of the ileum, biliary and pancreatic ducts occurs
Ⓓ malabsorption is the usual presentation
Ⓔ levamisole in a single dose eradicates the disease

101.
The typical features of strongyloidiasis include
Ⓐ skin penetration with migration to the gut via the lungs
Ⓑ larval penetration of the duodenal and jejunal mucosa
Ⓒ abdominal pain, diarrhoea and malabsorption
Ⓓ penetration of perianal skin producing a migrating linear weal
Ⓔ systemic spread in the immunosuppressed resulting in pneumonia

102.
The clinical features of infection with *Toxocara canis include*
Ⓐ larval penetration of the gastric mucosa after contact with dogs
Ⓑ development of adult worms throughout the body tissues
Ⓒ hepatosplenomegaly and visual impairment
Ⓓ pulmonary and peripheral blood eosinophilia
Ⓔ effectively treated with diethylcarbamazine

103.
Typical features of *Trichinella spiralis* infestation include
Ⓐ infection resulting from contact with the urine of rodents
Ⓑ larval migration from the small bowel to skeletal muscle
Ⓒ oedema of the eyelids with muscle pain and tenderness
Ⓓ acute myocarditis and encephalitis
Ⓔ response to corticosteroid and albendazole therapy

104.
In infection with Loa loa
Ⓐ transmission of microfilaria is by the mosquito *Culex fatigans*
Ⓑ the incubation period is usually 1–2 weeks
Ⓒ intermittent Calabar swellings in the subdermis are typical
Ⓓ adult worms are visible traversing the eye beneath the conjunctiva
Ⓔ diethylcarbamazine therapy is curative

105.
In onchocerciasis
Ⓐ larval infection is transmitted by the Simulium fly
Ⓑ worms mature over 2–4 weeks and persist for up to 1 year
Ⓒ cutaneous nodules and eosinophilia commonly develop
Ⓓ conjunctivitis, iritis and keratitis are characteristic
Ⓔ diethylcarbamazine or ivermectin therapy are curative

106.
Incubation periods of less than 1 week are characteristic of
Ⓐ syphilis
Ⓑ gonorrhoea
Ⓒ amoebiasis
Ⓓ diphtheria
Ⓔ cholera

107.
Children are no longer an infectious risk to others
Ⓐ 1 week after the last crop of chickenpox lesions
Ⓑ 5 days after the start of antibiotic therapy for scarlet fever
Ⓒ 1 week after the onset of a measles rash
Ⓓ 1 day after the onset of salivary gland swelling due to mumps
Ⓔ 1 week after the onset of a rubella rash

108.
In patients with *Helicobacter pylori* (HP) infection
Ⓐ the diagnosis can be confirmed by decreased urease concentrations in the gastric mucosa
Ⓑ the presence of oesophagitis indicates the need for HP eradication therapy
Ⓒ HP eradication is enhanced by sustained elevation of gastric pH
Ⓓ amoxycillin plus metronidazole therapy is more effective than amoxycillin alone
Ⓔ HP eradication reduces recurrence rates of both duodenal and gastric ulcers

109.
The following statements about viral infections are correct

Ⓐ Rubella is due to an RNA togavirus
Ⓑ Parvovirus B19 is an RNA virus causing bullous skin eruptions
Ⓒ Molluscum contagiosum is an RNA virus producing pericarditis
Ⓓ Echoviruses are RNA picornaviruses producing gastroenteritis and meningitis
Ⓔ Measles and mumps are DNA paramyxoviruses

110.
The typical features of Yersinia infections include

Ⓐ water-borne infection
Ⓑ exudative pharyngitis and enterocolitis
Ⓒ acute ileitis and mesenteric adenitis
Ⓓ erythema nodosum and reactive arthritis
Ⓔ clinical response to benzyl penicillin

5 DISEASES OF THE CARDIOVASCULAR SYSTEM

ANSWERS BEGIN ON P. 160

1.
The pain of myocardial ischaemia
- Ⓐ is typically induced by exercise and relieved by rest
- Ⓑ radiates to the neck and jaw but not the teeth
- Ⓒ rarely lasts longer than 10 seconds after resting
- Ⓓ is easily distinguished from oesophageal pain
- Ⓔ invariably worsens as exercise continues

2.
Syncope
- Ⓐ followed by facial flushing suggests a tachyarrhythmia
- Ⓑ without warning suggests a vaso-vagal episode
- Ⓒ on exercise is a typical feature of mitral regurgitation
- Ⓓ is the commonest cause of falls amongst elderly patients
- Ⓔ is a recognised presenting feature of pulmonary embolism

3.
Recognised features of severe cardiac failure include
- Ⓐ tiredness
- Ⓑ weight loss
- Ⓒ epigastric pain
- Ⓓ nocturia
- Ⓔ nocturnal cough

4.
In the normal human heart
- Ⓐ the atrio-ventricular node is usually supplied by the left circumflex coronary artery
- Ⓑ beta-1 adrenoceptors mediate chronotropic responses
- Ⓒ pulmonary artery systolic pressure normally varies between 90 and 140 mmHg
- Ⓓ the annulus fibrosus aids conduction of impulses from the atria to the ventricles
- Ⓔ cardiac output is the product of heart rate and ventricular end-diastolic volume

5.
In the normal electrocardiogram
- Ⓐ the PR interval is measured from the end of the P wave to the beginning of the R wave
- Ⓑ each small square represents 40 milliseconds at a standard paper speed of 25 mm/sec
- Ⓒ the heart rate is 75 per minute if the R-R interval measures 4 cm
- Ⓓ R waves become progressively larger from leads V1 to V6
- Ⓔ the P wave represents sinoatrial node depolarisation

6.
The following pulse characteristics are typical features of the disorders listed below
- Ⓐ pulsus bisferiens — combined mitral stenosis and regurgitation
- Ⓑ pulsus paradoxus — aortic regurgitation
- Ⓒ collapsing pulse — severe anaemia
- Ⓓ pulsus alternans — extrasystoles every alternate beat
- Ⓔ slow rising pulse — mitral stenosis

7.

The following statements about the jugular venous pressure (JVP) are true

Ⓐ The external jugular vein is a reliable guide to right atrial pressure

Ⓑ The JVP is conventionally measured from the suprasternal notch

Ⓒ The normal JVP, unlike the blood pressure, does not rise with anxiety

Ⓓ The normal JVP does not rise on abdominal compression

Ⓔ The normal JVP falls during inspiration

8.

These abnormalities of the jugular venous pulse are associated with the disorders listed below

Ⓐ cannon waves = pulmonary hypertension

Ⓑ giant 'a' waves = tricuspid stenosis

Ⓒ 'v' waves = tricuspid regurgitation

Ⓓ inspiratory rise in jugular venous pressure = pericardial tamponade

Ⓔ absent 'a' waves = atrio-ventricular dissociation

9.

Abnormalities on palpation of the praecordium are associated with the following disorders

Ⓐ 'tapping' apex beat = right ventricular hypertrophy

Ⓑ left parasternal heave = right ventricular hypertrophy

Ⓒ lower left parasternal systolic thrill = mitral regurgitation

Ⓓ impalpable apex beat = emphysema

Ⓔ double apical impulse = left ventricular aneurysm

10.

The following auscultatory findings are associated with the phenomena shown below

Ⓐ third heart sound = opening of mitral valve

Ⓑ varying intensity of first heart sound = AV dissociation

Ⓒ soft first heart sound = mitral stenosis

Ⓓ reversed splitting of second heart sound = left bundle branch block

Ⓔ fourth heart sound = atrial fibrillation

11.

A third heart sound (S3) is a typical finding in

Ⓐ mitral stenosis

Ⓑ healthy young athletes

Ⓒ constrictive pericarditis

Ⓓ left ventricular failure

Ⓔ lone atrial fibrillation

12.

The following statements about cardiac murmurs are true

Ⓐ diastolic murmurs are a recognised feature of normal pregnancy

Ⓑ ventricular septal defects produce pansystolic murmurs

Ⓒ an early high-pitched diastolic murmur suggests mitral stenosis

Ⓓ late-systolic murmurs suggest mitral valve prolapse

Ⓔ mitral diastolic murmurs are best heard at the left sternal edge with the patient leaning forwards

13.

Features that suggest a ventricular tachycardia rather than supraventricular tachycardia include

Ⓐ a ventricular rate > 160/minute

Ⓑ termination of the arrhythmia with carotid sinus pressure

Ⓒ variable intensity of the first heart sound

Ⓓ the presence of cardiac failure

Ⓔ QRS complexes < 0.14 sec in duration on ECG

14.

In the investigation of patients with suspected heart disease

ⓐ the normal upper limit for the cardiothoracic ratio on chest X-ray is 0.75

ⓑ a negative exercise ECG excludes the diagnosis of ischaemic heart disease

ⓒ a 'step-up' in oxygen saturation at cardiac catheterisation suggests an intracardiac shunt

ⓓ doppler echocardiography reliably assesses pressure gradients between cardiac chambers

ⓔ radionuclide blood pool scanning accurately quantifies left ventricular function

15.

The following statements about cardiac rhythms are true

ⓐ Cardiac rate falls with inspiration in autonomic neuropathy

ⓑ Re-entry tachyarrhythmias arise from anomalous AV conduction

ⓒ Sinus bradycardia < 60/min is a normal occurrence during sleep

ⓓ Sinus arrest is defined on ECG by P waves which do not elicit QRS complexes

ⓔ Episodes of both bradycardias and tachycardias suggest the sick sinus syndrome

16.

In a patient with a recurrent AV nodal re-entry tachycardia

ⓐ adenosine is the prophylactic therapy of first choice

ⓑ the cardiac rate is often 160–220 beats per minute

ⓒ polyuria after a prolonged episode is characteristic

ⓓ symptoms are invariably present during episodes

ⓔ transient bundle branch block on ECG indicates coexistent myocardial ischaemia

17.

Typical features of the Wolff–Parkinson–White (WPW) syndrome include

ⓐ tachyarrhythmias resulting from re-entry phenomenona

ⓑ ventricular pre-excitation via an accessory AV pathway

ⓒ atrial fibrillation with a ventricular response of > 160/min

ⓓ ECG between bouts showing prolonged PR interval with narrow QRS complexes

ⓔ useful therapeutic response to verapamil or digoxin

18.

Atrial tachycardia with AV block is typically associated with

ⓐ an irregularly irregular pulse

ⓑ slowing of the atrial rate on carotid sinus massage

ⓒ presence of P waves identical to those found during sinus rhythm

ⓓ digoxin toxicity and intracellular potassium depletion

ⓔ bizarre broad QRS complexes on ECG

19.

Atrial fibrillation is

ⓐ present in 10% of the elderly population over the age of 75 years

ⓑ usually readily converted to permanent sinus rhythm using DC cardioversion

ⓒ associated with an annual stroke risk of 5% if structural heart disease is present

ⓓ a common presenting feature of the sick sinus syndrome

ⓔ usually associated with a ventricular rate < 100 /min even before therapy is introduced

20.
In patients with atrial fibrillation
Ⓐ aspirin therapy alone does not reduce the risk of stroke
Ⓑ the radial pulse is typically irregularly irregular
Ⓒ the response in cardiac output to exercise is reduced due to the absence of atrial systole
Ⓓ elective DC cardioversion is contraindicated during anticoagulant therapy
Ⓔ alcohol abuse should be considered as a likely cause

21.
Ventricular ectopic beats
Ⓐ produce a clinically detectable reduction in stroke volume
Ⓑ which are symptomatic usually indicate underlying heart disease
Ⓒ secondary to cardiac disease typically disappear on exercise
Ⓓ are likely to be escape beats when there is underlying bradycardia
Ⓔ following acute myocardial infarction indicate the need for antiarrhythmic treatment

22.
In ventricular tachycardia
Ⓐ underlying cardiac disease is usually present
Ⓑ amiodarone is useful in the prevention of recurrent episodes
Ⓒ a shortened QT interval on ECG predisposes to recurrent episodes
Ⓓ carotid sinus massage usually slows the cardiac rate transiently
Ⓔ complicated by acute cardiac failure, cardioversion should be avoided

23.
In ventricular fibrillation
Ⓐ the radial pulse is extremely rapid and thready
Ⓑ unresponsive to treatment, profound hypokalaemia should be suspected
Ⓒ ECG confirmation is vital before DC shock is administered
Ⓓ cardioversion should be synchronised with the R wave on ECG
Ⓔ immediate lignocaine therapy avoids the need for cardioversion

24.
In cardiopulmonary resuscitation
Ⓐ a sharp blow to the praecordium helps restore sinus rhythm
Ⓑ asystole is the commonest finding on ECG
Ⓒ a normal ECG suggests profound hypovolaemia
Ⓓ if cardioversion fails intracardiac adrenaline should be given
Ⓔ the compression to ventilation ratio should be 5 : 1

25.
In the management of cardiac arrhythmias
Ⓐ moderation of alcohol consumption should be advised
Ⓑ symptoms are a reliable guide to the efficacy of drug treatment
Ⓒ endocardial pacing should be considered for refractory paroxysmal tachycardias
Ⓓ combination drug therapy is often better than monotherapy
Ⓔ treatment of the causative disease is of no proven benefit

26.
Digoxin
Ⓐ shortens the refractory period of conducting tissue
Ⓑ usually converts atrial flutter to sinus rhythm
Ⓒ acts primarily on cell membrane ionic pumps
Ⓓ effects are potentiated by hyperkalaemia
Ⓔ is a recognised cause of ventricular arrhythmias

27.

The cardiac drugs listed below are associated with the following adverse effects

Ⓐ digoxin — acute confusional state
Ⓑ verapamil — constipation
Ⓒ amiodarone — photosensitivity
Ⓓ propafenone — corneal microdeposits
Ⓔ lignocaine — convulsions

28.

In the classification of antiarrhythmic drugs, the following statements are true

Ⓐ class I agents inhibit the fast sodium channel
Ⓑ class II agents are beta-adrenoceptor antagonists
Ⓒ class III agents prolong the action potential
Ⓓ class IV agents inhibit the slow calcium channel
Ⓔ many antiarrhythmic agents have actions in more than one class

29.

The following class II antiarrhythmic drugs selectively block the beta 1-adrenoceptor

Ⓐ sotalol
Ⓑ atenolol
Ⓒ acebutolol
Ⓓ metoprolol
Ⓔ timolol

30.

Amiodarone therapy

Ⓐ prolongs the plateau phase of the action potential
Ⓑ potentiates the effect of warfarin
Ⓒ is useful in the prevention of VT but not SVT
Ⓓ should be withdrawn if corneal deposits occur
Ⓔ has a significant negative inotropic action

31.

The following statements about atrioventricular block are true

Ⓐ first degree block produces a soft first heart sound
Ⓑ the PR interval is fixed in Mobitz type I second degree block
Ⓒ decreasing PR intervals suggests Wenckebach's phenomenon
Ⓓ irregular cannon waves in the JVP suggest complete heart block
Ⓔ the QRS complex in complete heart block is always broad and bizarre

32.

Absolute indications for permanent endocardial pacing include

Ⓐ asymptomatic congenital complete heart block
Ⓑ asymptomatic Mobitz type I second degree heart block
Ⓒ Adams–Stokes attacks in the elderly
Ⓓ complete heart block due to rheumatic mitral valve disease
Ⓔ symptomatic second degree heart block following acute inferior myocardial infarction

33.

The following statements about bundle branch block (BBB) are true

Ⓐ Right BBB is most often the result of left ventricular hypertrophy
Ⓑ Right BBB produces right axis deviation with a QRS > 0.12 sec on ECG
Ⓒ Right BBB produces fixed splitting of the second heart sound
Ⓓ Left BBB produces reversed splitting of the second heart sound
Ⓔ Left posterior hemiblock produces left axis deviation on ECG

34.
Typical clinical features of acute circulatory failure due to anaphylactic shock include
Ⓐ elevated jugular venous pressure
Ⓑ warm dry skin
Ⓒ stridor
Ⓓ confusion
Ⓔ polyuria

35.
Acute circulatory failure with an elevated central venous pressure are typical findings in
Ⓐ acute pancreatitis
Ⓑ massive pulmonary embolism
Ⓒ ruptured ectopic pregnancy
Ⓓ acute right ventricular infarction
Ⓔ pericardial tamponade

36.
In a patient with cardiogenic shock due to acute myocardial infarction
Ⓐ the absence of pulmonary oedema suggests right ventricular infarction
Ⓑ the central venous pressure is the best index of left ventricular filling pressure
Ⓒ dopamine in low dose increases renal blood flow
Ⓓ high flow, high concentration oxygen is indicated
Ⓔ colloid infusion is indicated if oliguria and pulmonary oedema develop

37.
In the treatment of cardiac failure associated with acute pulmonary oedema
Ⓐ controlled oxygen therapy should be restricted to 28% oxygen in patients who smoke
Ⓑ morphine reduces angor animi and dyspnoea
Ⓒ frusemide therapy given intravenously reduces preload and afterload
Ⓓ nitrates should be avoided if the systolic blood pressure < 140 mmHg
Ⓔ ACE inhibitors decrease the afterload but increase the preload

38.
Right ventricular hypertrophy is a recognised finding in the following cardiac disorders
Ⓐ tricuspid stenosis
Ⓑ constrictive pericarditis
Ⓒ cor pulmonale
Ⓓ atrial septal defect
Ⓔ mitral stenosis

39.
Left ventricular hypertrophy is a typical finding in the following cardiac disorders
Ⓐ mitral stenosis
Ⓑ aortic stenosis
Ⓒ Addison's disease
Ⓓ left atrial myxoma
Ⓔ hypertrophic cardiomyopathy

40.
In chronic biventricular cardiac failure
Ⓐ angiotensin II contributes to renal salt and water retention
Ⓑ excess ADH is the major cause of oedema
Ⓒ hyponatraemia usually indicates total body sodium depletion
Ⓓ cardiac sympathetic neural activity is markedly diminished
Ⓔ atrial natriuretic peptide is released

41.
In the management of chronic heart failure
Ⓐ ACE inhibitor therapy reduces subsequent hospitalisation rates
Ⓑ coagulation is impaired and thromboembolic risk therefore declines
Ⓒ drug suppression of ventricular arrhythmia improves prognosis
Ⓓ the value of diuretic therapy is principally attributable to sodium depletion
Ⓔ digoxin is only of benefit if atrial fibrillation coexists

42.
The diagnosis of rheumatic fever in a patient with an elevated ASO titre is confirmed by

Ⓐ fever with an elevated erythrocyte sedimentation rate

Ⓑ arthralgia and a previous history of rheumatic fever

Ⓒ chorea and a prolonged PR interval on ECG

Ⓓ erythema nodosum and arthritis

Ⓔ rheumatic nodules and pancarditis

43.
In patients with significant mitral stenosis

Ⓐ the mitral valve orifice is reduced from 5 cm^2 to about 1 cm^2

Ⓑ a history of rheumatic fever or chorea is elicited in over 90%

Ⓒ left atrial enlargement cannot be detected on the chest X-ray

Ⓓ the risk of systemic emboli is trivial in sinus rhythm

Ⓔ mitral balloon valvuloplasty is not advisable if there is also significant mitral regurgitation

44.
Expected findings in a patient with significant mitral stenosis include

Ⓐ a soft early diastolic murmur

Ⓑ a quiet first sound and absence of an opening snap

Ⓒ left parasternal heave suggesting pulmonary hypertension

Ⓓ a displaced apex beat

Ⓔ the opening snap occurring just before the second heart sound

45.
Recognised features of chronic mitral regurgitation include

Ⓐ soft first heart sound and loud third heart sound

Ⓑ presentation with signs of right ventricular failure

Ⓒ the severity of regurgitation is increased by afterload reduction

Ⓓ a pansystolic murmur and hyperdynamic displaced apex beat

Ⓔ atrial fibrillation requiring anticoagulation

46.
Disorders typically producing the sudden onset of symptomatic mitral regurgitation include

Ⓐ Marfan's syndrome

Ⓑ acute myocardial infarction

Ⓒ acute rheumatic fever

Ⓓ infective endocarditis

Ⓔ diphtheria

47.
Clinical features suggesting severe aortic stenosis include

Ⓐ late-systolic ejection click

Ⓑ pulsus bisferiens

Ⓒ heaving, displaced apex beat

Ⓓ syncope associated with angina

Ⓔ loud second heart sound

48.
Disorders associated with aortic regurgitation include

Ⓐ ankylosing spondylitis

Ⓑ Marfan's syndrome

Ⓒ syphilitic aortitis

Ⓓ persistent ductus arteriosus

Ⓔ Takayasu's disease

49.

In a patient with aortic regurgitation in normal sinus rhythm

Ⓐ a mid-diastolic murmur is usually due to concomitant mitral stenosis

Ⓑ a systolic murmur is often due to coexistent aortic stenosis

Ⓒ a left parasternal heave and displaced apex beat are expected findings

Ⓓ systemic diastolic arterial pressure is usually low

Ⓔ a short early diastolic murmur suggests mild regurgitation

50.

The following statements about tricuspid valve disease are true

Ⓐ murmurs are best heard in mid-sternum at the end of expiration

Ⓑ ascites occur with tricuspid regurgitation but not stenosis

Ⓒ tricuspid stenosis produces cannon waves in the JVP

Ⓓ both stenosis and regurgitation produce systolic hepatic pulsation

Ⓔ endocarditis suggests the possibility of intravenous drug abuse

51.

The typical features of congenital pulmonary stenosis include

Ⓐ breathlessness and central cyanosis

Ⓑ giant 'a' waves in the JVP

Ⓒ loud second heart sound preceded by an ejection systolic click

Ⓓ left parasternal heave and systolic thrill

Ⓔ enlargement of the pulmonary artery visible on chest X-ray

52.

In infective endocarditis

Ⓐ streptococci and staphylococci account for over 80% of cases

Ⓑ left heart valves are more frequently involved than right heart valves

Ⓒ normal cardiac valves are not affected

Ⓓ glomerulonephritis usually occurs due to immune complex disease

Ⓔ a normal echocardiogram excludes the diagnosis

53.

In the management of infective endocarditis

Ⓐ blood cultures are best obtained when the fever peaks

Ⓑ antibiotic therapy should be delayed pending bacteriological confirmation

Ⓒ parenteral antibiotic therapy should be continued for 6 weeks

Ⓓ persistent fever suggests the possibility of antibiotic allergy

Ⓔ cardiac surgery should be considered if the vegetations are very large

54.

The risks of developing clinical evidence of coronary artery disease are

Ⓐ increased by exogenous oestrogen use in postmenopausal females

Ⓑ diminished by stopping smoking

Ⓒ reduced by the moderate consumption of alcohol

Ⓓ increased in hyperfibrinogenaemia

Ⓔ increased by hypercholesterolaemia but not hypertriglyceridaemia

55.

In the investigation of suspected angina pectoris

Ⓐ the resting ECG is usually abnormal

Ⓑ exercise-induced elevation in blood pressure indicates significant ischaemia

Ⓒ a normal ECG during exercise excludes angina pectoris

Ⓓ coronary angiography is only indicated if an exercise test is abnormal

Ⓔ physical examination is of no clinical value

56.

In the treatment of patients with angina pectoris

Ⓐ aspirin reduces the frequency of anginal attacks

Ⓑ glyceryl trinitrate is equally effective when swallowed as when taken sublingually

Ⓒ calcium antagonists are more effective for coronary artery spasm than beta-blockers

Ⓓ tissue levels of nitrates must be consistently high for maximum therapeutic effect

Ⓔ beta blockers are more effective than other anti-anginal agents

57.

In the management of angina pectoris

Ⓐ coronary angioplasty improves symptoms and subsequent mortality

Ⓑ coronary angioplasty should not be performed on stenotic arterial grafts

Ⓒ 90% of patients undergoing coronary artery grafting are pain free 5 years post-operation

Ⓓ coronary artery grafts improve prognosis in patients with stenosis of the left main coronary artery

Ⓔ the natural history of coronary artery disease is of progressively severe pain

58.

Unstable angina is

Ⓐ invariably preceded by a history of effort angina

Ⓑ associated with progression to myocardial infarction in 15%

Ⓒ due to plaque rupture, thrombosis or coronary artery spasm

Ⓓ an indication for immediate exercise testing to assess prognosis

Ⓔ best managed by emergency coronary artery bypass surgery

59.

The clinical features of acute myocardial infarction include

Ⓐ nausea and vomiting

Ⓑ breathlessness and angor animi

Ⓒ hypotension and peripheral cyanosis

Ⓓ sinus tachycardia or sinus bradycardia

Ⓔ absence of any symptoms or physical signs

60.

Findings consistent with anterior myocardial infarction occurring within the previous 6 hours include

Ⓐ hypertension and raised JVP

Ⓑ pericardial friction rub

Ⓒ ST elevation > 2 mm in leads II, III and AVF on ECG

Ⓓ gallop rhythm and soft first heart sound

Ⓔ serum lactate dehydrogenase activity > 3000 i.u./L

61.

The following drug therapies improve the long-term prognosis after acute myocardial infarction

Ⓐ aspirin

Ⓑ nitrates

Ⓒ calcium antagonists

Ⓓ ACE inhibitors

Ⓔ beta blockers

62.

Coronary artery thrombolysis with streptokinase therapy is

Ⓐ of no proven benefit to patients over the age of 75 years

Ⓑ more beneficial in patients with ST depression than ST elevation

Ⓒ relatively contraindicated in patients with uncontrolled hypertension

Ⓓ best avoided in patients with chest pain without elevation of serum creatine kinase activity

Ⓔ more likely to cause anaphylactic shock than therapy with tissue plasminogen activator

63.
In the treatment of acute myocardial infarction

Ⓐ aspirin given within 6 hours of onset reduces the mortality

Ⓑ streptokinase therapy reduces infarct size and mortality by > 25%

Ⓒ diamorphine is better given intravenously than by any other route

Ⓓ immediate calcium channel blocker therapy reduces the early mortality rate

Ⓔ mobilisation should be deferred until cardiac enzymes normalise

64.
In the treatment of arrhythmias following acute myocardial infarction

Ⓐ atropine should be given for all sinus bradycardias

Ⓑ frequent ventricular ectopics usually require lignocaine therapy

Ⓒ complete heart block in inferior infarcts usually requires endocardial pacing

Ⓓ lignocaine therapy should be given before cardioversion for ventricular fibrillation

Ⓔ cardioversion is indicated for all tachyarrhythmias inducing acute circulatory collapse

65.
The following statements about the prognosis of acute myocardial infarction are true

Ⓐ 75% of all deaths occur within the first 24 hours

Ⓑ Survivors of early VF have a worse prognosis

Ⓒ Stress and social isolation adversely affect the prognosis

Ⓓ 5 year survival is 75% for those who leave hospital

Ⓔ Late mortality is determined by the extent of myocardial damage

66.
The following statements about systemic hypertension are true

Ⓐ Casual blood pressure recordings correlate poorly with life expectancy

Ⓑ Systolic hypertension alone is of little prognostic value

Ⓒ Most patients have a normal plasma renin concentration

Ⓓ 15% of the adult UK population have essential hypertension

Ⓔ 15% of hypertensives have hypertension secondary to other disorders

67.
Recognised causes of secondary hypertension include

Ⓐ persistent ductus arteriosus

Ⓑ primary hyperaldosteronism

Ⓒ acromegaly

Ⓓ oestrogen-containing oral contraceptives

Ⓔ thyrotoxicosis

68.
In a patient with systemic hypertension, the following findings suggest the diagnoses shown

Ⓐ symmetrical small joint polyarthritis: hyperparathyroidism

Ⓑ radio-femoral delay in the pulses: renovascular disease

Ⓒ left ventricular failure: phaeochromocytoma

Ⓓ epigastric bruit: coarctation of the aorta

Ⓔ palpably enlarged kidneys: renovascular disease

69.
Complications of systemic hypertension include

Ⓐ retinal microaneurysms

Ⓑ dissecting aneurysm of the ascending aorta

Ⓒ renal artery stenosis

Ⓓ lacunar strokes of the internal capsule

Ⓔ subdural haemorrhage

70.

In the investigation of systemic hypertension

Ⓐ hyperkalaemic metabolic acidosis indicates hyperaldosteronism

Ⓑ excretion urography is useful in the diagnosis of renal artery stenosis

Ⓒ normal urinary 5-HIAA excretion excludes phaeochromocytoma

Ⓓ urine analysis for blood, protein and glucose is essential

Ⓔ the commonest cause of electrolyte abnormalities is diuretic treatment

71.

Accelerated phase or malignant hypertension is suggested by hypertension and

Ⓐ a loud second heart sound

Ⓑ a heaving apex beat

Ⓒ headache

Ⓓ retinal soft exudates or haemorrhages

Ⓔ renal or cardiac failure

72.

In the emergency treatment of accelerated hypertension

Ⓐ the aim is to lower the systolic blood pressure to normal within 60 minutes

Ⓑ intravenous sodium nitroprusside is usually necessary to control the severe hypertension

Ⓒ parenteral therapy is preferable to oral therapy

Ⓓ vasodilator therapy to reduce the afterload should be used

Ⓔ ACE inhibitors are indicated if renal artery stenosis is suspected

73.

In the treatment of mild to moderate systemic hypertension

Ⓐ treatment has more effect on the risk of stroke than the risk of coronary heart disease

Ⓑ weight reduction is more important to prognosis than stopping smoking

Ⓒ treatment is less likely to be of benefit if cardiac or renal disease are present

Ⓓ there are no proven benefits of therapy in patients aged over 70 years

Ⓔ moderation of alcohol consumption is likely to improve blood pressure control

74.

Important explanations for hypertension refractory to medical therapy include

Ⓐ poor compliance with drug therapy

Ⓑ inadequate drug therapy

Ⓒ phaeochromocytoma

Ⓓ primary hyperaldosteronism

Ⓔ renal artery stenosis

75.

Recognised causes of pulmonary arterial hypertension include

Ⓐ mitral stenosis

Ⓑ atrial septal defect

Ⓒ chronic obstructive pulmonary disease

Ⓓ pulmonary thromboembolism

Ⓔ persistent ductus arteriosus

76.

Typical clinical features of primary pulmonary hypertension include

Ⓐ male preponderance

Ⓑ exertional syncope

Ⓒ systemic arterial emboli

Ⓓ giant 'a' waves in the JVP and right parasternal heave

Ⓔ loud second heart sound and early diastolic murmur

77.
Clinical features characteristic of massive pulmonary embolism include
Ⓐ central and peripheral cyanosis
Ⓑ pleuritic chest pain and haemoptysis
Ⓒ breathlessness and syncope
Ⓓ tachycardia and elevated JVP
Ⓔ Q waves in leads I, II and AVL on ECG

78.
Recognised features of pulmonary infarction include
Ⓐ peripheral blood leucocytosis and fever
Ⓑ pleuro-pericardial friction rub
Ⓒ blood-stained pleural effusion
Ⓓ development of a lung abscess
Ⓔ ipsilateral elevation of the hemidiaphragm

79.
In the treatment of acute pulmonary thromboembolism
Ⓐ streptokinase therapy should be given immediately
Ⓑ 24% oxygen therapy should correct hypoxaemia
Ⓒ diamorphine therapy should be avoided if the patient is severely hypoxic
Ⓓ heparin infusion should be given until warfarin therapy has become effective
Ⓔ warfarin therapy should be continued for 4 weeks

80.
Dilated (congestive) cardiomyopathy is
Ⓐ usually idiopathic
Ⓑ associated with pathognomonic ECG changes
Ⓒ a recognised complication of cytotoxic chemotherapy
Ⓓ associated with chronic alcohol abuse
Ⓔ caused by coxsackie A infection

81.
The clinical features of restrictive (obliterative) cardiomyopathy include
Ⓐ a presentation which mimics that of constrictive pericarditis
Ⓑ primarily characterised by impaired diastolic function
Ⓒ association with primary or secondary amyloidosis
Ⓓ complication of conditions inducing a marked peripheral blood eosinophilia
Ⓔ gross cardiomegaly on chest X-ray

82.
Clinical features compatible with idiopathic dilated cardiomyopathy include
Ⓐ absence of a previous history of angina or myocardial infarction
Ⓑ deep Q waves in anterior ECG leads
Ⓒ biventricular dilatation with an ejection fraction < 20%
Ⓓ dyskinetic segment of left ventricle on echocardiography
Ⓔ functional mitral regurgitation

83.
Clinical features compatible with hypertrophic cardiomyopathy include
Ⓐ family history of sudden death
Ⓑ angina pectoris and exertional syncope
Ⓒ jerky pulse and heaving apex beat
Ⓓ murmurs suggesting both aortic stenosis and mitral regurgitation
Ⓔ soft or absent second heart sound

84.
Typical features of acute pericarditis include
Ⓐ chest pain resembling that of myocardial infarction
Ⓑ a friction rub that is best heard in the axilla in mid-expiration
Ⓒ ST elevation on the ECG that is concave upwards
Ⓓ elevation of the serum creatine kinase
Ⓔ ECG changes that are only seen in the chest leads

85.

In a 20-year-old woman with acute pericarditis, the following disorders should be excluded

Ⓐ Hodgkin's disease

Ⓑ systemic lupus erythematosus

Ⓒ coxsackie A virus infection

Ⓓ acute rheumatic fever

Ⓔ rubella virus infection

86.

The typical features of constrictive pericarditis include

Ⓐ severe breathlessness

Ⓑ a normal chest X-ray

Ⓒ a previous history of tuberculosis

Ⓓ tachycardia and a loud third heart sound

Ⓔ marked elevation of the JVP with a steep 'x' and 'y' descent

87.

Central cyanosis in infancy is an expected finding in the following congenital heart diseases

Ⓐ persistent ductus arteriosus

Ⓑ transposition of the great arteries

Ⓒ coarctation of the aorta

Ⓓ Fallot's tetralogy

Ⓔ atrial septal defect

88.

The following statements about persistent ductus arteriosus are true

Ⓐ Blood usually passes from the pulmonary artery to the aorta

Ⓑ The onset of heart failure usually occurs in early infancy

Ⓒ A systolic murmur around the scapulae is typical

Ⓓ Shunt reversal is indicated by cyanosis of the lower limbs

Ⓔ Prophylactic antibiotic therapy to prevent endocarditis is indicated

89.

Typical clinical features of coarctation of the aorta include

Ⓐ an association with a bicuspid aortic valve

Ⓑ cardiac failure developing in male adolescents

Ⓒ palpable collateral arteries around the scapulae

Ⓓ rib notching on chest X-ray associated with weak femoral pulses

Ⓔ ECG showing right ventricular hypertrophy

90.

In atrial septal defect

Ⓐ the lesion is usually of secundum type

Ⓑ the initial shunt is right to left

Ⓒ splitting of the second heart sound increases in expiration

Ⓓ the ECG typically shows right bundle branch block

Ⓔ surgery should be deferred until shunt reversal occurs

91.

In small ventricular septal defects

Ⓐ the murmur is confined to late systole

Ⓑ the heart is usually enlarged

Ⓒ there is a risk of infective endocarditis

Ⓓ surgical repair before adolesence is usually indicated

Ⓔ most patients are asymptomatic

92.

In right-to-left shunt reversals of congenital heart disease (Eisenmenger's syndrome)

Ⓐ pulmonary arterial hypertension is usually present

Ⓑ closure of the underlying lesion produces symptomatic relief

Ⓒ the chest X-ray is typically normal

Ⓓ central cyanosis and finger clubbing are often present

Ⓔ physical signs of the underlying lesion persist unchanged

93.
In Fallot's tetralogy

Ⓐ pulmonary and aortic stenosis are combined with a VSD

Ⓑ finger clubbing and central cyanosis are present from birth

Ⓒ the second heart sound is loud and widely split on inspiration

Ⓓ the chest X-ray and ECG are typically normal

Ⓔ cyanotic spells occur due to episodes of dysrhythmia

94.
Cardiovascular changes in normal pregnancy include

Ⓐ an increase in cardiac output by 150% by 12 weeks

Ⓑ tachycardia, elevated JVP and third heart sound

Ⓒ reduction in systemic diastolic pressure

Ⓓ pulmonary systolic murmur

Ⓔ increased blood coagulability

95.
Recognised causes of deep vein thrombosis include

Ⓐ pregnancy

Ⓑ polycythaemia

Ⓒ prolonged travelling

Ⓓ cardiac failure

Ⓔ carcinomatosis

96.
Clinical features of deep venous thrombosis include

Ⓐ cold, painful, blue limb with altered sensation

Ⓑ the absence of any abnormal physical sign

Ⓒ warm, painless, oedematous, white limb

Ⓓ calf tenderness and fever

Ⓔ syncopal episode during defecation

97.
In intermittent claudication due to atherosclerosis

Ⓐ pain is typically relieved by rest and elevation of the leg

Ⓑ secondary ischaemic ulcers are usually painless

Ⓒ pedal pulses are often still palpable

Ⓓ exercise which causes pain should be avoided

Ⓔ the risk of progression is lessened by warfarin

98.
Recognised causes of Raynaud's phenomenon include

Ⓐ beta-blocker therapy

Ⓑ cryoglobulinaemia

Ⓒ progressive systemic sclerosis

Ⓓ vibration trauma

Ⓔ giant cell arteritis

99.
Arterial embolism is a recognised complication of

Ⓐ left atrial myxoma

Ⓒ atrial septal defect

Ⓒ myocardial infarction

Ⓓ infective endocarditis

Ⓔ persistent ductus arteriosus

100.
Clinical presentations of acute systemic arterial embolism include

Ⓐ a warm, painful, swollen leg

Ⓑ left pleuritic chest pain

Ⓒ a painful, cold leg with altered sensation

Ⓓ hypogastric pain with watery diarrhoea

Ⓔ expressive dysphasia after myocardial infarction

101.
The risk of dissecting aortic aneurysm is increased in

Ⓐ Marfan's syndrome

Ⓑ coarctation of the aorta

Ⓒ pregnancy

Ⓓ calcific aortic stenosis

Ⓔ syphilitic aortitis

102.
Characteristic features of dissecting aortic aneurysm include
Ⓐ haemopericardium
Ⓑ acute paraparesis
Ⓒ interscapular back pain
Ⓓ early diastolic murmur
Ⓔ pleural effusion

103.
In the New York Heart Association grading of dyspnoea or angina
Ⓐ Grade 0 = asymptomatic
Ⓑ Grade 1 = symptoms on moderate exertion with minor restriction of activity
Ⓒ Grade 2 = symptoms on mild exertion with major restriction of activity
Ⓓ Grade 3 = symptoms on moderate exertion with major restriction of activity
Ⓔ Grade 4 = symptoms occur even at rest

104.
Components of the jugular venous pulse are explained on the basis of the following events
Ⓐ 'c' wave = closure of the tricuspid valve
Ⓑ 'a' wave = atrial systole
Ⓒ 'v' wave = onset of ventricular systole
Ⓓ 'x' descent = atrial relaxation
Ⓔ 'y' descent = opening of tricuspid valve and onset of ventricular diastole

105.
The following statements about the measurement of the blood pressure (BP) are true
Ⓐ An arm cuff smaller than recommended lowers BP recordings
Ⓑ Appearance of the first Korotkov sound denotes systolic pressure
Ⓒ Muffling of the sound denotes phase V diastolic pressure
Ⓓ Inter-observer variation is less with phase IV than phase V
Ⓔ Resting BP should be recorded, as random BP recordings do not correlate with morbidity

106.
In the normal ECG
Ⓐ depolarisation proceeds from epicardium to endocardium
Ⓑ depolarisation away from the positive electrode produces a positive deflection
Ⓒ depolarisation of the interventricular septum is recorded by the Q wave in V5 + V6
Ⓓ the AVR lead = right arm positive with respect to the other limb leads
Ⓔ voltage amplitudes vary with the thickness of cardiac muscle

DISEASES OF THE RESPIRATORY SYSTEM

6

ANSWERS BEGIN ON P. 172

1.
Central cyanosis is an expected finding in
- Ⓐ SVC obstruction
- Ⓑ fibrosing alveolitis
- Ⓒ polycythaemia
- Ⓓ hypothermia
- Ⓔ chronic bronchitis

2.
Finger clubbing is a typical finding in
- Ⓐ chronic bronchitis
- Ⓑ bronchiectasis
- Ⓒ primary biliary cirrhosis
- Ⓓ cryptogenic fibrosing alveolitis
- Ⓔ ventricular septal defect

3.
Hyperinflation of the chest is suggested by
- Ⓐ pectus excavatum
- Ⓑ AP diameter equals the lateral diameter chest
- Ⓒ increased cricosternal distance
- Ⓓ intercostal muscle indrawing
- Ⓔ an obtuse subcostal angle

4.
Typical chest findings in a large right pleural effusion include
- Ⓐ normal chest expansion
- Ⓑ dull percussion note
- Ⓒ absent breath sounds
- Ⓓ decreased vocal resonance
- Ⓔ pleural friction rub

5.
Typical chest findings in right lower lobe consolidation include
- Ⓐ decreased chest expansion
- Ⓑ dull percussion note
- Ⓒ decreased breath sounds
- Ⓓ increased vocal resonance
- Ⓔ rhonchi and crepitations

6.
Typical chest findings in right lower lobe collapse include
- Ⓐ decreased chest expansion
- Ⓑ stony dull percussion note
- Ⓒ bronchial breath sounds
- Ⓓ decreased vocal resonance
- Ⓔ crepitations

7.
Typical chest findings in a large right pneumothorax include
- Ⓐ decreased chest expansion
- Ⓑ normal percussion note
- Ⓒ increased breath sounds
- Ⓓ increased vocal resonance
- Ⓔ absence of added sounds

8.
Dyspnoea is usually due to decreased pulmonary compliance in
- Ⓐ pulmonary embolism
- Ⓑ ankylosing spondylitis
- Ⓒ chronic bronchitis and emphysema
- Ⓓ pneumococcal pneumonia
- Ⓔ pulmonary oedema

9.
In the normal adult
- Ⓐ the transverse fissure separates the right middle lobe from the right lower lobe
- Ⓑ the left main bronchus is more vertical than the right
- Ⓒ the left upper lobe lies anterior to the left lower lobe
- Ⓓ the oblique fissure extends from the thoracic vertebral level T3
- Ⓔ pulmonary surfactant is secreted by Type I pneumocytes

10.

In the normal resting adult

Ⓐ pulmonary ventilation is 10 litres per minute

Ⓑ alveolar ventilation is 5 litres per minute

Ⓒ pulmonary blood flow is 10 litres per minute

Ⓓ the PaO_2 is 11–13 kPa and $PaCO_2$ is 4.8–6.0 kPa

Ⓔ pulmonary blood flow is higher at the lung base

11.

During ventilation, the work done against elastic resistance is increased by

Ⓐ ankylosing spondylitis

Ⓑ chronic bronchitis

Ⓒ bronchial asthma

Ⓓ pulmonary oedema

Ⓔ obstruction of a main bronchus

12.

In the central control of breathing

Ⓐ fever reduces the sensitivity of the respiratory centre

Ⓑ only central chemoreceptors are sensitive to arterial PCO_2

Ⓒ peripheral chemoreceptors are sensitive only to arterial PO_2

Ⓓ chronic alveolar hypoventilation decreases sensitivity to arterial PCO_2

Ⓔ chest wall and pulmonary stretch receptors stimulate ventilation during exercise

13.

Alveolar hypoventilation is typically associated with

Ⓐ pulmonary embolism

Ⓑ severe chest wall deformity

Ⓒ salicylate intoxication

Ⓓ pulmonary fibrosis

Ⓔ severe chronic bronchitis

14.

The following statements about pulmonary function tests are true

Ⓐ Over 80% of vital capacity can normally be expelled in one second

Ⓑ The transfer factor is measured using inspired oxygen

Ⓒ Residual volume is increased in chronic bronchitis and emphysema

Ⓓ The FEV/FVC ratio is usually normal in ankylosing spondylitis

Ⓔ Peak expiratory flow rates accurately reflect the severity of restrictive lung disorders

15.

Typical clinical features in patients with type II ventilatory failure

Ⓐ retinal venous distension

Ⓑ drowsiness

Ⓒ cold clammy skin

Ⓓ headache

Ⓔ muscle twitching

16.

The following disorders characteristically produce type I respiratory failure

Ⓐ kyphoscoliosis

Ⓑ Guillain–Barré polyneuropathy

Ⓒ adult respiratory distress syndrome

Ⓓ extrinsic allergic alveolitis

Ⓔ inhaled foreign body in a major airway

17.

The following disorders characteristically produce type II respiratory failure

Ⓐ heroin overdose

Ⓑ poliomyelitis

Ⓒ pulmonary embolism

Ⓓ cryptogenic fibrosing alveolitis

Ⓔ bronchial asthma

18.

The following statements about oxygen therapy are true

Ⓐ At sea level, the pressure of oxygen in inspired air is 20 kPa

Ⓑ Chronic domiciliary oxygen therapy is indicated only when PO_2 is < 6 kPa

Ⓒ Dissolved oxygen contributes to tissue oxygenation in anaemia

Ⓓ Oxygen toxicity in adults can produce retrolental fibroplasia

Ⓔ Central cyanosis unresponsive to 100% oxygen indicates right to left shunting of > 20%

19.

In the delivery of oxygen therapy, the following statements are true

Ⓐ MC masks are most valuable in chronic type II failure

Ⓑ Ventimasks help prevent re-breathing of carbon dioxide

Ⓒ Nasal cannulae deliver inspired oxygen concentration of 30% at 2 L/min

Ⓓ Ventimasks require that the oxygen should be humidified by passage through water

Ⓔ Oxygen toxicity will not occur until after > 48 hours of > 40% oxygen

20.

In mechanical respiratory support

Ⓐ cardiac output increases with positive end-expiratory pressure (PEEP)

Ⓑ PEEP helps correct V/Q mismatch

Ⓒ continuous positive airways pressure (CPAP) requires intubation

Ⓓ barotrauma only occurs with PEEP

Ⓔ intermittent ventilation is useful in the transition to non-assisted ventilation

21.

In the treatment of chronic bronchitis associated with type II respiratory failure

Ⓐ oxygen should be given using an MC mask at 2 L/min

Ⓑ nebulised doxapram improves small airways obstruction

Ⓒ cough disturbing sleep should be treated with pholcodeine

Ⓓ corticosteroid therapy is usually contraindicated

Ⓔ continuous oxygen therapy reduces pulmonary hypertension

22.

Adult respiratory distress syndrome is associated with

Ⓐ alveolar oedema with a protein content 20 g/L

Ⓑ hypoxaemia and systemic hypotension

Ⓒ severe dyspnoea with rhonchi rather than crepitations

Ⓓ widespread `fluffy or soft` opacification on chest X-ray

Ⓔ thrombocytopenia and disseminated intravascular coagulation

23.

The following respiratory disorders are commonly due to the viral infections listed below

Ⓐ laryngotracheobronchitis (croup)— coxsackie A virus

Ⓑ epiglottitis—rhinoviruses

Ⓒ bronchiolitis—respiratory syncytial virus

Ⓓ viral pneumonia—enteroviruses

Ⓔ pharyngoconjunctival fever—echoviruses

24.

Influenza A and B viral infections are associated with

Ⓐ short-lived type-specific immunity following infection

Ⓑ an incubation period of 7–10 days

Ⓒ leucopenia

Ⓓ acute tracheobronchitis

Ⓔ staphylococcal bronchopneumonia

25.

Typical clinical features of acute tracheobronchitis include

Ⓐ an irritating unproductive cough at onset

Ⓑ superinfection with *Staphylococcus aureus*

Ⓒ retrosternal chest pain

Ⓓ pyrexia and neutrophil leucocytosis

Ⓔ crepitations rather than rhonchi on auscultation

26.

Characteristic features of pneumococcal pneumonia include

Ⓐ sudden onset of rigors and pleuritic pain

Ⓑ peak frequency in childhood and old age

Ⓒ lobar collapse and diminished breath sounds

Ⓓ bacteraemia and neutrophil leucocytosis

Ⓔ herpes labialis

27.

Recognised complications of pneumococcal pneumonia include

Ⓐ bronchial carcinoma

Ⓑ pericarditis

Ⓒ peripheral circulatory failure

Ⓓ pleural effusion and empyema

Ⓔ subphrenic abscess

28.

Typical features of staphylococcal pneumonia include

Ⓐ an illness clinically indistinguishable from pneumococcal pneumonia

Ⓑ multiple lung abscesses appearing as thin-walled cysts

Ⓒ association with influenza A infection

Ⓓ staphylococcal sepsis elsewhere in the body

Ⓔ penicillin resistance

29.

Typical features of klebsiella pneumonia include

Ⓐ upper lobe collapse on chest X-ray

Ⓑ severe systemic disturbance and high mortality

Ⓒ copious chocolate-coloured sputum

Ⓓ organisms resistant to chloramphenicol and gentamicin

Ⓔ occurrence in previously healthy individuals

30.

Recognised features of mycoplasmal pneumonia include

Ⓐ institutional outbreaks in young adults

Ⓑ haemolytic anaemia and cold agglutinins in the serum

Ⓒ fever and malaise preceding respiratory symptoms by several days

Ⓓ inconspicuous physical signs in the chest

Ⓔ response to tetracycline or erythromycin therapy

31.

Typical features of legionella pneumonia include

Ⓐ oro-faecal spread of infection

Ⓑ vomiting and diarrhoea

Ⓒ hyponatraemia and confusion

Ⓓ inconspicuous physical signs in the chest

Ⓔ response to rifampicin and/or erythromycin therapy

32.

A non-pneumococcal pneumonia should be suspected if the clinical features include

Ⓐ respiratory symptoms preceding systemic upset by several days

Ⓑ chest signs less dramatic than the chest X-ray appearances

Ⓒ the development of a pleural effusion

Ⓓ the absence of a neutrophil leucocytosis

Ⓔ palpable splenomegaly and proteinuria

33.
Pneumonia in the immunocompromised is best treated with the following drug regimes
Ⓐ *Pneumocystis carinii* — co-trimoxazole
Ⓑ *Pseudomonas aeruginosa* — azlocillin or ciprofloxacin
Ⓒ Cytomegalovirus — ganciclovir
Ⓓ Herpes simplex — acyclovir
Ⓔ Respiratory syncytial virus — tribavirin

34.
Typical features of acute bronchopneumonia include
Ⓐ occurrence in middle-aged adults
Ⓑ occurrence after debilitating illness and influenza
Ⓒ absence of a neutrophil leucocytosis
Ⓓ acute onset with pleuritic chest pain
Ⓔ bronchiectasis and fibrosis are recognised complications

35.
The following statements about aspiration pneumonias are true
Ⓐ Bronchiectasis is a recognised complication
Ⓑ Chest X-ray abnormalities are typically bilateral
Ⓒ Lobar collapse predisposes to the development of lung abscess
Ⓓ Systemic upset is usually marked
Ⓔ Adult respiratory distress syndrome may be a complication

36.
The clinical features of suppurative pneumonia and lung abscess include
Ⓐ prior pulmonary infarction
Ⓑ the presence of an inhaled foreign body
Ⓒ rigors and pleuritic chest pain
Ⓓ bronchial breathing if there is an underlying bronchial carcinoma
Ⓔ radiological features of cavitation

37.
Post-primary tuberculosis in the UK is associated with
Ⓐ occurrence in childhood rather than old age
Ⓑ an increased prevalence in diabetic patients
Ⓒ human rather than bovine strains of Mycobacteriae
Ⓓ alcohol abuse and malnutrition
Ⓔ air-borne re-infection rather than reactivation of infection

38.
Typical features of primary tuberculosis include
Ⓐ a sustained pyrexial illness
Ⓑ caseation within the regional lymph nodes
Ⓒ bilateral hilar lymphadenopathy on chest X-ray
Ⓓ erythema nodosum
Ⓔ pleural effusion with a negative tuberculin skin test

39.
Recognised features of miliary tuberculosis include
Ⓐ severe systemic upset with fever in childhood
Ⓑ blood dyscrasias and hepatosplenomegaly
Ⓒ normal chest X-ray and negative tuberculin test
Ⓓ inconspicuous physical signs in the chest
Ⓔ characteristic granulomata on liver and bone biopsy

40.
Typical features of post-primary tuberculosis include
Ⓐ purulent sputum negative for TB on microscopy
Ⓑ bilateral upper lobe opacities on chest X-ray
Ⓒ conspicuous physical signs in the chest
Ⓓ haematogenous dissemination in most cases
Ⓔ cavitation of pulmonary lesions

41.
Recognised complications of post-primary tuberculosis include
Ⓐ aspergilloma
Ⓑ amyloidosis
Ⓒ miliary tuberculosis
Ⓓ bronchiectasis
Ⓔ paraplegia

42.
The following statements about tuberculin tine testing are true
Ⓐ false positives are common in sarcoidosis and acute exanthemata
Ⓑ the skin reaction is best assessed 3 days after innoculation
Ⓒ tuberculin-positive family contacts do not require BCG vaccination
Ⓓ grade III and IV reactions are characterised by 4 discrete papules
Ⓔ tuberculin-positive children are immune to tuberculosis

43.
In the treatment of post-primary pulmonary tuberculosis
Ⓐ combination drug therapy is always indicated
Ⓑ sputum remains infectious for at least 4 weeks after the onset of therapy
Ⓒ at least 12 months daily therapy is required for 100% effectiveness
Ⓓ isoniazid and pyrazinamide do not cross the blood-brain barrier
Ⓔ treatment failure is invariably due to multiple drug resistance

44.
Recognised adverse reactions to anti-tuberculous drugs include
Ⓐ streptomycin — renal failure
Ⓑ isoniazid — hypothyroidism
Ⓒ rifampicin — optic neuritis
Ⓓ pyrazinamide — hepatitis
Ⓔ ethambutol — vestibular neuronitis

45.
Prophylactic anti-TB drug therapy is indicated in the following tuberculin-positive individuals
Ⓐ insulin-dependent diabetics
Ⓑ patients receiving long-term immunosuppressant drug
Ⓒ HIV antibody-positive subjects
Ⓓ children aged < 3 years old who have not had BCG immunisation
Ⓔ adults who have recently become tuberculin-positive

46.
Pulmonary infection with *Aspergillus fumigatus* is a recognised cause of the following
Ⓐ bullous emphysema
Ⓑ mycetoma
Ⓒ necrotising pneumonitis
Ⓓ bronchopulmonary eosinophilia
Ⓔ extrinsic allergic alveolitis

47.
Typical features of seasonal allergic rhinitis include
Ⓐ cell-mediated delayed hypersensitivity response to pollens
Ⓑ sneezing and lacrimation
Ⓒ purulent nasal discharge
Ⓓ positive skin sensitivity tests
Ⓔ response to ipratropium nasal spray

48.
Typical features of early onset bronchial asthma include
Ⓐ individuals are usually atopic
Ⓑ a single allergen is often identifiable
Ⓒ paroxysmal expiratory wheeze and dyspnoea
Ⓓ a strong family history of allergic disorders
Ⓔ *Aspergillus fumigatus* is usually present in the sputum

49.
Typical features of late-onset bronchial asthma include
Ⓐ invariable history of cigarette smoking
Ⓑ multiple allergens are often identifiable
Ⓒ exposure to aspirin and certain chemicals induces attacks
Ⓓ asthma is more often chronic than episodic
Ⓔ serum IgE concentrations are often normal

50.
Features indicative of severe acute asthma include
Ⓐ pulse rate = 120 per minute
Ⓑ peak expiratory flow rate = 350 L per minute
Ⓒ pulsus paradoxus = 30 mmHg
Ⓓ arterial PaO_2 = 10 kPa
Ⓔ arterial $PaCO_2$ = 6 kPa

51.
The initial management of severe acute asthma should include
Ⓐ 28% oxygen delivered by a Ventimask
Ⓑ salbutamol 2.5 mg–5 mg by inhalation
Ⓒ ampicillin 500 mg orally and cromoglycate 10 mg by inhalation
Ⓓ hydrocortisone 200 mg i.v. and prednisolone 40 mg orally
Ⓔ arterial blood gas analysis and chest X-ray

52.
The typical features of asthmatic pulmonary eosinophilia include
Ⓐ immediate hypersensitivity and immune complex reactions
Ⓑ positive skin and serum tests for *Aspergillus fumigatus*
Ⓒ isolation of *Aspergillus clavatus* in the sputum
Ⓓ recurrent upper lobe collapse
Ⓔ chronic asthma and bronchiectasis

53.
Mediastinal opacification on the chest X-ray is a typical feature of
Ⓐ thymoma
Ⓑ retrosternal goitre
Ⓒ Pancoast tumour
Ⓓ hiatus hernia
Ⓔ neurofibroma

54.
In a patient with hoarseness
Ⓐ a bovine cough suggests a functional cause
Ⓑ stridor suggests bilateral cord paralysis
Ⓒ inhaled corticosteroids are often beneficial
Ⓓ the finding of a left hilar mass is likely to explain the symptom
Ⓔ teflon injection of the paralysed vocal cord aids functional improvement

55.
Characteristic features of pulmonary eosinophilia include
Ⓐ an association with ascariasis and microfilariasis
Ⓑ eosinophilic pneumonia without peripheral blood eosinophilia
Ⓒ prominent asthmatic features
Ⓓ induction by exposure to sulphonamide drugs
Ⓔ opacities on chest X-ray

56.
Clinical features compatible with a diagnosis of extrinsic allergic alveolitis include
Ⓐ expiratory rhonchi and sputum eosinophilia
Ⓑ dry cough, dyspnoea and pyrexia
Ⓒ end-inspiratory crepitations
Ⓓ FEV_1/FVC ratio = 50%
Ⓔ positive serum precipitin tests

57.
Pathognomonic features of chronic bronchitis include
Ⓐ decreased residual volume
Ⓑ increase in the gas transfer factor
Ⓒ decreased mucus secretion
Ⓓ increased FEV$_1$/FVC ratio
Ⓔ cough and breathlessness for more than 2 months in the previous year

58.
Typical features of pulmonary emphysema include
Ⓐ normal FEV/FVC ratio indicating the absence of airways obstruction
Ⓑ central cyanosis occurring as an early manifestation
Ⓒ reduced carbon monoxide transfer factor
Ⓓ dyspnoea more prominent than in chronic bronchitis
Ⓔ alpha$_1$-antitrypsin deficiency in young adults

59.
Characteristic findings in pulmonary emphysema during inspiration include
Ⓐ elevation of the JVP during inspiration
Ⓑ tracheal descent
Ⓒ indrawing of the intercostal muscles
Ⓓ contraction of the scalene muscles
Ⓔ widespread rhonchi

60.
Typical chest X-ray findings in chronic bronchitis and emphysema include
Ⓐ prominent pulmonary arteries at the hila
Ⓑ low flat diaphragms
Ⓒ prominent peripheral vascular markings
Ⓓ upper lobe pulmonary venous congestion
Ⓔ Kerley B lines and cardiomegaly

61.
Recognised causes of bronchiectasis include
Ⓐ primary hypogammaglobulinaemia
Ⓑ an inhaled foreign body
Ⓒ cystic fibrosis
Ⓓ asthmatic pulmonary eosinophilia
Ⓔ sarcoidosis

62.
Typical clinical features of bronchiectasis include
Ⓐ chronic cough with scanty sputum volumes
Ⓑ recurrent pleurisy
Ⓒ haemoptysis
Ⓓ empyema thoracis
Ⓔ crepitations on auscultation

63.
In the treatment of bronchiectasis
Ⓐ postural drainage is best undertaken twice daily
Ⓑ failure of medical therapy is a clear indication for surgery
Ⓒ antibiotic therapy is indicated if sputum purulence persists
Ⓓ thoracic CT is advisable before surgery is undertaken
Ⓔ pulmonary emphysema is a contraindication to surgery

64.
The following statements about bronchial obstruction are true
Ⓐ Lobar emphysema develops in the lung distal to a partial obstruction
Ⓑ Mediastinal displacement is invariably towards the affected side
Ⓒ Infection is inevitable especially in partial obstruction
Ⓓ A collapsed right middle lobe is best detected radiologically
Ⓔ Inhaled foreign bodies usually lodge in the left main bronchus

65.
Typical features of bronchial adenoma include
Ⓐ occurrence in elderly females
Ⓑ carcinoid syndrome if liver metastases are present
Ⓒ recurrent haemoptysis
Ⓓ lobar emphysema
Ⓔ recurrent pneumonia

66.
Bronchial carcinoma
Ⓐ accounts for 10% of all male deaths from cancer
Ⓑ typically presents with massive haemoptysis
Ⓒ histology reveals adenocarcinoma in 50%
Ⓓ is associated with asbestos exposure
Ⓔ is 40 times more common in smokers than non-smokers

67.
Bronchial carcinoma is
Ⓐ surgically resectable in approximately 40%
Ⓑ reliably excluded by the finding of a normal chest X-ray
Ⓒ associated with a 50% 5 year survival after surgical resection
Ⓓ only diagnosable reliably by bronchoscopy
Ⓔ usually small cell in origin if associated with finger clubbing

68.
Non-metastatic manifestations of bronchial carcinoma include
Ⓐ cerebellar degeneration
Ⓑ myasthenia
Ⓒ gynaecomastia
Ⓓ polyneuropathy
Ⓔ dermatomyositis

69.
Typical presentations of small cell bronchial carcinoma include
Ⓐ nephrotic syndrome
Ⓑ inappropriate ADH secretion
Ⓒ ectopic ACTH secretion
Ⓓ ectopic parathyroid hormone secretion
Ⓔ hypertrophic pulmonary osteoarthropathy

70.
Typical features of cryptogenic fibrosing alveolitis include
Ⓐ hypercapnic respiratory failure
Ⓑ positive antinuclear and rheumatoid factors
Ⓒ finger clubbing
Ⓓ recurrent wheeze and haemoptysis
Ⓔ increased neutrophil and eosinophil count in bronchial washings

71.
In coal-worker's pneumoconiosis
Ⓐ the disease usually progresses despite avoidance of coal dust
Ⓑ certification for compensation depends upon the clinical features
Ⓒ upper lobe opacities suggest progressive massive fibrosis
Ⓓ accompanying chronic bronchitis is not due to coal dust exposure
Ⓔ confirmatory physical findings are often present

72.
Typical findings in silicosis include
Ⓐ chest X-ray abnormalities similar to those found in coal workers
Ⓑ 'egg-shell' calcification of the hilar lymph nodes
Ⓒ progression of the disease arrested when dust exposure ceases
Ⓓ fibrotic peripheral nodules in patients with rheumatoid disease
Ⓔ occupational history of coal, tin and mineral mining

73.
The following statements about asbestos-related disease are true
Ⓐ Pleural plaques usually progress to become mesotheliomas
Ⓑ Benign pleural effusions are not blood-stained
Ⓒ Finger clubbing and basal crepitations suggest pulmonary asbestosis
Ⓓ The FEV_1/FVC ratio is typically decreased
Ⓔ mesothelioma can only be reliably diagnosed at thoracotomy

74.

Occupational exposure to the following substances produces an extrinsic allergic alveolitis

Ⓐ cotton dust — bagassosis
Ⓑ mouldy hay — farmer's lung
Ⓒ tin dioxide — siderosis
Ⓓ avian protein — bird fancier's lung
Ⓔ mouldy barley — bysinnosis

75.

The following statements about sarcoidosis are true

Ⓐ pulmonary lesions typically cavitate
Ⓑ the tuberculin tine test is usually positive
Ⓒ erythema marginatum is a characteristic finding
Ⓓ spontaneous resolution is unusual
Ⓔ hypercalcaemia suggests skeletal involvement

76.

Typical features of subacute sarcoidosis include

Ⓐ hilar lymphadenopathy on chest X-ray
Ⓑ cranial neuropathies
Ⓒ conjunctivitis
Ⓓ erosive polyarthritis
Ⓔ swollen parotid glands

77.

A pleural effusion with a protein content of 50 g/L would be compatible with

Ⓐ congestive cardiac failure
Ⓑ pulmonary infarction
Ⓒ subphrenic abscess
Ⓓ pneumonia
Ⓔ nephrotic syndrome

78.

In a patient with a symptomatic pleural effusion

Ⓐ physical signs in the chest are invariably present
Ⓑ pleural biopsy should be avoided given a protein content of 50 g/L
Ⓒ TB can be excluded if the chest X-ray is otherwise normal
Ⓓ lymphocytosis in the pleural fluid is pathognomonic of pleural TB
Ⓔ milky pleural fluid suggests thoracic duct obstruction

79.

Typical features of an empyema thoracis include

Ⓐ bilateral effusions on chest X-ray
Ⓑ a fluid level on chest X-ray suggests a bronchopleural fistula
Ⓒ persistent pyrexia despite antibiotic therapy
Ⓓ recent abdominal surgery
Ⓔ bacteriological culture of the organism despite antibiotic therapy

80.

The following statements about spontaneous pneumothorax are true

Ⓐ Breathlessness and pleuritic chest pain are usually present
Ⓑ Bronchial breathing is audible over the affected hemithorax
Ⓒ Absent peripheral lung markings on chest X-ray suggests tension
Ⓓ Surgical referral is required if there is a bronchopleural fistula
Ⓔ Pleurodesis should be considered for recurrent pneumothoraces

DISEASES OF THE ALIMENTARY TRACT AND PANCREAS

ANSWERS BEGIN ON P. 180

1.

The following statements about gastrointestinal motility are true

Ⓐ the lower oesophageal sphincter is controlled solely by neural factors

Ⓑ the upper oesophageal sphincter is closed except during swallowing

Ⓒ initial gastric relaxation on eating is vagally mediated

Ⓓ normally, 50% of gastric solids are emptied within 30 minutes of ingestion

Ⓔ vagotomy delays gastric emptying of liquids more than solids

2.

In the neuroendocrine control of the alimentary tract

Ⓐ neural control is mediated by mucosal hormone secretion

Ⓑ the initial release of gastrin occurs in reponse to food intake

Ⓒ sympathetic nerve fibres run in the splanchnic nerves

Ⓓ parasympathetic nerves mediate the inhibition of hormone secretion

Ⓔ exocrine pancreatic secretion is controlled solely by hormonal factors

3.

In the normal alimentary tract

Ⓐ the small bowel surface epithelium is replaced every 48 hours

Ⓑ secretory IgA protects the gut from bacterial invasion

Ⓒ fat-soluble drugs and vitamins are transported via the lymphatics

Ⓓ folic acid is chiefly absorbed in the distal jejunum and ileum

Ⓔ approximately 1.5 L of fluid passes into the caecum daily

4.

Recognised causes of stomatitis include

Ⓐ lichen planus

Ⓑ psoriasis

Ⓒ erythema multiforme

Ⓓ herpes simplex

Ⓔ candidiasis

5.

Recognised causes of dysphagia include

Ⓐ iron deficiency anaemia

Ⓑ pharyngeal pouch

Ⓒ Barrett's oesophagus

Ⓓ myasthenia gravis

Ⓔ African trypanosomiasis

6.

The following statements about pharyngeal pouch are true

Ⓐ upper gastrointestinal endoscopy is the investigation of choice

Ⓑ recurrent episodes of stridor are common

Ⓒ presentation typically occurs in adolescence

Ⓓ recurrent pneumonia is a recognised complication

Ⓔ dysphagia typically progresses over several months

7.

Typical features of sideropenic dysphagia include

Ⓐ glossitis

Ⓑ hyperchlorhydria

Ⓒ splenomegaly

Ⓓ hysterical personality

Ⓔ mid-oesophageal web

8.

Typical features of oesophageal achalasia include

Ⓐ recurrent pneumonia

Ⓑ spasm of the lower oesophageal sphincter

Ⓒ heartburn and acid reflux

Ⓓ predisposition to oesophageal carcinoma

Ⓔ symptomatic response to pneumatic balloon dilatation

9.

Paraoesophageal hiatus hernia

Ⓐ is commoner than oesophagogastric hiatus hernia

Ⓑ usually presents with symptoms of acid reflux

Ⓒ typically presents with iron deficiency anaemia

Ⓓ often causes incompetence of the lower oesophageal sphincter

Ⓔ usually progresses to produce an oesophageal stricture

10.

Oesophagogastric hiatus hernia

Ⓐ occurs more frequently in elderly women than men

Ⓑ usually presents with slowly progressive dysphagia

Ⓒ invariably results in peptic oesophagitis

Ⓓ associated with odynophagia suggests oesophageal carcinoma

Ⓔ is best treated surgically when oesophagitis is severe

11.

In diffuse oesophageal spasm

Ⓐ Auerbach's plexus is normal

Ⓑ most patients are over the age of 60 years at presentation

Ⓒ strong uncoordinated contractions occur unrelated to swallowing

Ⓓ dysphagia is most often due to an associated oesophagitis

Ⓔ acid-lowering drug therapy typically reduces the frequency of chest pain

12.

Oesophageal carcinoma in the UK

Ⓐ is more common in men than women

Ⓑ is most often due to adenocarcinoma

Ⓒ typically produces dysphagia with a poorly localised level

Ⓓ predominantly affects the upper third of the oesophagus

Ⓔ is associated with alcohol and tobacco consumption

13.

Typical features of oesophageal carcinoma at presentation include

Ⓐ acid reflux and odynophagia

Ⓑ painless obstruction to the passage of a food bolus

Ⓒ weight loss attributable to metastatic disease

Ⓓ metastatic spread in over 75%

Ⓔ overall survival rates at 5 years of approximately 33%

14.

The following factors are significantly associated with chronic duodenal ulcer disease

Ⓐ oral contraceptive therapy

Ⓑ duodenogastric reflux

Ⓒ pernicious anaemia

Ⓓ Helicobacter pylori infection

Ⓔ tobacco consumption

15.

Typical features of peptic ulcer dyspepsia include

Ⓐ pain relieved by eating

Ⓑ well-localised pain relieved by vomiting

Ⓒ pain-free remissions lasting many weeks

Ⓓ nausea and retrosternal pain relieved by belching

Ⓔ nocturnal pain causing frequent night waking

16.
The following statements about peptic ulcer disease are true
Ⓐ freedom from symptoms invariably indicates ulcer healing
Ⓑ ulcer healing is delayed by tobacco consumption
Ⓒ ulcer healing is promoted by the use of a bland diet
Ⓓ endoscopy is advisable if a gastric ulcer is seen on barium meal
Ⓔ relapse after acid-lowering drug therapy usually indicates malignancy

17.
In the investigation and treatment of chronic dyspepsia
Ⓐ most patients aged < 45 years have an underlying peptic ulcer
Ⓑ 25% of duodenal ulcers relapse unless *H. pylori* has been eradicated
Ⓒ magnesium-containing antacids produce constipation
Ⓓ bismuth compounds should not be used for maintenance therapy
Ⓔ gastric ulcers associated with NSAID therapy are less likely to be associated with *H. pylori* gastritis than gastric ulcers occurring in patients not taking NSAIDs

18.
Gastroduodenal haemorrhage in the UK is
Ⓐ more often due to chronic gastric ulcer than oesophageal varices
Ⓑ associated with a 5% mortality when due to chronic peptic ulceration
Ⓒ a recognised complication of severe head injury
Ⓓ best investigated by endoscopy within 24 hours of admission
Ⓔ significantly associated with anti-inflammatory drug therapy

19.
Typical features of major acute gastroduodenal haemorrhage include
Ⓐ severe abdominal pain
Ⓑ angor animi and restlessness
Ⓒ syncope preceding other evidence of bleeding
Ⓓ elevated blood urea and creatinine concentrations
Ⓔ peripheral blood microcytosis

20.
When acute gastroduodenal haemorrhage is suspected
Ⓐ a pulse rate of 120/minute is most likely to be due to anxiety
Ⓑ hypotension without a tachycardia suggests an alternative diagnosis
Ⓒ the absence of anaemia suggests the volume of blood loss is modest
Ⓓ naso-gastric aspiration provides an accurate estimate of blood loss
Ⓔ endoscopy is best deferred pending blood volume replacement

21.
In resuscitating a patient with an acute gastrointestinal bleed
Ⓐ sedation is mandatory before endoscopy
Ⓑ transfusion requires whole blood rather than packed red cells
Ⓒ volume replacement with colloids is preferable to crystalloids
Ⓓ monitoring central venous pressure and/or urine output is advisable
Ⓔ surgical intervention should be deferred in younger patients

22.
Perforation of a peptic ulcer is typically associated with
Ⓐ acute rather than chronic ulcers
Ⓑ duodenal more often than gastric ulcers
Ⓒ abdominal pain unrelated to the extent of peritoneal soiling
Ⓓ the absence of nausea and vomiting
Ⓔ symptomatic improvement several hours following onset

23.
Characteristic features of gastric outlet obstruction include
Ⓐ metabolic acidosis
Ⓑ bile vomiting
Ⓒ urinary pH < 5
Ⓓ symptomatic relief after vomiting
Ⓔ absent gastric peristalsis

24.
Typical features of a gastrinoma (Z–E syndrome) include
Ⓐ a small gastric tumour
Ⓑ hepatic metastases at presentation
Ⓒ parathyroid adenomas
Ⓓ constipation
Ⓔ absent acid secretory response to pentagastrin stimulation

25.
Following gastric surgery for peptic ulcer disease
Ⓐ osteoporosis develops within 5 years
Ⓑ postprandial discomfort is common
Ⓒ anaemia does not occur after vagotomy alone
Ⓓ iron deficiency is commoner than folate deficiency
Ⓔ diarrhoea usually responds to tetracycline therapy

26.
In the typical early post-cibal or dumping syndrome
Ⓐ symptoms develop 1–2 hours after meals
Ⓑ gastric emptying of liquids is delayed
Ⓒ weakness, palpitation and sweating are due to hypoglycaemia
Ⓓ small, iso-osmolar meals produce symptomatic improvement
Ⓔ peripheral vasoconstriction is often marked

27.
Acute gastritis is typically associated with
Ⓐ *Helicobacter pylori* infection
Ⓑ pathognomonic appearances on barium radiology
Ⓒ alcohol abuse
Ⓓ elemental iron poisoning
Ⓔ significant bleeding in renal failure

28.
Chronic gastritis is typically associated with
Ⓐ significant dyspepsia
Ⓑ pernicious anaemia
Ⓒ specific histopathology
Ⓓ post gastric surgery
Ⓔ gastric carcinoma

29.
Carcinoma of the stomach is
Ⓐ commoner in the Western than the Eastern hemisphere
Ⓑ 100 times more common in patients with pernicious anaemia
Ⓒ associated with blood group O
Ⓓ a recognised cause of diarrhoea due to rapid gastric emptying
Ⓔ a recognised long-term complication of gastric surgery

30.
Typical features of gastric carcinoma in the UK include
Ⓐ progression to involve the duodenum
Ⓑ origin within a chronic peptic ulcer
Ⓒ overall 5 year survival rate of 25%
Ⓓ folate deficiency anaemia
Ⓔ supraclavicular lymphadenopathy

31.
Recognised features of gastric carcinoma include
Ⓐ presentation with ascites or an ovarian tumour mass
Ⓑ characteristic peripheral blood tumour markers
Ⓒ more favourable prognosis when arising in the gastric fundus
Ⓓ acanthosis nigricans
Ⓔ linitis plastica more obvious radiologically than endoscopically

32.
The following statements about pancreatic function are true
Ⓐ the islets of Langerhans comprise 10% of pancreatic cell mass
Ⓑ 4–5 L of pancreatic exocrine fluid enters the duodenum daily
Ⓒ secretin stimulates pancreatic trypsin secretion
Ⓓ pancreatic polypeptide decreases pancreatic and biliary secretion
Ⓔ pancreatic enzyme activity depends on an alkaline medium

33.
In the investigation of chronic pancreatic disease
Ⓐ glucose tolerance is typically normal in pancreatic carcinoma
Ⓑ duodenal ileus is a characteristic feature of chronic pancreatitis
Ⓒ ultrasound scanning is more sensitive than CT scanning
Ⓓ ERCP can reliably distinguish carcinoma from chronic pancreatitis
Ⓔ pancreatic calcification suggests that chronic pancreatitis is the result of alcohol abuse

34.
Recognised causes of acute pancreatitis include
Ⓐ mumps and coxsackie B viral infections
Ⓑ hypothermia and hyperlipidaemia
Ⓒ gallstones in the common bile duct
Ⓓ azathioprine therapy
Ⓔ alcohol abuse

35.
The following are characteristic of acute pancreatitis
Ⓐ abdominal guarding develops soon after the onset of pain
Ⓑ normal serum amylase concentration in the first 4 hours after onset
Ⓒ persistent serum hyperamylasaemia suggests a developing pseudocyst
Ⓓ hypercalcaemia develops 5–7 days after onset
Ⓔ hyperactive loud bowel sounds

36.
In the management of acute pancreatitis
Ⓐ early laparotomy is advisable to exclude alternative diagnoses
Ⓑ opiates should be avoided because of spasm of the sphincter of Oddi
Ⓒ intravenous fluids are unnecessary in the absence of a tachycardia
Ⓓ the PaO_2 and the central venous pressure should be monitored
Ⓔ nasogastric aspiration is required since an ileus is inevitable

37.
Typical features of chronic pancreatitis include
Ⓐ back pain persisting for days or weeks
Ⓑ decreased vitamin B_{12} absorption
Ⓒ increased sodium concentration in the sweat
Ⓓ abdominal pain occurring 12–24 hours after alcohol intake
Ⓔ pancreatic calcification on plain X-ray or ultrasound scan

38.
Pancreatic carcinoma in the UK is associated with
Ⓐ an incidence which has decreased in the last 20 years
Ⓑ occurrence in males rather than females
Ⓒ tobacco consumption
Ⓓ an overall 5 year survival rate of 20%
Ⓔ metastatic spread in 33% at presentation

39.
The typical features of pancreatic carcinoma include
Ⓐ adenocarcinomatous histology
Ⓑ origin in the body of the pancreas in 60% of cases
Ⓒ abdominal pain when arising in the ampulla of Vater
Ⓓ back pain and weight loss indicate a poor prognosis
Ⓔ presentation with painless jaundice

40.
The following statements about small bowel absorption are true
Ⓐ fat is chiefly absorbed in the terminal ileum
Ⓑ fructose is absorbed by simple diffusion
Ⓒ breath hydrogen concentration reflects small bowel lactase activity
Ⓓ stool/serum alpha$_1$ antitrypsin ratios reflect protein absorption
Ⓔ the absorption of SeHCAT bile acid reflects ileal function

41.
The following statements about small bowel malabsorption are true
Ⓐ gastroenterostomy impairs intraluminal digestive processes
Ⓑ bacterial small bowel colonisation reduces bile acid deconjugation
Ⓒ 10 g of stool nitrogen per day indicates protein malabsorption
Ⓓ cholestyramine is useful in the control of bile salt diarrhoea
Ⓔ steatorrhoea is a recognised feature of small bowel resection

42.
In gluten enteropathy (coeliac disease)
Ⓐ the typical onset is in adolescence
Ⓑ there is a predisposition to gut lymphoma and carcinoma
Ⓒ the toxic agent is the polypeptide alpha-gliadin
Ⓓ gluten-free diets improve absorption but not the villous atrophy
Ⓔ serum anti-endomysium IgA antibody titres are characteristically elevated

43.
In the stagnant loop syndrome
Ⓐ diabetic autonomic neuropathy is a recognised cause
Ⓑ anaemia is typically due to folate deficiency
Ⓒ sclerodactyly suggests that the underlying cause is carcinoid syndrome
Ⓓ treatment with intravenous antibiotics is advisable
Ⓔ creation of an ileo-colic fistula should be considered

44.
Characteristic features of Crohn's disease include
Ⓐ familial association with ulcerative colitis
Ⓑ onset after the age of 70 years
Ⓒ disease confined to the ileum and colon
Ⓓ predisposition to biliary calculi
Ⓔ giant cell granulomata indistinguishable from TB

45.
The typical clinical features of Crohn's disease include
Ⓐ association with tobacco consumption
Ⓑ diarrhoea is more severe than in ulcerative colitis
Ⓒ presentation with sub-acute intestinal obstruction
Ⓓ segmental involvement of the colon and rectum
Ⓔ inflammation confined to the mucosa on histology

46.
Recognised complications of Crohn's disease include
Ⓐ pernicious anaemia
Ⓑ erythema nodosum
Ⓒ enteropathic arthritis
Ⓓ aphthous mouth ulcers
Ⓔ small bowel lymphoma

47.
In the treatment of ileo-caecal Crohn's disease
Ⓐ surgical bypass is preferable to localised resection
Ⓑ antibiotic therapy should be avoided
Ⓒ corticosteroid therapy is contraindicated in the acute phase
Ⓓ cholestyramine reduces the diarrhoea but increases steatorrhoea
Ⓔ sulphasalazine reduces the risk of small bowel obstruction

48.
Intestinal obstruction
Ⓐ of mechanical type is a complication of inguinal hernia
Ⓑ of paralytic type is a feature of peripheral circulatory failure
Ⓒ from peritonitis is typically mechanical in type
Ⓓ associated with strangulation is invariably mechanical in type
Ⓔ of paralytic type eventually progresses to a mechanical type

49.
In patients with intestinal obstruction
Ⓐ vomiting is an invariable feature
Ⓑ the finding of an empty rectum usually excludes faecal impaction
Ⓒ hyperactive loud bowel sounds suggest mechanical obstruction
Ⓓ persisting diarrhoea excludes obstruction
Ⓔ abdominal tenderness suggests strangulation or peritonitis

50.
Acute generalised peritonitis
Ⓐ complicating appendicitis is typically caused by *Esch. coli*
Ⓑ carries an overall mortality rate < 1% in the UK
Ⓒ due to tuberculosis is usually blood-borne arising from pulmonary TB
Ⓓ is invariably due to infection
Ⓔ causes increasing abdominal rigidity as paralytic ileus develops

51.
The following statements about intra-abdominal abscess are true
Ⓐ Pelvic abscess typically presents with urinary retention
Ⓑ Constipation is a typically early feature of pelvic abscess
Ⓒ Lower posterior chest tenderness suggests subphrenic abscess
Ⓓ Abscesses are best localised by abdominal ultrasonography
Ⓔ Antibiotic therapy alone should resolve a subphrenic abscess

52.
Acute appendicitis
Ⓐ typically commences with right iliac fossa pain
Ⓑ is often associated with luminal obstruction of the appendix
Ⓒ produces urinary symptoms simulating acute pyelonephritis
Ⓓ typically produces rigors and persistent vomiting
Ⓔ is usually associated with a temperature > 39 degrees C

53.
Characteristic features of ulcerative colitis include
Ⓐ invariable involvement of the rectal mucosa
Ⓑ segmental involvement of the colon and rectum
Ⓒ pseudo-polyposis following healing of mucosal damage
Ⓓ inflammation extending from the mucosa to the serosa
Ⓔ entero-cutaneous and entero-enteric fistulae

54.
Ulcerative colitis differs from Crohn's colitis in that
Ⓐ the disease occurs at any age
Ⓑ tobacco consumption is not associated with ulcerative colitis
Ⓒ toxic dilatation only occurs in ulcerative colitis
Ⓓ aphthous stomatitis is less common than in Crohn's disease
Ⓔ colonic strictures do not occur in ulcerative colitis

55.
Recognised complications of ulcerative colitis include
Ⓐ pyoderma gangrenosum
Ⓑ pericholangitis
Ⓒ venous thromboembolism
Ⓓ colonic carcinoma
Ⓔ enteropathic arthritis

56.

In the treatment of severe acute ulcerative colitis

ⓐ antibiotic therapy is mandatory if the patient is febrile

ⓑ codeine phosphate increases the risk of toxic dilatation

ⓒ systemic corticosteroids induce a remission in the majority

ⓓ hypoproteinaemia indicates the need for albumin infusion

ⓔ failure of medical therapy indicates the need for surgery

57.

In the maintenance treatment of ulcerative colitis

ⓐ corticosteroid therapy should be given orally rather than rectally

ⓑ sulphasalazine therapy reduces the risk of colonic carcinoma

ⓒ azathioprine will reduce corticosteroid maintenance therapy requirements

ⓓ the onset of urticaria suggests an allergy to sulphasalazine

ⓔ unlike sulphasalazine, mesalazine produces headache and diarrhoea

58.

Typical features of colonic diverticulosis in the UK include

ⓐ predominantly involvement of the right hemicolon

ⓑ predisposition to the development of colonic carcinoma

ⓒ better diagnosed by colonoscopy than by barium enema radiology

ⓓ reduction in the number of diverticula with a high fibre diet

ⓔ the absence of symptoms in the absence of complications

59.

Typical features of colonic diverticulitis include

ⓐ severe rectal bleeding

ⓑ chronic iron deficiency anaemia

ⓒ septicaemia and paralytic ileus

ⓓ right iliac fossa pain

ⓔ vesico-colic fistula

60.

The following statements about colonic polyps are true

ⓐ 75% of polyps occur in the right hemicolon

ⓑ the typical histology is that of tubular adenoma

ⓒ polyps > 2 cm in diameter are usually malignant

ⓓ intussusception is a recognised complication

ⓔ presentation with constipation is typical

61.

Familial adenomatous polyposis

ⓐ is inherited as an autosomal recessive trait

ⓑ is usually clinically apparent before the age of 10 years

ⓒ left untreated, progresses to carcinoma before the age of 40 years

ⓓ is associated with gastric and small bowel polyps

ⓔ under the age of 20 years is best treated with immunosuppressant therapy

62.

The following statements about colonic carcinoma are true

ⓐ It is the commonest of all gastrointestinal carcinomas

ⓑ The majority of carcinomas arise in the right hemicolon

ⓒ After resection, there is a recognised risk of a second carcinoma

ⓓ Dukes' A classifies tumour extending to the serosa only

ⓔ Only a minority of rectal tumours are palpable per rectum

63.

In colonic carcinoma

Ⓐ of the caecum, presentation with iron deficiency anaemia is typical

Ⓑ obstruction is typically an early event in carcinoma of the sigmoid

Ⓒ metastatic spread is to the lungs rather than the liver

Ⓓ concomitant multiple tumours are present in 20% of patients

Ⓔ rising serum CEA levels post-resection suggest recurrent tumour

64.

In Hirschsprung's disease of the colon

Ⓐ there is a family history in 90%

Ⓑ presentation typically occurs between the ages of 3 and 5 years

Ⓒ there is a segmental absence of the myenteric nerve plexus

Ⓓ the rectum is typically loaded on digital examination

Ⓔ the surgical treatment of choice is a defunctioning colostomy

65.

The typical features of acute small bowel ischaemia include

Ⓐ occlusion of the inferior mesenteric artery

Ⓑ the recent onset of atrial fibrillation

Ⓒ the sudden onset of abdominal pain, vomiting and diarrhoea

Ⓓ peripheral circulatory failure and signs of peritonitis

Ⓔ gaseous distension of the small bowel on plain abdominal X-rays

66.

The typical features of acute ischaemic colitis include

Ⓐ rigors, abdominal pain and constipation

Ⓑ occlusion of the superior mesenteric artery

Ⓒ profuse bloody diarrhoea and abdominal tenderness

Ⓓ mucosal oedema with 'thumb-printing' on barium enema radiology

Ⓔ resolution with the later development of a colonic stricture

67.

The typical features of the irritable bowel syndrome include

Ⓐ nocturnal diarrhoea and weight loss

Ⓑ onset after the age of 45 years

Ⓒ history of abdominal pain in childhood

Ⓓ right iliac fossa pain and urinary frequency

Ⓔ abdominal distension, flatulence and pellety stools

68.

The management of functional bowel disorders should include

Ⓐ explanation and reassurance after a detailed clinical examination

Ⓑ barium enema and barium follow-through examinations in all patients

Ⓒ evaluation of social and emotional factors

Ⓓ referral for psychiatric assessment and therapy

Ⓔ dihydrocodeine for abdominal pain and diarrhoea

8 DISEASES OF THE LIVER & BILIARY SYSTEM

ANSWERS BEGIN ON P. 188

1.
In the normal liver
Ⓐ the space of Disse separates the hepatocytes from sinusoidal endothelium
Ⓑ the hepatic artery supplies 50% of the total hepatic oxygen supply
Ⓒ portal blood flow falls postprandially
Ⓓ all hepatocytes are capable of performing all metabolic functions
Ⓔ the macrophages (Kupffer cells) comprise 2% of hepatic cell mass

2.
In hepatic carbohydrate metabolism
Ⓐ hepatic glycogen reserves can withstand 7 days of fasting
Ⓑ insulin stimulates the hepatic uptake of glucose absorbed after meals
Ⓒ insulin suppresses hepatic lipolysis and glycogenolysis
Ⓓ hepatic gluconeogenesis utilises pyruvate, glycerol and alanine
Ⓔ hypoglycaemia is a common early feature of liver disease

3.
Bilirubin is
Ⓐ derived exclusively from the breakdown of haemoglobin
Ⓑ bound in the unconjugated form to plasma beta-globulin
Ⓒ conjugated in the microsomes of the hepatocytes
Ⓓ water-soluble as bilirubin diglucuronide and reabsorbed in the small bowel
Ⓔ normally excreted as stercobilinogen in the faeces and as urobilinogen in the urine

4.
The concentration of conjugated bilirubin in the
Ⓐ serum in haemolytic anaemia is typically increased
Ⓑ urine of healthy subjects is typically undetectable
Ⓒ serum normally constitutes most of the total serum bilirubin
Ⓓ serum in Gilbert's syndrome is typically increased
Ⓔ urine in viral hepatitis parallels that of urobilinogen

5.
The serum alanine aminotransferase (ALT) concentration is
Ⓐ derived from a microsomal enzyme specific to hepatocytes
Ⓑ typically more than five times normal in alcoholic hepatitis
Ⓒ usually normal in both obstructive and haemolytic jaundice
Ⓓ likely to rise and fall in parallel with the serum bilirubin in viral hepatitis
Ⓔ likely to increase in response to the intake of enzyme-inducing drugs

6.
The serum alkaline phosphatase concentration
Ⓐ is derived from the liver, bone, small bowel and placenta
Ⓑ usually increases to more than five times normal in viral hepatitis
Ⓒ derives mainly from hepatic sinusoidal and canalicular membranes
Ⓓ is of particular prognostic value in chronic liver disease
Ⓔ increases more in extrahepatic than intrahepatic cholestasis

7.
When monitoring serum liver function values in liver disease
Ⓐ the albumin concentration falls rapidly in acute fulminant liver failure
Ⓑ persistent hypergammaglobulinaemia indicates hepatocyte necrosis
Ⓒ an increased IgA concentration is typical of alcoholic hepatitis
Ⓓ the prothrombin time increases rapidly in severe acute hepatitis
Ⓔ an increased IgG concentration suggests primary biliary cirrhosis

8.
In the investigation of suspected liver disease
Ⓐ ultrasonography reliably distinguishes solid from cystic masses
Ⓑ radioisotope scanning reliably excludes liver disease
Ⓒ the anterior liver surface is not usually visible at laparoscopy
Ⓓ the mortality rate of percutaneous liver biopsy is about 5%
Ⓔ ascitic protein concentrations > 30 g/L are compatible with diagnosis of carcinomatosis

9.
The following statements about liver disease are true
Ⓐ alcohol is a recognised cause of intrahepatic cholestasis
Ⓑ night sweats are a recognised feature of hepatic metastases
Ⓒ osteomalacia is a recognised feature of chronic obstructive jaundice
Ⓓ jaundice and a palpable gallbladder suggest common bile duct stones
Ⓔ serum unconjugated and conjugated bilirubin concentrations are increased in acute hepatitis

10.
In haemolytic jaundice in an adult
Ⓐ the finding of a serum bilirubin > 100 μmol/L is typical
Ⓑ jaundice is often not evident unless the serum bilirubin > 50 μmol/L
Ⓒ the urine is usually dark brown due to the presence of urobilinogen
Ⓓ the majority of patients have palpable splenomegaly
Ⓔ the stools are characteristically pale

11.
Characteristic features of Gilbert's syndrome include
Ⓐ an autosomal recessive mode of inheritance
Ⓑ decreased hepatic glucuronyl transferase activity
Ⓒ unconjugated hyperbilirubinaemia < 100 μol/L
Ⓓ serum bilirubin concentration increased by fasting
Ⓔ increased serum bile acid concentrations

12.
Drug-induced cholestatic jaundice is a typical adverse effect of
Ⓐ chlorpropamide
Ⓑ salicylates
Ⓒ chlorpromazine
Ⓓ methyl testosterone
Ⓔ ethinyl oestradiol

13.
The histopathological characteristics of viral hepatitis include
Ⓐ polymorph leucocyte infiltration of the lobules
Ⓑ sparing of the centrilobular areas
Ⓒ collapse of the reticulin architecture
Ⓓ hepatocyte necrosis with eosinophilic bodies
Ⓔ fatty infiltration

14.

The typical features of type A viral hepatitis (HAV) include

Ⓐ RNA virus infection associated with seafood poisoning

Ⓑ an incubation period of 3 months

Ⓒ a greater risk of fulminant liver failure in the young than the old

Ⓓ headache, right hypochondrial pain and tenderness

Ⓔ progression to chronic active hepatitis if cholestasis is prolonged

15.

The following statements about type A viral hepatitis are true

Ⓐ persistent viraemia produces the post-hepatitis syndrome

Ⓑ relapsing hepatitis usually indicates a poorer prognosis

Ⓒ the virus is not usually transmitted via infected blood

Ⓓ drug-induced acute hepatitis produces identical liver histology

Ⓔ travellers given immune serum globulin are protected for 3 months

16.

The following features suggest extrahepatic cholestasis rather than viral hepatitis

Ⓐ a palpable gallbladder and hepatomegaly

Ⓑ right hypochondrial tenderness

Ⓒ serum alkaline phosphatase concentration > 3 times normal

Ⓓ marked pruritus and rigors

Ⓔ peripheral blood polymorph leucocytosis

17.

Circulating hepatitis B surface antigen (HBsAg)

Ⓐ is detectable during the prodrome of acute type B hepatitis

Ⓑ envelops a DNA viral particle transmissible in all body fluids

Ⓒ persists in about 25% of adults following acute type B hepatitis

Ⓓ disappears before jaundice develops in some individuals

Ⓔ is commoner in asymptomatic subjects in the Western rather than the Eastern hemisphere

18.

The typical features of type B viral hepatitis (HBV) include

Ⓐ an incubation period of 1 month

Ⓑ history of exposure to unsafe sex or drug abuse

Ⓒ prodromal illness with polyarthralgia

Ⓓ hepatitic illness more severe than with type A virus

Ⓔ absence of progression to chronic active hepatitis

19.

In non-A, non-B viral hepatitis (NANBV)

Ⓐ the clinical features are similar to other viral hepatitides

Ⓑ there are distinct parenteral and enteric forms (types C + E)

Ⓒ the disease does not progress to chronic active hepatitis

Ⓓ 1 month and 3 month incubation forms of the disease occur

Ⓔ the viruses responsible produce 90% of all post-transfusion hepatitis

20.

In delta or type D viral hepatitis (HDV)

Ⓐ the infective agent is an RNA virus

Ⓑ enteral and parenteral modes of transmission occur

Ⓒ replication of the virus requires the presence of type B virus

Ⓓ simultaneous infection with HBV often produces severe hepatitis

Ⓔ pre-existing HBV carriage predisposes to the progression to chronic active hepatitis

21.

The typical features of fulminant hepatic failure include

Ⓐ onset within 8 weeks of the initial illness

Ⓑ hepatosplenomegaly and ascites

Ⓒ encephalopathy and fetor hepaticus

Ⓓ nausea, vomiting and renal failure

Ⓔ cerebral oedema without papilloedema

22.

Typical liver function values in fulminant hepatic failure include

Ⓐ hypoalbuminaemia

Ⓑ hypoglycaemia

Ⓒ prolonged prothrombin time

Ⓓ serum alkaline phosphatase > three times normal

Ⓔ peripheral blood lymphocytosis

23.

The management of fulminant liver failure includes

Ⓐ avoidance of dietary protein

Ⓑ acid-lowering drug therapy to prevent erosive gastritis

Ⓒ fresh frozen plasma to correct coagulation disorders

Ⓓ parenteral dextrose 10% to correct hypoglycaemia

Ⓔ parenteral mannitol 20% to control cerebral oedema

24.

The typical histopathology of persistent hepatitis includes

Ⓐ lymphocytic infiltration limited to portal tracts

Ⓑ prominent hepatocytic changes with fatty infiltration

Ⓒ destruction of the lobular architecture

Ⓓ piecemeal necrosis of the liver parenchyma

Ⓔ clinical correlation with chronic active hepatitis

25.

Typical clinical features of chronic persistent hepatitis include

Ⓐ persistently severe nausea, anorexia and abdominal pain

Ⓑ jaundice with hepatosplenomegaly

Ⓒ normal serum concentrations of bilirubin and alkaline phosphatase

Ⓓ progression to chronic active hepatitis and cirrhosis

Ⓔ liver histology shows an abnormal lobular architecture

26.

The clinical features of chronic active hepatitis include

Ⓐ predominance of females aged 20–40

Ⓑ acute onset simulating viral hepatitis in 25% of patients

Ⓒ arthralgia, fever and amenorrhoea

Ⓓ spider telangiectasia and hepatosplenomegaly

Ⓔ Cushingoid facies, hirsutism and acne

27.

Hepatitis B-associated chronic active hepatitis (CAH) differs from autoimmune CAH in that it

Ⓐ typically affects males over 30 years of age

Ⓑ often produces fulminant hepatic failure

Ⓒ is often characterised by florid physical signs

Ⓓ typically progresses slowly without exacerbations

Ⓔ is less likely to be complicated by hepatoma

28.

Diseases associated with chronic active hepatitis include

Ⓐ autoimmune haemolytic anaemia
Ⓑ Hashimoto's thyroiditis
Ⓒ type I diabetes mellitus
Ⓓ Sjögren's syndrome
Ⓔ rheumatoid arthritis

29.

8 weeks after the onset of the illness, the following serum tests strongly support a diagnosis of autoimmune chronic active hepatitis

Ⓐ antinuclear and smooth muscle antibodies in high titres
Ⓑ persistent alanine aminotransferase activity > 10 times normal
Ⓒ hypoalbuminaemia with gammaglobulin > 2 times normal
Ⓓ decreased caeruloplasmin concentration
Ⓔ antimitochondrial antibodies in titres > 640

30.

In the management of patients with chronic active hepatitis

Ⓐ liver biopsy soon after the onset of the illness is vital
Ⓑ remissions and relapses are characteristic
Ⓒ associated with autoantibodies, 50% die within 5 years despite treatment
Ⓓ corticosteroid and azathioprine therapy is life-saving
Ⓔ interferon is of value in chronic HBV hepatitis

31.

The typical features of adult hepatic cirrhosis include

Ⓐ progressive hepatomegaly
Ⓑ massive splenomegaly
Ⓒ peripheral blood macrocytosis
Ⓓ parotid gland enlargement
Ⓔ gaseous abdominal distension

32.

Hepatic cirrhosis in adults is

Ⓐ cryptogenic in aetiology in 60% of patients
Ⓑ an early complication of severe acute type B viral hepatitis
Ⓒ a recognised complication of acute paracetamol poisoning
Ⓓ more likely if alcohol abuse is chronic rather than in episodic binges
Ⓔ a recognised complication of kwashiorkor

33.

In patients with hepatic cirrhosis

Ⓐ central cyanosis results from pulmonary veno-arterial shunting
Ⓑ increasing jaundice suggests progressive liver failure
Ⓒ the peripheral blood flow is typically reduced
Ⓓ the glomerular filtration rate is decreased
Ⓔ oesophageal varices indicate portal hypertension

34.

Hepatic encephalopathy due to progressive liver failure is suggested by

Ⓐ dysarthria and chorea
Ⓑ focal neurological signs
Ⓒ yawning and hiccoughing
Ⓓ serum aminotransferase activity > 10 times normal
Ⓔ epilepsy and disorientation

35.

Hepatic encephalopathy in cirrhosis is typically precipitated by

Ⓐ infection
Ⓑ hypokalaemia
Ⓒ abdominal surgery
Ⓓ gastrointestinal bleeding
Ⓔ lactulose therapy

36.

In the management of hepatic cirrhosis with ascites

Ⓐ the dietary sodium intake should be restricted to 80 mmol/day

Ⓑ paracentesis with salt-poor albumin improves the survival rate

Ⓒ the daily calorie intake should be restricted to 1500 calories

Ⓓ diuretic therapy should achieve a weight loss of 2 kg/day

Ⓔ protein intake should be at least 60 g/day unless encephalopathy is suspected

37.

The management of severe hepatic encephalopathy should include

Ⓐ withdrawal of dietary protein intake

Ⓑ sedatives to minimise neuropsychiatric symptoms

Ⓒ neomycin to reduce colonic bacterial flora

Ⓓ diuretic therapy with potassium supplementation

Ⓔ enteral or parenteral glucose 300 g/day

38.

The hepatorenal syndrome in cirrhosis is characterised by

Ⓐ acute renal tubular necrosis

Ⓑ proteinuria and an abnormal urinary sediment

Ⓒ urinary sodium concentration < 10 mmol/L

Ⓓ urine/plasma osmolality ratio < 1

Ⓔ an elevated central venous pressure in most patients

39.

In the management of acute bleeding from oesophageal varices due to hepatic cirrhosis

Ⓐ there is a 50% mortality rate

Ⓑ variceal banding or sclerotherapy are contraindicated

Ⓒ vasopressin and somatostatin both reduce portal venous pressure

Ⓓ balloon tamponade is best deferred until endoscopic confirmation of bleeding varices

Ⓔ oesophageal transection is contraindicated in hepatic failure

40.

Prevention of recurrent variceal bleeding is achievable using

Ⓐ somatostatin (octreotide) therapy

Ⓑ transjugular intrahepatic portasystemic stent shunting

Ⓒ beta-adrenoceptor antagonist treatment

Ⓓ variceal banding

Ⓔ sclerotherapy

41.

In primary biliary cirrhosis

Ⓐ middle-aged males are affected predominantly

Ⓑ pruritus is invariably accompanied by jaundice

Ⓒ osteomalacia and osteoporosis are often present

Ⓓ rigors and abdominal pain are a typical presentation

Ⓔ serum smooth muscle antibodies are present in high titres

42.

The typical features of primary biliary cirrhosis include

Ⓐ xanthomata of the palmar creases and eyelids

Ⓑ poor prognosis even in asymptomatic patients

Ⓒ hepatomegaly preceding splenomegaly

Ⓓ dilated bile ducts on ultrasonography

Ⓔ improved survival rate with immunosuppressant therapy

43.

The typical features of primary haemochromatosis include

Ⓐ association with HLA A3 in 75%

Ⓑ male predominance

Ⓒ hepatic cirrhosis and diabetes mellitus

Ⓓ hypertrophic cardiomyopathy

Ⓔ grey skin pigmentation due to ferritin deposition

44.
The typical features of Wilson's disease include
Ⓐ acute haemolytic anaemia
Ⓑ acute hepatitis and chronic active hepatitis
Ⓒ parkinsonian syndrome and hepatic cirrhosis
Ⓓ osteomalacia and raised serum copper concentration
Ⓔ renal tubular acidosis and Kayser–Fleischer rings

45.
Recognised causes of portal hypertension include
Ⓐ polycystic disease of the liver
Ⓑ myeloproliferative disease
Ⓒ hepatic schistosomiasis
Ⓓ neonatal umbilical sepsis
Ⓔ hepatic vein obstruction (Budd–Chiari syndrome)

46.
Primary hepatocellular carcinoma is associated with
Ⓐ hepatic cirrhosis in 80% of patients in the UK
Ⓑ ingestion of aflatoxin-contaminated food in the tropics
Ⓒ haemochromatosis
Ⓓ hepatitis A virus infection
Ⓔ androgen and oestrogen ingestion

47.
The typical features of hepatocellular carcinoma include
Ⓐ fever, weight loss and abdominal pain
Ⓑ ascites and intra-abdominal bleeding
Ⓒ venous hum over the liver
Ⓓ serum alpha-fetoprotein in high titre
Ⓔ surgically resectable disease in 50% of patients

48.
Pyogenic liver abscess is a recognised complication of
Ⓐ ascending cholangitis
Ⓑ Crohn's disease
Ⓒ pancreatitis
Ⓓ septicaemia
Ⓔ subphrenic abscess

49.
The typical features of pyogenic liver abscess include
Ⓐ obstructive jaundice and weight loss
Ⓑ tender hepatomegaly without splenomegaly
Ⓒ pleuritic pain and pleural effusion
Ⓓ multiple abscesses especially in ascending cholangitis
Ⓔ *Escherichia coli*, anaerobes and streptococci present in pus

50.
The following statements about biliary anatomy are true
Ⓐ The right and left hepatic ducts join to form the common bile duct
Ⓑ The normal common bile duct measures 20 mm in diameter
Ⓒ The bile and pancreatic ducts usually join the duodenum separately
Ⓓ The gallbladder is chiefly innervated by sympathetic nerves
Ⓔ 1–2 litres of bile is secreted daily and concentrated tenfold in the gall bladder

51.
Gallstones are
Ⓐ more common in black Africans and Indians than Caucasians
Ⓑ demonstrable in over 80% of UK patients > 60 years of age
Ⓒ predominantly composed of cholesterol in 75% of gallstones in the UK
Ⓓ usually pigment stones in hepatic cirrhosis
Ⓔ usually the result of reduced hepatic bile acid secretion

52.
Gallstones are a recognised complication of
Ⓐ obesity
Ⓑ oral contraceptive therapy
Ⓒ chronic haemolytic anaemia
Ⓓ terminal ileal disease
Ⓔ total parenteral nutrition

53.
The typical features of acute cholecystitis include
Ⓐ absence of obstruction of the cystic duct
Ⓑ sterile culture of bile 72 hours after onset
Ⓒ invariable association with gallstones
Ⓓ exacerbation of pain following morphine analgesics
Ⓔ radio-opaque gallstones on plain X-ray

54.
The typical clinical features of acute cholecystitis include
Ⓐ jaundice, nausea and vomiting
Ⓑ colicky abdominal pain in spasms lasting about 5 minutes
Ⓒ right hypochondrial tenderness worse on inspiration
Ⓓ air in the biliary tree on plain X-ray
Ⓔ peripheral blood leucocytosis

55.
The typical features of cholangiocarcinoma include
Ⓐ association with hepatic cirrhosis
Ⓑ abdominal pain and obstructive jaundice
Ⓒ serum alpha-fetoprotein in high titre
Ⓓ serum alkaline phosphatase > three times normal
Ⓔ surgically resectable in the majority

56.
Carcinoma of the gallbladder is
Ⓐ much commoner in males than females
Ⓑ usually squamous in cell type
Ⓒ associated with gallstones and calcification of the gallbladder
Ⓓ suggested by the presence of a palpable non-tender abdominal mass
Ⓔ surgically curable in most instances

9 NUTRITIONAL FACTORS IN DISEASE

ANSWERS BEGIN ON P. 194

1.

The daily essential nutrient requirements in man include

Ⓐ 1–2 mg vitamins D, K, and B_{12}
Ⓑ 1–2 mg vitamins A, B_1 and B_6
Ⓒ 50 g protein
Ⓓ 50 mg vitamin C
Ⓔ 100 mg calcium and phosphate

2.

The following statements about adult dietary energy resources are true

Ⓐ Carbohydrates have a calorific value of 4 kcal/g
Ⓑ Fats have a calorific value of 5 kcal/g
Ⓒ Sucrose, lactose and maltose are monosaccharides
Ⓓ Linoleic and linolenic acids are essential fatty acids
Ⓔ Proteins provide 4 kcal/g and all nine essential amino acids

3.

A healthy daily diet for a slim, active man should include

Ⓐ 1700 kcal (8.4 MJ)
Ⓑ 50 g of carbohydrate
Ⓒ 15 mg of both iron and zinc
Ⓓ 60 g of protein of good biological value
Ⓔ 50 mg of folic acid

4.

The following statements about the basal metabolic rate (BMR) and energy balance are true

Ⓐ The BMR is the largest single component of energy expenditure
Ⓑ The BMR increases with lean body mass and age
Ⓒ The BMR is greater in females than males
Ⓓ Children require 2500 kcal per day
Ⓔ The normal BMI range = 20–25 and is calculated from the formula Weight (kg)/Height (m)^2

5.

Clinical features of protein-energy malnutrition in adults include

Ⓐ a body mass index = 20–25
Ⓑ oedema in the absence of hypoalbuminaemia
Ⓒ nocturia, cold intolerance and diarrhoea
Ⓓ skin depigmentation, hair loss and covert infection
Ⓔ cerebral atrophy and sinus tachycardia

6.

Expected laboratory findings in protein-energy malnutrition in adults include

Ⓐ decreased plasma free fatty acid concentrations
Ⓑ increased plasma cortisol and reverse T3 concentrations
Ⓒ impaired delayed skin sensitivity to tuberculin
Ⓓ decreased plasma insulin, glucose and T3 concentrations
Ⓔ decreased urinary osmolality and creatinine excretion

7.

The following statements about protein-energy malnutrition (PEM) in children are true

Ⓐ Kwashiorkor is a combined protein and calorie deficiency state

Ⓑ Nutritional marasmus occurs in isolated total calorie deficiency

Ⓒ Nutritional dwarfism is usually associated with a body mass index of < 16

Ⓓ There is an increased susceptibility to all types of infection

Ⓔ Premature weaning and childhood illnesses predispose to PEM

8.

The clinical features of protein-energy malnutrition include

Ⓐ marked muscle wasting and abdominal distension in marasmus

Ⓑ weight loss more than growth retardation in marasmus

Ⓒ hepatic steatosis and hypoproteinaemic oedema in kwashiorkor

Ⓓ desquamative dermatosis, stomatitis and anorexia in marasmus

Ⓔ associated zinc deficiency in kwashiorkor

9.

The following statements about the treatment of severe protein-energy malnutrion are true

Ⓐ Mortality rates of about 20% occur even in hospitalised patients

Ⓑ Correction of fluid and electrolyte balance is vital

Ⓒ Calorie and protein intake restoration worsens the oedema

Ⓓ Fatty liver leads to cirrhosis if calorie intakes remain poor

Ⓔ Childhood mortality rates would be halved by oral rehydration, breast feeding and immunisation

10.

The following statements about calcium balance in adult man are true

Ⓐ Total body calcium is about 1.2 kg of which 99% is in bone

Ⓑ The UK recommended adult intake is 800 mg daily

Ⓒ 70% of dietary calcium is excreted in the faeces

Ⓓ Dietary phytates and oxalates enhance calcium absorption

Ⓔ The serum calcium is a sensitive index of total body calcium

11.

The following statements about iron balance in a healthy young adult female are true

Ⓐ The healthy daily diet should provide 15 mg of iron

Ⓑ 60% of dietary inorganic iron is absorbed

Ⓒ Organic iron is better absorbed than inorganic iron

Ⓓ Daily iron losses of 1 mg result from desquamated cells

Ⓔ 500 ml of blood contains 25 μg of iron

12.

The following statements about deficiency states are true

Ⓐ Iodine deficiency produces goitre and thyrotoxicosis

Ⓑ Soft drinking water contains more fluoride than hard water

Ⓒ Zinc deficiency produces dermatitis, hair loss and diarrhoea

Ⓓ Copper deficiency in children produces anaemia and poor growth

Ⓔ Phosphate deficiency occurs in neonates fed on cow's milk

13.

Vitamin A is

Ⓐ a fat-soluble vitamin

Ⓑ present as retinol in carrots and certain green vegetables

Ⓒ the treatment of choice in xerophthalmia and keratomalacia

Ⓓ recommended in minimum dietary requirements of 50 mg daily for adults

Ⓔ present in high concentrations in fish liver oils

14.

Vitamin D

Ⓐ is present in high concentrations in dairy products

Ⓑ is non-essential in the diet given adequate sunlight exposure

Ⓒ like vitamin A is stored mainly in the liver

Ⓓ is converted from cholecalciferol to 1,25 dihydroxycholecalciferol

Ⓔ enhances calcium absorption by the induction of specific enterocyte transport proteins

15.

Rickets

Ⓐ results from vitamin D deficiency before epiphyseal fusion

Ⓑ in the UK occurs principally in children of Asiatic origin

Ⓒ is suggested by delayed motor milestones and dental eruption

Ⓓ produces cranio-tabes and epiphyseal swelling of the ribs

Ⓔ produces chest wall deformities and kyphosis if untreated

16.

Characteristic findings in severe rickets include

Ⓐ epiphyseal expansion of the lower radius on X-ray

Ⓑ hypophosphataemia due to secondary hyperparathyroidism

Ⓒ hyperphosphaturia and an increased serum alkaline phosphatase

Ⓓ deformities of the spine, pelvis and long bones

Ⓔ undetectable plasma concentrations of 25-hydroxycholecalciferol

17.

Characteristic findings in osteomalacia in adults include

Ⓐ a significant reduction in total bone mass and bone osteoid

Ⓑ presentation with persistent skeletal pain and bone tenderness

Ⓒ difficulty climbing stairs and a waddling gait

Ⓓ rib, scapular and pelvic pseudo-fractures

Ⓔ predisposing factors including anti-convulsant therapy or renal impairment

18.

Characteristic findings in generalised osteoporosis include

Ⓐ chronic bone pain and impaired healing of bone fractures

Ⓑ an association with alcohol abuse and malnutrition

Ⓒ X-ray changes more marked in the limbs than the axial skeleton

Ⓓ normal bone mineralisation but abnormal bone mass

Ⓔ decreased serum calcium and phosphate concentrations

19.
Vitamin K is
Ⓐ a fat-soluble vitamin found in leafy vegetables
Ⓑ synthesised in the liver by the conversion of vitamin K_2
Ⓒ vital for the synthesis of clotting factors 2, 7, 9, 10
Ⓓ often deficient in neonates due to the absence of normal gut flora
Ⓔ absorbed by an active process which is inhibited by warfarin therapy

20.
Vitamin C deficiency
Ⓐ impairs wound healing due to defective collagen synthesis
Ⓑ would develop within 4 months given a daily intake of 5 mg
Ⓒ produces bleeding gums in edentulous individuals
Ⓓ produces perifollicular haemorrhages and 'corkscrew' hairs
Ⓔ in childhood produces anaemia and bone and joint pains

21.
In thiamin deficiency
Ⓐ anaerobic glycolysis is impaired resulting in lactic acidosis
Ⓑ the diet is deficient in green vegetables and dairy products
Ⓒ sudden death results from low output cardiac failure
Ⓓ peripheral neuropathy results in marked muscle wasting
Ⓔ Wernicke's encephalopathy is usually suggested by ataxia, nystagmus and gaze palsies

22.
Deficiency of the following B vitamins is associated with the clinical syndromes listed below
Ⓐ niacin — pellagra
Ⓑ pyridoxine — isoniazid-induced peripheral neuropathy
Ⓒ pyridoxine — haemolytic anaemia
Ⓓ riboflavin — angular stomatitis and naso-labial seborrhoea
Ⓔ riboflavin — cheilosis

23.
The following statements about vitamin B_{12} and folic acid are true
Ⓐ The serum vitamin B_{12} level is lower in vegetarians than omnivores
Ⓑ Both vitamin B_{12} and folate are essential for DNA synthesis
Ⓒ A daily intake of 1–2 μg of vitamin B_{12} is recommended
Ⓓ A daily intake of 1–2 mg of folic acid is recommended
Ⓔ Deficiency of either vitamin produces a peripheral blood macrocytosis and pancytopenia

24.
In the nutritional support of hospital patients
Ⓐ vitamin K deficiency is associated with antibiotic use
Ⓑ polymeric feeds are indicated in inflammatory bowel disease
Ⓒ 2.5 L of 10% dextrose provides 1000 kcal
Ⓓ solutions of up to 20% dextrose can safely be given by peripheral vein
Ⓔ the use of dextrose alone as a calorie source produces muscle wasting

25.
The following statements about dietary fibre are true
Ⓐ Cereals increase stool bulk due to water-holding effects
Ⓑ Pulses increase stool bulk due to colonic bacterial growth
Ⓒ Pectins and gums retard gastric emptying
Ⓓ Monosaccharides produced by bacterial digestion are absorbed
Ⓔ Average daily intakes of 15 g are inadequate

26.
Patients with the following characteristics are at increased risk of malnutrition
Ⓐ alcoholism
Ⓑ major burns
Ⓑ leukaemia receiving chemotherapy
Ⓑ weight loss of 10% or more in the past 6 months
Ⓔ steroid therapy

27.

In the assessment of nutritional deficiency in hospital patients

Ⓐ nutritional supplementation is not required until clinical signs are apparent

Ⓑ 1 kg of weight loss approximates to 6000 kcal of energy

Ⓒ plasma albumin is a reliable index of visceral protein depletion

Ⓓ elevated serum methyl malonate suggests vitamin B_{12} deficiency

Ⓔ lymphocytosis suggests protein depletion

28.

Characteristic findings in simple obesity in adults include

Ⓐ a body mass index > 30

Ⓑ increased plasma cortisol and insulin concentrations

Ⓒ a family history of obesity of similar degree and distribution

Ⓓ onset in females at the menarche, in pregnancy or menopause

Ⓔ basal metabolic rates and thermic responses to food are similar to lean subjects

29.

Recognised associations of obesity include

Ⓐ hyperuricaemia

Ⓑ depression

Ⓒ gallstones

Ⓓ type II diabetes mellitus

Ⓔ hyperlipoproteinaemia

30.

Ideal weight reducing diets in the treatment of moderate obesity should

Ⓐ provide no more than 500 kcal (2.1 MJ)

Ⓑ theoretically achieve a weight loss of at least 2 kg per week

Ⓒ be accompanied by anorectic drug therapy in most

Ⓓ maintain nitrogen balance given a daily intake of 25 g protein

Ⓔ reduce carbohydrate intake much more than total fat intake

31.

The following statements about the management of obesity are correct

Ⓐ The long-term results of therapeutic starvation are no better than conventional dieting

Ⓑ Jogging for 20 minutes five times per week will expend an additional 900 kcal per week

Ⓒ Effective calorie restriction usually produces symptomatic ketosis

Ⓓ The calorie content of 200 ml of wine or 500 ml of beer = 150 kcal

Ⓔ D-fenfluramine and fluoxetine increase satiety rather than suppress the appetite

32.

The mechanical disabilities associated with obesity include

Ⓐ pes planus

Ⓑ osteoarthrosis of the hips and knees

Ⓒ increased proneness to accidents

Ⓓ temporo-mandibular arthritis

Ⓔ atlanto-axial subluxation

33.

Drug therapies known to increase appetite and body weight include

Ⓐ oral contraceptives

Ⓑ chlorpromazine

Ⓒ amitriptyline

Ⓓ fluoxetine

Ⓔ glipizide

DISTURBANCES IN WATER, ELECTROLYTE AND ACID-BASE BALANCE

10

ANSWERS BEGIN ON P. 198

1.

In a normal 70 kg man, the following statements are true

Ⓐ Total body water is approximately 42 litres

Ⓑ 70% of the total body water is intracellular

Ⓒ 70% of extracellular water is intravascular

Ⓓ Sodium, bicarbonate and chloride ions are mainly intracellular

Ⓔ Potassium, magnesium, phosphate and sulphate ions are mainly extracellular

2.

In a healthy man living in a temperate climate

Ⓐ 500 ml of water per day are derived from metabolic processes

Ⓑ water loss from the skin and lungs is about 250 ml per day

Ⓒ obligatory urinary water loss is about 500 ml per day

Ⓓ faecal water loss is about 750 ml per day

Ⓔ urinary sodium losses should be < 10 mmol per day in response to sodium depletion

3.

Typical causes of combined salt and water depletion include

Ⓐ inadequate sodium intake

Ⓑ chronic diuretic drug therapy

Ⓒ uncontrolled diabetes mellitus

Ⓓ primary hypoadrenalism

Ⓔ acute pancreatitis

4.

Typical causes of hyponatraemia include

Ⓐ diabetes insipidus

Ⓑ hepatocellular failure

Ⓒ psychogenic polydipsia

Ⓓ Cushing's syndrome

Ⓔ diuretic drug therapy

5.

In the treatment of moderately severe combined sodium and water depletion

Ⓐ the pulse and BP are reliable indices of the severity of losses

Ⓑ 5% dextrose should be used to replace the extracellular fluid volume losses

Ⓒ 2–4 litres of isotonic saline should be given in the first 12 hours of therapy

Ⓓ potassium and hydrogen ion balance are often disturbed

Ⓔ 1.26% sodium bicarbonate should be given parenterally if metabolic acidosis is present and there is evidence of pre-existing renal disease

6.

Primary water depletion is a recognised complication of

Ⓐ primary hyperparathyroidism

Ⓑ toxic confusional states

Ⓒ oesophageal carcinoma

Ⓓ lithium therapy

Ⓔ acute pancreatitis

7.

Expected features of severe primary water depletion include

Ⓐ urine osmolality of 300 mosm/kg

Ⓑ plasma sodium of 130 mmol/L

Ⓒ marked thirst and oliguria

Ⓓ hypotension and peripheral circulatory failure

Ⓔ muscle weakness and a 'doughy' consistency of skin tissue

8.

In the treatment of moderately severe water depletion

Ⓐ the use of isotonic sodium chloride should be avoided

Ⓑ 5–10 litres of isotonic dextrose should be given within the first 12 hours

Ⓒ the urine volume reliably indicates the volume of fluid required

Ⓓ cerebral oedema is the principal risk of the use of hypotonic fluids

Ⓔ peripheral circulatory failure would suggest that there is also significant sodium depletion

9.

The following statements about potassium balance are true

Ⓐ 85% of the daily potassium intake is excreted in the urine

Ⓑ Intracellular potassium ion concentrations are about 140 mmol/L

Ⓒ Cellular uptake of potassium is enhanced by adrenaline and insulin

Ⓓ Bicarbonate ions impair cellular uptake of potassium

Ⓔ The normal dietary potassium intake is about 2–3 g (50–80 mmol) per day

10.

Recognised causes of potassium depletion include

Ⓐ metabolic alkalosis

Ⓑ cardiac failure

Ⓒ corticosteroid treatment

Ⓓ renal tubular acidosis

Ⓔ triamterene diuretic therapy

11.

The clinical features of severe potassium depletion include

Ⓐ polyuria due to renal tubular dysfunction

Ⓑ muscle weakness, paraesthesiae and depressed tendon reflexes

Ⓒ flattening of the T wave, ST depression and U waves on ECG

Ⓓ abdominal distension and paralytic ileus

Ⓔ sinus bradycardia and decreased digoxin sensitivity

12.

Hyperkalaemia is a recognised finding in

Ⓐ severe untreated diabetic ketoacidosis

Ⓑ primary hypoadrenalism

Ⓒ rhabdomyolysis

Ⓓ prostaglandin inhibitor therapy in renal impairment

Ⓔ angiotensin-converting enzyme inhibitor therapy

13.

Clinical features of hyperkalaemia include

Ⓐ tall peaked T waves and ST depression on ECG

Ⓑ asystole and ventricular fibrillation

Ⓒ peripheral paraesthesiae

Ⓓ widening of the QRS and conduction defects on ECG

Ⓔ symptoms and signs indistinguishable from those induced by hypokalaemia

14.

The emergency treatment of severe hyperkalaemia should include

Ⓐ dietary restriction of coffee and fruit juices

Ⓑ parenteral dextrose and glucagon therapy

Ⓒ parenteral calcium gluconate therapy

Ⓓ restoration of sodium and water balance

Ⓔ calcium resonium orally and/or rectally

15.
Magnesium deficiency is
Ⓐ a cause of confusion, depression and epilepsy
Ⓑ usually due to prolonged vomiting and diarrhoea
Ⓒ found in uncontrolled diabetes mellitus and alcoholism
Ⓓ found in primary hyperparathyroidism and hyperaldosteronism
Ⓔ best treated with oral magnesium sulphate

16.
The renal excretion of water is dependent on
Ⓐ the glomerular filtration rate
Ⓑ the proximal tubular reabsorption of solute
Ⓒ solute concentrations in the thick ascending limb of the loop of Henle
Ⓓ the absence of antidiuretic hormone arginine-vasopressin
Ⓔ the integrity of the distal convoluted tubules

17.
Expected findings in acute water intoxication include
Ⓐ serum sodium concentration < 130 mmol/L
Ⓑ urinary osmolality 290 mosm/kg
Ⓒ nausea, headache and confusion
Ⓓ prompt response to 1 L of normal sodium chloride
Ⓔ clinical evidence of increased ECF volume

18.
Dilutional hyponatraemia due to inappropriate ADH secretion is associated with the following
Ⓐ abdominal surgery
Ⓑ meningoencephalitis
Ⓒ hypothyroidism
Ⓓ morphine and phenothiazine therapy
Ⓔ pulmonary tuberculosis

19.
Sodium and water retention should be expected following drug therapy with
Ⓐ triamterene
Ⓑ indomethacin
Ⓒ an oestrogen
Ⓓ thyroxine
Ⓔ captopril

20.
The following statements about diuretic therapy are true
Ⓐ Frusemide reduces sodium reabsorption in the proximal tubules
Ⓑ Thiazides aggravate hyperglycaemia and hyperuricaemia
Ⓒ Triamterene antagonises aldosterone in the distal tubules
Ⓓ Amiloride is contraindicated in oliguric renal failure
Ⓔ Bumetanide produces hyponatraemia even when oedema is still present

21.
The following statements about hydrogen ion balance are true
Ⓐ $[H+]$ = dissociation constant $(K) \times [CO_2] / [HCO_3]$
Ⓑ the normal plasma hydrogen ion concentration is 36–44 nmol/L
Ⓒ the plasma bicarbonate concentration is predominantly regulated by the renal tubules
Ⓓ phosphates and sulphates are excreted principally in the bile
Ⓔ carbon dioxide is principally transported in the blood as carbaminohaemoglobin

22.

The following statements about acid-base regulation in healthy subjects are true

Ⓐ The blood pH is calculated from the measured arterial $PaCO_2$

Ⓑ $H^+ + HCO_3^- \Leftrightarrow H_2CO_3 \Leftrightarrow H_2O + CO_2$

Ⓒ the normal anion gap = plasma $Na^+ - (Cl^- + HCO_3^-)$

Ⓓ the blood $PaCO_2$ correlates closely with alveolar $PaCO_2$

Ⓔ the normal plasma bicarbonate concentration is 36–44 mmol/L

23.

The metabolic acidosis induced by the following disorders is typically associated with

Ⓐ increased plasma bicarbonate concentration in lactic acidosis

Ⓑ increased anion gap in starvation acidosis

Ⓒ increased blood $PaCO_2$ in diabetic ketoacidosis

Ⓓ low plasma chloride concentration in renal tubular acidosis

Ⓔ increased red cell carbonic acid production during acetazolamide therapy

DISEASES OF THE KIDNEY AND GENITO-URINARY SYSTEM

11

ANSWERS BEGIN ON P. 201

1.
The following statements about resting renal blood flow in health are correct

ⓐ A total of about 10 000 nephrons receive 1.2 L of blood per minute

ⓑ The afferent arterioles supply blood direct to the distal tubules

ⓒ The glomerular capillaries are supplied by the afferent arterioles

ⓓ The blood supply of the medulla arises from efferent arterioles

ⓔ The glomerular capillary filtration pressure is about 80 mmHg

2.
Within the normal kidney

ⓐ 33% of the filtered water is reabsorbed in the proximal tubules

ⓑ ADH increases the water permeability of the distal tubules

ⓒ the glomerular filtrate contains about 200 mg protein per litre

ⓓ 33% of the filtered sodium is reabsorbed in the proximal tubules

ⓔ the juxtaglomerular apparatus comprises specialised cells of the efferent arterioles and proximal convoluted tubules

3.
In the proximal convoluted tubules of the normal kidney

ⓐ 33% of filtered chloride is actively reabsorbed

ⓑ > 90% of filtered potassium is actively reabsorbed

ⓒ 66% of the filtered sodium is passively reabsorbed

ⓓ most of the filtered glucose is actively reabsorbed

ⓔ 33% of the filtered bicarbonate is passively reabsorbed

4.
In the distal convoluted tubules of the normal kidney

ⓐ sodium ions are reabsorbed with chloride ions

ⓑ sodium ions are reabsorbed in exchange for potassium or hydrogen

ⓒ the active secretion of potassium is controlled by aldosterone

ⓓ passive water loss is controlled by the effects of ADH

ⓔ ammonium is secreted once most of the bicarbonate is reabsorbed

5.
The kidney produces the following substances

ⓐ erythropoietin

ⓑ 25-hydroxycholecalciferol

ⓒ prostaglandins PGE_2 and PGI_2

ⓓ angiotensin-converting enzyme

ⓔ aldosterone

6.
Urinary protein excretion

ⓐ comprising light chains is detectable by dipstix

ⓑ > 3 g/day is invariably due to glomerular disease

ⓒ in childhood is greater during the night than the day

ⓓ comprising myoglobin produces a positive dipstix test for blood

ⓔ comprises albumin alone in early diabetic nephropathy

7.
Proteinuria in excess of 3 g per day is a typical feature of
Ⓐ cardiac failure
Ⓑ polycystic renal disease
Ⓒ renal vein thrombosis
Ⓓ minimal lesion glomerulonephritis
Ⓔ chronic pyelonephritis

8.
Microscopic haematuria is an expected finding in
Ⓐ renal amyloidosis
Ⓑ papillary necrosis
Ⓒ membranous glomerulonephritis
Ⓓ infective endocarditis
Ⓔ renal infarction

9.
In the investigation of renal disease
Ⓐ urine pH in health ranges from 4.3 to 8.0
Ⓑ renal clearance (C)=UV/P measures glomerular function
Ⓒ healthy adult kidneys measure 11–14 cm in length
Ⓓ 75% of IVU contrast is excreted in the first hour
Ⓔ renal biopsy is mandatory in chronic renal failure

10.
Typical features of the acute glomerulonephritis syndrome include
Ⓐ bilateral renal angle pain and tenderness
Ⓑ hypertension and periorbital facial oedema
Ⓒ oliguria < 800 ml and haematuria
Ⓓ highly selective proteinuria
Ⓔ history of allergy with oedema of the lips

11.
Typical features of the nephrotic syndrome include
Ⓐ bilateral renal angle pain
Ⓑ generalised oedema and pleural effusions
Ⓒ hypoalbuminaemia and proteinuria > 3 g/day
Ⓓ hypertension and polyuria
Ⓔ urinary sodium concentration > 20 mmol/L

12.
Immune-complex glomerulonephritis is an expected feature of
Ⓐ acute pyelonephritis
Ⓑ acute hepatitis B virus infection
Ⓒ systemic lupus erythematosus
Ⓓ IgA nephropathy
Ⓔ renal amyloidosis

13.
Proliferative glomerulonephritis occurs in association with
Ⓐ immune complex deposition on the glomerular basement membrane
Ⓑ bacterial rather than viral infections
Ⓒ infection with haemolytic streptococci more than any other bacteria
Ⓓ haemoptysis in Goodpasture's syndrome
Ⓔ a poorer prognosis in childhood than in adulthood

14.
The following statements about acute proliferative glomerulonephritis are true
Ⓐ A rise in diastolic blood pressure is found in < 25% of patients
Ⓑ Impaired urinary concentration is a typical early feature
Ⓒ Hypocomplementaemia is typical of post-streptococcal nephritis
Ⓓ Prognosis is worse if glomerulosclerosis is seen
Ⓔ Microscopic haematuria is invariable despite normal renal function

15.
In the treatment of acute proliferative glomerulonephritis
Ⓐ recovery is accelerated by dietary protein restriction
Ⓑ corticosteroid therapy is contraindicated
Ⓒ sodium restriction is usually unnecessary
Ⓓ fluid restriction is mandatory when oedema is present
Ⓔ hypertension usually responds to sodium restriction alone

16.

IgA nephropathy is characterised by

Ⓐ recurrent macroscopic haematuria in young adult males

Ⓑ onset 14–21 days following respiratory tract infections

Ⓒ nephrotic syndrome in 20% of patients

Ⓓ progression to chronic renal failure occurs in 10% of patients

Ⓔ diffuse mesangial proliferative glomerulonephritis on renal biopsy

17.

Typical features of mesangiocapillary glomerulonephritis include

Ⓐ presentation at age 15–25 years

Ⓑ hypertension and renal impairment at presentation

Ⓒ good response to immunosuppressant therapy

Ⓓ 10% progress to chronic renal failure

Ⓔ elevated complement levels

18.

The characteristic features of crescentic glomerulonephritis are

Ⓐ presentation with a nephrotic syndrome

Ⓑ clinical course rapidly progressing to renal failure

Ⓒ systemic lupus erythematosus is often present

Ⓓ mesangial proliferation is usually absent on renal biopsy

Ⓔ immunosuppressant therapy is successful in the majority

19.

The typical features of Goodpasture's syndrome include

Ⓐ circulating anti-glomerular basement membrane antibodies

Ⓑ crescentic glomerulonephritis

Ⓒ presentation in young adult males during the springtime

Ⓓ haemoptysis and pulmonary infiltrates on chest X-ray

Ⓔ no response to immunosuppressant therapy

20.

The characteristic features of membranous glomerulonephritis are

Ⓐ absence of glomerular or mesangial cell proliferation histologically

Ⓑ presentation with a nephrotic syndrome in middle aged males

Ⓒ progression to renal failure in 50% of patients

Ⓓ association with HLA B8 and DRw3 confers a good prognosis

Ⓔ treatment with immunosuppression is useful in the majority

21.

Characteristic features of minimal lesion glomerulonephritis are

Ⓐ occurrence in adults after intercurrent infections

Ⓑ marked mesangial cell proliferation on renal biopsy

Ⓒ nephrotic syndrome with unselective proteinuria

Ⓓ hypertension and microscopic haematuria

Ⓔ association with HLA B12 and DRw7

22.

In the treatment of minimal lesion glomerulonephritis

Ⓐ therapy should be deferred in childhood pending renal biopsy

Ⓑ diuretics should be avoided to minimise the risk of renal impairment

Ⓒ following corticosteroid therapy, 30% relapse within 3 years

Ⓓ immunosuppressant therapy is indicated for frequent relapses

Ⓔ deterioration in renal function commonly develops in the long term

23.

Renal involvement in systemic lupus erythematosus (SLE) is

Ⓐ clinically apparent in 40% at presentation

Ⓑ invariably present on renal biopsy in patients with SLE

Ⓒ usually apparent as a diffuse proliferative glomerulonephritis

Ⓓ associated with a poor prognosis in patients with membranous glomerulonephritis

Ⓔ characteristically present in drug-induced SLE

24.

Renal amyloidosis is characteristically associated with

Ⓐ acute proliferative glomerulonephritis syndrome

Ⓑ nephrogenic diabetes insipidus

Ⓒ renal tubular acidosis

Ⓓ progression to renal failure in 50% within 6 months

Ⓔ myelomatosis

25.

The typical features of lower urinary tract infections include

Ⓐ rigors, loin pain and renal impairment

Ⓑ suprapubic pain, dysuria and haematuria

Ⓒ progression to acute pyelonephritis if untreated

Ⓓ midstream urine culture producing *Escherichia coli* > 100 000/ml

Ⓔ the drug of choice for the majority is ciprofloxacin

26.

The typical features of acute pyelonephritis in adults include

Ⓐ normal anatomy of the urinary tract

Ⓑ vomiting, rigors and renal angle tenderness

Ⓒ renal angle pain is usually bilateral

Ⓓ evidence of reflux on isotope renography

Ⓔ loin pain and fullness in the flank

27.

During pregnancy

Ⓐ asymptomatic bacteriuria is present in 20% of patients

Ⓑ ureteric atonia predisposes to the onset of acute pyelonephritis

Ⓒ treatment of asymptomatic bacteriuria prevents symptom onset

Ⓓ intravenous urography is mandatory if there is an acute pyelonephritis

Ⓔ co-trimoxazole is the treatment of choice in acute cystitis

28.

Chronic pyelonephritis is

Ⓐ a recognised association of nephrocalcinosis

Ⓑ usually symptomatic from the onset of the condition

Ⓒ associated with a poorer prognosis in paraplegic or diabetic patients

Ⓓ likely to present with renal impairment only after the age of 60 years

Ⓔ a recognised cause of chronic sodium depletion

29.

Chronic pyelonephritis in adults

Ⓐ accounts for 80% of patients requiring chronic dialysis in the UK

Ⓑ is usually attributable to vesico-ureteric reflux in childhood

Ⓒ has pathognomonic histopathological features on renal biopsy

Ⓓ is usually associated with demonstrable ureteric reflux

Ⓔ producing hypotension should be treated with oral sodium salts

30.

Recognised complications of chronic renal failure include

Ⓐ macrocytic anaemia

Ⓑ peripheral neuropathy

Ⓒ bone pain

Ⓓ pericarditis

Ⓔ metabolic alkalosis

31.
Typical biochemical features of chronic renal failure include
Ⓐ impaired urinary concentrating ability
Ⓑ hypophosphataemia
Ⓒ hypercalcaemia
Ⓓ metabolic acidosis
Ⓔ proteinuria > 3 g/L

32.
Adverse prognostic features in chronic renal failure include
Ⓐ papilloedema
Ⓑ urinary granular casts
Ⓒ enterocolitis
Ⓓ renal osteodystrophy
Ⓔ serum creatinine > 300 μmol/L

33.
The following statements about dialysis and transplantation are true
Ⓐ Peritoneal dialysis is preferable to haemodialysis in childhood
Ⓑ Peritoneal instillation of 2 L of fluid for 6 hours a day is adequate
Ⓒ Peritoneal dialysis (CAPD) is contraindicated in diabetic patients
Ⓓ Renal graft survival is influenced more by ABO than HLA compatibility
Ⓔ The 3 year renal graft survival is approximately 25%

34.
The typical features of established acute renal failure include
Ⓐ oliguria < 800 ml per day indicates irreversibilty
Ⓑ systemic hypertension with significant renal ischaemia
Ⓒ urinary osmolality > 600 mosm/kg indicates acute tubular necrosis
Ⓓ urinary sodium concentration < 20 mmol/L indicates irreversibility
Ⓔ anaemia with a haemoglobin concentration < 80 g/L

35.
Treatment of the oliguric phase of acute renal failure includes
Ⓐ restriction of dietary protein to 40 g per day
Ⓑ calcium resonium orally and/or rectally to reduce hyperkalaemia
Ⓒ restriction of fluid intake to the total volume of daily losses
Ⓓ tetracycline therapy if enterocolitis supervenes
Ⓔ avoidance of dialysis if pulmonary oedema supervenes

36.
Haemofiltration in the oliguric phase of acute renal failure is
Ⓐ particularly useful when parenteral nutrition is required
Ⓑ contraindicated in patients with cardiac failure
Ⓒ preferable to peritoneal dialysis in young children
Ⓓ usually undertaken on a 24-hour basis for 10–20 days
Ⓔ less effective than peritoneal dialysis in restoring acid-base balance

37.
During the diuretic phase of acute renal failure
Ⓐ the blood urea concentration decreases rapidly
Ⓑ increases in the dietary protein intake should be avoided
Ⓒ sodium and bicarbonate supplementation is required
Ⓓ fluid restriction should be maintained
Ⓔ renal medullary dysfunction typically persists for 2–3 months

38.
In post-renal acute renal failure
Ⓐ unilateral obstruction suggests non-function of the other kidney
Ⓑ anuria is less common than in acute tubular necrosis
Ⓒ surgical intervention should be deferred until the blood urea falls
Ⓓ ultrasound examination may confirm the diagnosis
Ⓔ relief of the obstruction is usually followed by persistent oliguria

39.
Typical features of acute tubulo-interstitial nephritis include
Ⓐ skin rashes, arthralgia and bone marrow depression
Ⓑ absence of a peripheral blood eosinophilia
Ⓒ renal biopsy evidence of an eosinophilic interstitial nephritis
Ⓓ renal impairment typically follows withdrawal of the drug
Ⓔ onset following antibiotic or anti-inflammatory drug therapy

40.
Ureteric obstruction
Ⓐ predisposes to stone formation
Ⓑ is a recognised complication of cervical carcinoma
Ⓒ unlike bladder-neck obstruction, seldom causes haematuria
Ⓓ at the pelvi-ureteric junction in childhood is usually congenital
Ⓔ is typically pain-free if the onset is gradual

41.
Disorders predisposing to renal stone formation include
Ⓐ urinary tract infection
Ⓑ prolonged immobilisation
Ⓒ hypoparathyroidism
Ⓓ renal tubular acidosis
Ⓔ sarcoidosis

42.
In the treatment of renal calculi
Ⓐ anuria indicates the need for urgent surgical intervention
Ⓑ the urine should be alkalinised if the stone is radio-opaque
Ⓒ bendrofluazide increases urinary calcium excretion
Ⓓ allopurinol increases urinary urate excretion in gouty patients
Ⓔ renal pelvic stones require removal at open surgery

43.
The clinical features of adult polycystic renal disease include
Ⓐ an autosomal recessive mode of inheritance
Ⓑ cystic disease of the liver and pancreas
Ⓒ renal angle pain and haematuria
Ⓓ unilateral renal enlargement in the majority
Ⓔ aneurysms of the circle of Willis

44.
Characteristic features of renal tubular acidosis (RTA) include
Ⓐ normal anion gap
Ⓑ hyperchloraemic acidosis
Ⓒ inappropriately high urinary pH > 5.4
Ⓓ decreased glomerular filtration rate
Ⓔ normocytic normochromic anaemia

45.
Recognised causes of distal type 1 RTA include
Ⓐ lithium therapy
Ⓑ hyperparathyroidism
Ⓒ Sjögren's syndrome
Ⓓ renal transplant rejection
Ⓔ chronic pyelonephritis

46.
Renal excretion of the following drugs is impaired in renal failure
Ⓐ cimetidine
Ⓑ tetracycline
Ⓒ digoxin
Ⓓ morphine
Ⓔ gentamicin

47.

Recognised features of renal carcinoma include

Ⓐ persistent fever

Ⓑ bone metastases

Ⓒ renal colic with haematuria

Ⓓ polycythaemia

Ⓔ serum alpha-fetoprotein in high titre

48.

The following statements about the urinary bladder are true

Ⓐ Tabes dorsalis produces incontinence with painless bladder distension

Ⓑ Prolapsed lumbar vertebral disc usually produces urinary urgency

Ⓒ Pneumaturia is typically caused by severe bladder sepsis

Ⓓ Urinary stress incontinence suggests cerebrovascular disease

Ⓔ Urinary retention results from tricyclic antidepressant therapy

49.

Typical features of bladder carcinoma include

Ⓐ squamous cell rather than transitional cell in origin

Ⓑ presentation with urinary frequency and nocturia

Ⓒ unresponsive to radiotherapy

Ⓓ early metastatic spread to the liver and lungs

Ⓔ association with exposure to dyes and tobacco consumption

50.

Typical features of prostatic carcinoma include

Ⓐ slowly progressive obstructive uropathy

Ⓑ presentation with urinary frequency and nocturia

Ⓒ preservation of the normal anatomy on digital rectal examination

Ⓓ local spread along the lumbosacral nerve plexus

Ⓔ osteolytic rather than osteosclerotic bone metastases

51.

The typical features of benign prostatic hypertrophy include

Ⓐ peak incidence in the age group 40–60 years

Ⓑ acute urinary retention and haematuria

Ⓒ increased plasma testosterone concentration

Ⓓ normal serum prostatic acid phosphatase concentration

Ⓔ asymmetrical prostatic enlargement on rectal examination

52.

Characteristic features of testicular tumours include

Ⓐ testicular pain in seminoma of the testis

Ⓑ alpha-fetoprotein and chorionic gonadotrophin secretion in teratomas

Ⓒ absence of distant metastases

Ⓓ peak incidence in the age group 40–60 years

Ⓔ seminomas are both radio- and chemo-sensitive

12 ENDOCRINE AND METABOLIC DISEASES

ANSWERS BEGIN ON P. 206

1.
The following hypothalamic releasing factors stimulate the pituitary gland to secrete the hormones listed below
Ⓐ dopamine — prolactin
Ⓑ somatostatin — growth hormone
Ⓒ thyrotrophin releasing hormone (TRH) — TSH and prolactin
Ⓓ gonadotrophin releasing hormone (GnRH) — LH and FSH independently
Ⓔ corticotrophin releasing hormone (CRH) — beta-lipotrophin and ACTH

2.
The following statements about pituitary tumours are true
Ⓐ Chromophobe adenomas may cause pressure effects or hormone secretion
Ⓑ Diabetes insipidus usually indicates suprasellar extension
Ⓒ Cushing's disease is usually caused by acidophilic macroadenomas
Ⓓ Acromegaly is most often associated with basophilic microadenomas
Ⓔ Tumour enlargement with expansion of the pituitary fossa usually presents with headaches and/or a bi-temporal upper quadrantanopia

3.
The typical features of acromegaly include
Ⓐ thoracic kyphosis and myopathy
Ⓑ hypertension and diabetes mellitus
Ⓒ goitre and cardiomegaly
Ⓓ growth hormone suppression during a glucose tolerance test
Ⓔ hyperhydrosis

4.
Typical features of pituitary-dependent Cushing's disease include
Ⓐ enlargement of the pituitary fossa
Ⓑ amenorrhoea and depression
Ⓒ proximal myopathy and diabetes mellitus
Ⓓ suppression of plasma cortisol following dexamethasone
Ⓔ hypotension and hyperkalaemia

5.
Recognised causes of hyperprolactinaemia include
Ⓐ oestrogen therapy
Ⓑ chlorpromazine and haloperidol therapy
Ⓒ primary hypothyroidism
Ⓓ hypoadrenalism
Ⓔ Cushing's disease

6.
In childhood growth hormone deficiency
Ⓐ panhypopituitarism is a typical finding
Ⓑ most patients have a craniopharyngioma
Ⓒ a genetic deficiency of GH releasing factor is common
Ⓓ delayed bone development is a characteristic feature
Ⓔ treatment with human growth hormone produces precocious puberty

7.
Recognised causes of short stature in childhood include
Ⓐ Klinefelter's syndrome
Ⓑ Turner's syndrome
Ⓒ emotional deprivation
Ⓓ Cushing's syndrome
Ⓔ hyperthyroidism

8.
Recognised causes of hypopituitarism include
- Ⓐ post-partum haemorrhage
- Ⓑ Cushing's syndrome
- Ⓒ acromegaly
- Ⓓ autoimmune hypophysitis
- Ⓔ sarcoidosis

9.
The clinical features of hypopituitarism include
- Ⓐ hypotension with hyperkalaemia
- Ⓑ a normal increment in plasma cortisol 30 minutes after parenteral ACTH
- Ⓒ loss of libido, menstruation and secondary sexual hair
- Ⓓ hypoglycaemia without the typical symptoms
- Ⓔ coma and water intoxication

10.
The typical features of cranial diabetes insipidus include
- Ⓐ serum sodium concentration > 150 mmol/L with urine SG < 1.001
- Ⓑ increased polyuria following corticosteroid therapy for hypopituitarism
- Ⓒ onset following basal meningitis or hypothalamic trauma
- Ⓓ decreased renal responsiveness to ADH following carbamazepine therapy
- Ⓔ unlike psychogenic polydipsia, the response to ADH is invariably normal

11.
Recognised causes of nephrogenic diabetes insipidus include
- Ⓐ lithium therapy
- Ⓑ heavy metal poisoning
- Ⓒ congenital sex-linked recessive disorder
- Ⓓ chlorpropamide therapy
- Ⓔ hyperkalaemia and hypocalcaemia

12.
Recognised causes of inappropriate ADH secretion include
- Ⓐ meningitis
- Ⓑ head injury
- Ⓒ lobar pneumonia
- Ⓓ small cell bronchial carcinoma
- Ⓔ phenothiazine and amitriptyline therapy

13.
The following statements about thyroid hormones are true
- Ⓐ T_3 and T_4 are both stored in colloid vesicles as thyroglobulin
- Ⓑ T_4 is metabolically more active than T_3
- Ⓒ T_3 and T_4 are mainly bound to albumin in the serum
- Ⓓ 85% of the circulating T_3 arises from extra-thyroidal T_4
- Ⓔ conversion of T_4 to T_3 decreases in acute illness

14.
The finding of reduced serum total T3, total T4 and TSH concentrations is compatible with the following conditions
- Ⓐ hypopituitarism
- Ⓑ primary hypothyroidism
- Ⓒ nephrotic syndrome
- Ⓓ liver failure
- Ⓔ pregnancy

15.
The following invariably indicate significant thyroid gland disease
- Ⓐ decreased serum total T_4 and TSH concentrations
- Ⓑ increased serum free T_3 and decreased TSH concentrations
- Ⓒ decreased serum free T_4 without a rise in TSH in response to TRH
- Ⓓ decreased serum total T_4 and elevated TSH with TSH receptor antibodies
- Ⓔ increased total T_4 and T_3 with normal TSH

16.

The following statements about thyrotoxicosis are true

Ⓐ most cases are due to Graves' disease

Ⓑ multinodular goitre is more common than uninodular goitre

Ⓒ amiodarone treatment is occasionally responsible

Ⓓ the thyroid gland is diffusely hyperactive in Graves' disease

Ⓔ there is an increased prevalence of HLA DR3 in Grave's disease

17.

The clinical features of thyrotoxicosis include

Ⓐ atrial fibrillation with a collapsing pulse

Ⓑ weight loss and oligomenorrhoea

Ⓒ peripheral neuropathy

Ⓓ proximal myopathy and exophthalmos

Ⓔ decreased insulin requirements in type I diabetes mellitus

18.

In the treatment of thyrotoxicosis

Ⓐ propranolol should not be given in atrial fibrillation

Ⓑ carbimazole blocks the secretion of T_3 and T_4 by the thyroid

Ⓒ persistent suppression of the serum TSH is an indication for surgery

Ⓓ serum TSH receptor antibodies usually persist despite carbimazole

Ⓔ surgery is more likely to be necessary in young men than women

19.

Following ^{131}I radioiodine treatment for thyrotoxicosis

Ⓐ rising TSH suggests disease recurrence

Ⓑ at least 50% of patients develop hypothyroidism within 7 years

Ⓒ relapse is common in patients with a solitary 'hot' nodule

Ⓓ a clinical effect should be expected within 4–12 weeks

Ⓔ 70% of patients require further radioiodine therapy

20.

The following regimes would be appropriate in the management of a 30-year-old woman with severe thyrotoxic Graves' disease

Ⓐ carbimazole with ^{131}I radioiodine

Ⓑ potassium perchlorate with carbimazole

Ⓒ propranolol with carbimazole

Ⓓ subtotal thyroidectomy following thyrotoxic control

Ⓔ prednisolone with potassium iodide and propranolol

21.

Complications of subtotal thyroidectomy for thyrotoxicosis include

Ⓐ transient hypothyroidism

Ⓑ recurrent laryngeal nerve palsy

Ⓒ hypoparathyroidism

Ⓓ recurrent thyrotoxicosis

Ⓔ thyroid carcinoma

22.

In Graves' ophthalmopathy

Ⓐ diplopia is the most common presenting symptom

Ⓑ the patient is invariably thyrotoxic

Ⓒ serum eye muscle antibodies are pathognomonic

Ⓓ in 90% of patients the condition resolves spontaneously

Ⓔ hypothyroidism exacerbates the condition

23.

The clinical features of primary hypothyroidism include

Ⓐ carpal tunnel syndrome and proximal myopathy

Ⓑ cold sensitivity and menorrhagia

Ⓒ deafness and dizziness

Ⓓ puffy eyelids and malar flush

Ⓔ absent ankle tendon reflexes

24.
Biochemical findings in primary hypothyroidism include

Ⓐ low serum free T_3 preceding an increase in serum TSH concentration

Ⓑ increased serum prolactin concentration

Ⓒ inappropriate ADH secretion

Ⓓ increased serum alkaline phosphatase concentration

Ⓔ increased serum cholesterol concentration

25.
Clinical features of primary hypothyroidism in childhood include

Ⓐ malabsorption with diarrhoea

Ⓑ precocious puberty

Ⓒ retardation of growth and sexual development

Ⓓ epiphyseal dysgenesis on bone X-rays

Ⓔ permanent mental retardation

26.
Recognised causes of goitre include

Ⓐ acromegaly

Ⓑ lithium and amiodarone therapy

Ⓒ Hashimoto's thyroiditis

Ⓓ oral contraceptive therapy and pregnancy

Ⓔ Pendred's syndrome (thyroidal dyshormonogenesis)

27.
The following statements about goitre are true

Ⓐ Onset in later life favours a diagnosis of thyroid carcinoma

Ⓑ Hypothyroidism favours a diagnosis of Hashimoto's thyroiditis

Ⓒ Deafness in childhood suggests a diagnosis of dyshormonogenesis

Ⓓ Thyroxine treatment for associated hypothyroidism causes goitre enlargement

Ⓔ Serum thyroid antibodies favour a diagnosis of subacute thyroiditis

28.
Typical features of de Quervain's subacute thyroiditis include

Ⓐ a large painless goitre

Ⓑ giant cells on histopathology

Ⓒ clinical signs of hyperthyroidism

Ⓓ an elevated ESR and serum thyroid antibodies

Ⓔ long-term hypothyroidism in most patients

29.
The development of a simple colloid goitre is associated with

Ⓐ coxsackie B viral infection

Ⓑ dietary iodine deficiency

Ⓒ excess dietary calcium intake

Ⓓ cranial irradiation

Ⓔ dietary goitrogens

30.
Thyroid carcinoma of

Ⓐ lymphomatous type usually presents as a single 'hot' thyroid nodule

Ⓑ anaplastic type is usually cured by local radiotherapy

Ⓒ follicular type is best treated by ^{131}I radioiodine therapy alone

Ⓓ papillary type should be treated with total thyroidectomy

Ⓔ medullary type secretes calcitonin causing severe hypocalcaemia

31.
The serum calcium concentration is typically increased in

Ⓐ hypoalbuminaemia

Ⓑ pyloric stenosis

Ⓒ carcinomatosis

Ⓓ hypoparathyroidism

Ⓔ chronic sarcoidosis

32.
Typical clinical features of primary hyperparathyroidism include
Ⓐ recurrent acute pancreatitis and renal colic due to calculi
Ⓑ hyperplasia of all the parathyroid glands on histology
Ⓒ osteitis fibrosa on bone X-rays at presentation
Ⓓ the complications of pseudo-gout and hypertension
Ⓔ renal tubular acidosis and nephrogenic diabetes insipidus

33.
Typical biochemical findings in primary hyperparathyroidism include
Ⓐ increased serum calcium and phosphate concentrations
Ⓑ decreased serum 1,25-dihydroxycholecalciferol concentration
Ⓒ hypercalciuria and hyperphosphaturia
Ⓓ increased serum alkaline phosphatase with bony involvement
Ⓔ increased serum calcium and PTH concentrations

34.
Recognised features of secondary hyperparathyroidism include
Ⓐ calcification of the basal ganglia
Ⓑ complication of chronic renal failure
Ⓒ parathyroid enlargement is often palpable
Ⓓ development of parathyroid adenomas
Ⓔ complication of gluten enteropathy

35.
Recognised features in type I multiple endocrine neoplasia include
Ⓐ sex-linked recessive mode of inheritance
Ⓑ hypercalcaemia, hypergastrinaemia and hyperprolactinaemia
Ⓒ medullary thyroid carcinoma, phaeochromocytoma and parathyroid adenoma
Ⓓ neurofibromata, phaeochromocytoma and medullary thyroid carcinoma
Ⓔ insulinoma, pituitary adenoma and parathyroid adenoma

36.
Recognised causes of hypercalcaemia include
Ⓐ bone metastases
Ⓑ carcinomas secreting PTH-like peptides
Ⓒ severe Addison's disease
Ⓓ severe hypothyroidism
Ⓔ chronic sarcoidosis

37.
The clinical features of hypoparathyroidism include
Ⓐ carpopedal and laryngeal spasm
Ⓑ fungal infection of the fingernails
Ⓒ abdominal pain and constipation
Ⓓ peripheral paraesthesiae and psychosis
Ⓔ cataracts and epilepsy

38.
Recognised causes of hypoparathyroidism include
Ⓐ autoimmune disease often also involving other endocrine glands
Ⓑ Di George syndrome with congenital thymic aplasia
Ⓒ subtotal thyroidectomy for thyrotoxicosis
Ⓓ medullary carcinoma of the thyroid gland
Ⓔ metastatic disease within the thyroid gland

39.
The typical features of pseudohypoparathyroidism include
Ⓐ impaired coupling of adenyl cyclase with the renal PTH receptor
Ⓑ decreased serum PTH and calcitonin concentrations
Ⓒ decreased serum calcium and phosphate concentrations
Ⓓ family history of short stature and growth retardation
Ⓔ good response to parenteral PTH

40.
Recognised causes of tetany due to hypocalcaemia include
Ⓐ hyperventilation
Ⓑ pyloric stenosis
Ⓒ primary hyperaldosteronism
Ⓓ acute pancreatitis
Ⓔ gluten enteropathy

41.
In the treatment of primary hypoparathyroidism
Ⓐ intravenous calcium gluconate should be given if tetany develops
Ⓑ intranasal PTH therapy should be given long-term
Ⓒ calcitonin therapy prevents the onset of cataracts
Ⓓ oral 1 alpha-hydroxycholecalciferol restores calcium homeostasis
Ⓔ 5% carbon dioxide inhalation is required if tetany develops

42.
The following statements about adrenal gland physiology are true
Ⓐ ACTH normally controls the adrenal secretion of aldosterone
Ⓑ ACTH increases adrenal androgen and cortisol secretion
Ⓒ The plasma cortisol concentration normally peaks in the evening
Ⓓ Hyperglycaemia increases the rate of cortisol secretion
Ⓔ Cortisol enhances gluconeogenesis and lipogenesis from amino acids

43.
A cushingoid appearance is an expected finding in
Ⓐ chronic alcohol abuse
Ⓑ pituitary macroadenomas
Ⓒ ACTH-secreting bronchial carcinoma
Ⓓ adrenocortical adenoma
Ⓔ fludrocortisone therapy

44.
The typical clinical features of Cushing's syndrome include
Ⓐ generalised osteoporosis
Ⓑ systemic hypotension
Ⓒ hirsutism and amenorrhoea
Ⓓ proximal myopathy
Ⓔ hypoglycaemic episodes

45.
Expected findings in patients with benign adrenal adenomas include
Ⓐ preservation of the normal diurnal rhythm of cortisol secretion
Ⓑ plasma cortisol < 170 nmol/L 10 hours after 2 mg oral dexamethasone
Ⓒ increased free cortisol/creatinine ratios in early-morning urine
Ⓓ increased plasma dehydroepiandrosterone concentration
Ⓔ elevated ACTH at 0800 hours

46.
Adverse effects of oral corticosteroid therapy include
Ⓐ peptic ulceration
Ⓑ hypertension
Ⓒ avascular bone necrosis
Ⓓ pseudo-gout
Ⓔ insomnia

47.
In primary hyperaldosteronism (Conn's syndrome)
Ⓐ peripheral oedema is usually present
Ⓑ proximal myopathy is due to hypokalaemia
Ⓒ polyuria and polydipsia are characteristic
Ⓓ diabetes mellitus is often present
Ⓔ hypertension is associated with hyperreninaemia

48.
Recognised causes of primary adrenocortical insufficiency include
Ⓐ haemochromatosis
Ⓑ autoimmune adrenalitis
Ⓒ amyloidosis
Ⓓ sarcoidosis
Ⓔ tuberculosis

49.
Typical features of primary adrenocortical insufficiency include

Ⓐ anorexia, weight loss and diarrhoea
Ⓑ pigmentation of scars from surgery preceding hypoadrenalism
Ⓒ vitiligo, weakness and hypotension
Ⓓ increased insulin requirements in diabetic patients
Ⓔ amenorrhoea and loss of body hair

50.
Typical features of secondary adrenocortical insufficiency include

Ⓐ impaired gonadotrophin secretion usually precedes ACTH deficiency
Ⓑ impaired plasma cortisol response 30 minutes after ACTH stimulation
Ⓒ vitiligo and skin hyperpigmentation
Ⓓ hypotension and hyperkalaemia
Ⓔ preservation of the normal diurnal rhythm of cortisol secretion

51.
In the treatment of primary adrenocortical insufficiency

Ⓐ oral hydrocortisone is the glucocorticoid of choice
Ⓑ fludrocortisone is usually unnecessary unless there is hyperkalaemia
Ⓒ the dose of cortisol should not be increased without medical advice
Ⓓ adrenal crisis requires intravenous crystalloids and hydrocortisone
Ⓔ typical maintenance therapy comprises at least 50 mg cortisol daily

52.
Recognised features of congenital adrenal hyperplasia include

Ⓐ 21-hydroxylase enzyme deficiency
Ⓑ decreased plasma cortisol and aldosterone concentrations
Ⓒ increased mortality in male infants
Ⓓ growth acceleration and precocious puberty
Ⓔ increased plasma 17 alpha-hydroxyprogesterone concentration

53.
The insulin-induced hypoglycaemia stimulation test is

Ⓐ mandatory in the confirmation of secondary hypoadrenalism
Ⓑ best terminated when the plasma glucose falls below 2.2 mmol/L
Ⓒ contraindicated in ischaemic heart disease and epilepsy
Ⓓ contraindicated in advanced hypopituitarism
Ⓔ an unreliable test of hypothalamic function

54.
The typical features of phaeochromocytoma include

Ⓐ predominantly adrenaline rather than noradrenaline secretion
Ⓑ episodic nausea with sweating and marked skin pallor
Ⓒ underlying malignant tumour in the majority
Ⓓ presentation with hypertension and hypercalcaemia
Ⓔ control of symptoms following propranolol therapy alone

55.
Recognised causes of impotence include

Ⓐ pituitary microprolactinoma
Ⓑ psychological distress
Ⓒ peripheral vascular disease
Ⓓ diabetes mellitus
Ⓔ multiple sclerosis

56.
In male infertility associated with oligospermia

Ⓐ increased plasma FSH levels suggest testicular dysfunction
Ⓑ testicular biopsy should be undertaken to exclude malignancy
Ⓒ testicular production of sperm may be normal
Ⓓ gonadotrophin therapy usually restores normal fertility
Ⓔ low plasma FSH levels suggest obstruction is the cause

57.
Hypogonadotrophic hypogonadism is typically associated with
- Ⓐ atrophy of the testicular interstitial (Leydig) cells
- Ⓑ Klinefelter's syndrome (XXY)
- Ⓒ isolated GnRH deficiency (Kallmann's syndrome)
- Ⓓ haemochromatosis
- Ⓔ hepatic cirrhosis

58.
The clinical features of male hypogonadism include
- Ⓐ total absence of pubic hair if pre-pubertal in onset
- Ⓑ growth retardation if pre-pubertal in onset
- Ⓒ atrophy of the external genitalia if post-pubertal in onset
- Ⓓ impairment of strength, libido and erectile function
- Ⓔ sweating with hot flushes after post-pubertal castration

59.
Recognised causes of hypergonadotrophic hypogonadism include
- Ⓐ Klinefelter's syndrome
- Ⓑ Turner's syndrome
- Ⓒ autoimmune ovarian disease
- Ⓓ leprosy
- Ⓔ cryptorchidism

60.
In cryptorchidism with inguinal testes in a child
- Ⓐ the individual is usually otherwise normal
- Ⓑ hypogonadotrophic hypogonadism should be excluded
- Ⓒ the seminiferous tubules are typically normal
- Ⓓ testicular interstitial cell function is usually normal
- Ⓔ treatment with chorionic gonadotrophin or GnRH is contraindicated

61.
Recognised causes of primary amenorrhoea include
- Ⓐ endometriosis
- Ⓑ congenital adrenal hyperplasia
- Ⓒ Turner's syndrome
- Ⓓ gluten enteropathy
- Ⓔ craniopharyngioma

62.
Recognised causes of secondary amenorrhoea include
- Ⓐ pituitary microprolactinoma
- Ⓑ anorexia nervosa
- Ⓒ Cushing's syndrome
- Ⓓ renal failure
- Ⓔ Stein–Leventhal syndrome

63.
The typical features of idiopathic premature menopause include
- Ⓐ decreased plasma LH and FSH concentrations
- Ⓑ hirsutism and clitoral hypertrophy
- Ⓒ bone fractures due to osteomalacia
- Ⓓ superficial dyspareunia and dysuria
- Ⓔ age at onset 45–55 years

64.
The following statements about diabetes mellitus are true
- Ⓐ The UK prevalence is approximately 1%
- Ⓑ The disorder is more common in nulliparous than multiparous women
- Ⓒ Type I IDDM is typically inherited as an autosomal dominant trait
- Ⓓ Type II NIDDM increases in prevalence with advancing age
- Ⓔ Hyperglycaemia occurs only after 50% reduction in islet cell mass

65.

Type I insulin-dependent diabetes mellitus is associated with

Ⓐ 'insulitis' — mononuclear infiltrate of islets

Ⓑ cow's milk feeding of infants < 3 months old

Ⓒ serum islet cell antibodies in > 80% of newly-diagnosed patients

Ⓓ hypothyroidism

Ⓔ possession of HLA antigens DR3 and DR4

66.

Secondary diabetes mellitus is associated with

Ⓐ thiazide diuretic therapy

Ⓑ haemochromatosis

Ⓒ primary hyperaldosteronism

Ⓓ pancreatic carcinoma

Ⓔ thyrotoxicosis, phaeochromocytoma and acromegaly

67.

The following statements about type II diabetes mellitus are true

Ⓐ There is clear evidence of disordered autoimmunity in NIDDM

Ⓑ Monozygotic twins show approximately 100% concordance for NIDDM

Ⓒ Patients with NIDDM typically exhibit hypersensitivity to insulin

Ⓓ Obesity predisposes to NIDDM in genetically-susceptible individuals

Ⓔ Insulin secretion in response to amino acids is normal in NIDDM

68.

Biochemical consequences of diabetes mellitus include

Ⓐ extracellular fluid depletion

Ⓑ decreased glycogenolysis

Ⓒ decreased lipolysis

Ⓓ increased gluconeogenesis

Ⓔ increased urinary excretion of potassium and magnesium

69.

In decompensated diabetes mellitus

Ⓐ thirst results from the increased osmolality of glomerular filtrate

Ⓑ hyperpnoea is the result of acidosis due to lactic and ketoacids

Ⓒ water and electrolyte depletion is greater in the mentally confused

Ⓓ increases in lipolysis reflect the degree of insulin deficiency

Ⓔ insulin deficiency inhibits the peripheral utilisation of ketoacids

70.

In the diagnosis of diabetes mellitus

Ⓐ glycosylated haemoglobin (HbA_{1c}) is a screening test

Ⓑ absence of glycosuria excludes diabetes

Ⓒ glycosuria in young patients is usually due to reduced renal threshold

Ⓓ 5% have serious vascular disease at presentation

Ⓔ plasma glucose levels are higher than whole blood levels

71.

Latent rather than potential diabetes mellitus is suggested by

Ⓐ an abnormal glucose tolerance test (GTT) developing in pregnancy

Ⓑ an abnormal GTT returning to normal following weight reduction

Ⓒ a normal GTT which becomes abnormal during glucocorticoid therapy

Ⓓ a child with a normal GTT but whose parents both have type I IDDM

Ⓔ an identical twin with a normal GTT whose twin has type I IDDM

72.

The oral glucose tolerance test is

Ⓐ diabetic if the 2 hour blood glucose > 10 mmol/L

Ⓑ diabetic if the fasting blood glucose > 6.7 mmol/L

Ⓒ undertaken following 3 days of dietary carbohydrate restriction

Ⓓ best administered using 75 g glucose in 250 ml water

Ⓔ diabetic if any blood glucose exceeds 12 mmol/L

73.

The following statements about glucose estimations are true

Ⓐ The plasma glucose is 15% lower than whole blood concentrations

Ⓑ The urinary dipstix is glucose-specific

Ⓒ Positive urinary dipstix indicate urinary glucose concentrations > 5 mmol/L

Ⓓ Normal renal threshold for glucose reabsorption is 10 mmol/L

Ⓔ Renal glycosuria in healthy young adults increases the lifetime likelihood of NIDDM

74.

Typical presentations of diabetes mellitus include

Ⓐ weight loss and nocturia

Ⓑ balanitis or pruritus vulvae

Ⓒ epigastric pain and vomiting

Ⓓ limb pains with absent ankle reflexes

Ⓔ asymptomatic glycosuria in the elderly

75.

In the dietary management of diabetes mellitus

Ⓐ 75% of patients also require hypoglycaemic drug therapy

Ⓑ carbohydrate intakes should be 50% of total calorie intake

Ⓒ ice cream and chocolates should never be consumed

Ⓓ fat intakes should not exceed 35% of total calorie intake

Ⓔ in obese patients, calorie intake should not exceed 600 kcal/day

76.

Sulphonylurea drug therapy in diabetes mellitus

Ⓐ causes more weight gain when given with biguanide therapy

Ⓑ decreases plasma immunoreactive insulin concentrations

Ⓒ decreases the number of peripheral insulin receptors

Ⓓ decreases hepatic glycogenolysis and gluconeogenesis

Ⓔ causes alcohol-induced flushing as a dominantly-inherited trait

77.

The following statements about insulin therapy are true

Ⓐ The duration of action of unmodified insulins = 6 hours

Ⓑ The duration of action of depot insulins = 12 hours +

Ⓒ Obese individuals tend to require lower total doses

Ⓓ The standard UK solution strength = 100 i.u./ml

Ⓔ Human insulins are less potent than animal-derived insulins

78.

In the management of a newly-diagnosed 30-year-old diabetic

Ⓐ insulin-induced hypoglycaemia should be experienced as part of patient education

Ⓑ insulin requirements during the first 8 weeks often decrease

Ⓒ insulin should normally be administered once daily initially

Ⓓ glycosylated haemoglobin levels should be monitored weekly

Ⓔ 6-hourly urine testing is recommended during pregnancy

79.

Typical symptoms of hypoglycaemia in diabetic patients include

Ⓐ feelings of faintness and hunger

Ⓑ tremor, palpitation and dizziness

Ⓒ headache, diplopia and confusion

Ⓓ abnormal behaviour despite plasma glucose consistently > 5 mmol/L

Ⓔ nocturnal sweating, nightmares and convulsions

80.

In the treatment of severe hypoglycaemia in diabetic patients

Ⓐ 50 ml 50% glucose should be given intravenously

Ⓑ glucagon should be avoided if the episode was due to sulphonylurea therapy

Ⓒ an alternative explanation is likely if the patient is taking metformin therapy alone

Ⓓ recovery is invariably complete within an hour of therapy

Ⓔ hospital admission is usually unnecessary if due to chlorpropamide therapy

81.

In a comatose diabetic, features suggesting hypoglycaemia rather than ketoacidosis include

Ⓐ systemic hypotension

Ⓑ brisk tendon reflexes

Ⓒ air hunger

Ⓓ moist skin and tongue

Ⓔ abdominal pain

82.

The typical clinical features of diabetic ketoacidosis include

Ⓐ abdominal pain and air hunger

Ⓑ rapid, weak pulse and hypotension

Ⓒ profuse sweating and oliguria

Ⓓ vomiting and constipation

Ⓔ coma with extensor plantar responses

83.

Typical findings in diabetic ketoacidosis include

Ⓐ water deficit of 5–10 litres

Ⓑ both sodium and potassium deficits of > 400 mmol

Ⓒ arterial blood gas analysis $PaO_2 = 7$ kPa, $PaCO_2 = 7$ kPa and pH = 7.20

Ⓓ decreased serum potassium concentration at presentation

Ⓔ peripheral blood leucocytosis

84.

In the management of diabetic ketoacidosis

Ⓐ intracellular water deficit is best restored using normal saline

Ⓑ potassium should be given irrespective of the serum concentration

Ⓒ bicarbonate infusion is often only necessary in renal failure

Ⓓ dextrose should be avoided unless hypoglycaemia supervenes

Ⓔ circulatory failure requires colloid infusion initially

85.

In the long-term management of diabetes

Ⓐ retinal neovascularisation should be treated by improved glycaemic control

Ⓑ microaneurysms are only visible with fluorescein angiography

Ⓒ visual symptoms correlate well with severity of retinal disease

Ⓓ microalbuminuria suggests renal tubular dysfunction

Ⓔ neuropathy may present with sudden death

86.

In the management of diabetes mellitus during pregnancy

Ⓐ there is an increased perinatal mortality rate

Ⓑ the baby is usually smaller than expected from gestational age

Ⓒ delivery should be undertaken by caesarian section at week 36

Ⓓ mild diabetes responds well to sulphonylurea and diet therapy

Ⓔ insulin requirements usually decrease throughout pregnancy

87.

In the management of diabetics requiring elective surgery

Ⓐ patients should stop sulphonylureas 24 hours prior to surgery

Ⓑ usual insulin should be given preoperatively to prevent ketoacidosis

Ⓒ patients with NIDDM require insulin cover for major surgery

Ⓓ those undergoing cardiopulmonary bypass have lower insulin needs

Ⓔ glucose-insulin infusion is the optimal method perioperatively

88.

In the classification of hyperlipidaemias, the following findings are typical

Ⓐ chylomicronaemia in types I and V

Ⓑ hypertriglyceridaemia in types III, IV and V

Ⓒ hypercholesterolaemia in types II, III and IV

Ⓓ tendon xanthomata in type IIa hypercholesterolaemia

Ⓔ palmar xanthomata in type III hyperlipidaemia

89.

In the treatment of hyperlipidaemia in patients aged < 60 years

Ⓐ dietary fat restriction reduces the plasma cholesterol by 10%

Ⓑ lowering a plasma cholesterol > 6.5 mmol/L is of no proven value

Ⓒ drug therapy is usually necessary if plasma cholesterol > 7.8 mmol/L

Ⓓ high plasma HDL/LDL ratios indicate the need for drug therapy

Ⓔ fibrates reduce cholesterol synthesis by inhibiting HMG CoA reductase

90.

Hypoglycaemia is

Ⓐ confirmed by a plasma glucose level of 2.4 mmol/L

Ⓑ a recognised complication of acute alcoholic intoxication

Ⓒ best investigated using a 48-hour fast if unexplained

Ⓓ the cause of late dumping syndrome following partial gastrectomy

Ⓔ most obvious preprandially in patients with an insulinoma

91.

In the classification of acute and non-acute porphyrias

Ⓐ delta-ALA synthetase activity is increased in all porphyrias

Ⓑ porphobilinogen deaminase activity is reduced in acute porphyrias

Ⓒ neuropsychiatric features are typical of the non-acute porphyrias

Ⓓ photosensitivity is typical of the acute porphyrias

Ⓔ variegate porphyria and coproporphyria are acute porphyrias

92.

The typical features of acute intermittent porphyria include

Ⓐ increased porphobilinogen deaminase activity

Ⓑ the absence of clinical symptoms or signs

Ⓒ vomiting, constipation and abdominal pain

Ⓓ hypertension and tachycardia

Ⓔ exacerbation by diamorphine or chlorpromazine therapy

13 DISEASES OF THE BLOOD

ANSWERS BEGIN ON P. 215

1.
In the normal formation of blood cells
Ⓐ fetal haemopoiesis does not take place in bone marrow
Ⓑ all lymphocytes originate in the bone marrow
Ⓒ haemopoiesis in adults extends to the femoral and humeral heads
Ⓓ the proerythroblast precedes the development of the normoblast
Ⓔ erythropoietin is produced by renal glomerular mesangial cells

2.
Mature erythrocytes
Ⓐ contain blood group antigens in their cytoplasm
Ⓑ stain with methylene blue due to ribosomes producing haemoglobin
Ⓒ derive energy from glucose to fuel the Na^+/K^+ ionic pump
Ⓓ have a circulation half-life of about 120 days
Ⓔ contain carbonic anhydrase which facilitates carbon dioxide transport

3.
Haemoglobin
Ⓐ F comprises two alpha and two delta chains
Ⓑ A_2 comprises two alpha and two gamma chains
Ⓒ has four porphyrin rings each containing ferrous iron
Ⓓ is an important buffer of carbonic acid
Ⓔ oxygen binding is increased by RBC 2-3-diphosphoglycerate

4.
Mature neutrophil granulocytes
Ⓐ typically comprise > 50% of the total peripheral blood WBC in health
Ⓑ remain in the circulation for less than 12 hours
Ⓒ exhibit increased nuclear segmentation in infection
Ⓓ are derived from a different stem cell from that of monocytes
Ⓔ produce the vitamin B_{12} binding protein transcobalamin III

5.
Platelets (thrombocytes)
Ⓐ have a circulation life span of 10 hours in healthy subjects
Ⓑ are produced and regulated under the control of thrombopoietins
Ⓒ contain small nuclear remnants called Howell–Jolly bodies
Ⓓ decrease in number in response to aspirin therapy
Ⓔ release serotonin and thromboxanes

6.
The following statements about RBC morphology are true
Ⓐ Hypochromia is pathognomonic of iron deficiency
Ⓑ Polychromasia indicates active production of new RBCs
Ⓒ Poikilocytosis is invariably associated with anisocytosis
Ⓓ Punctate basophilia is a typical feature of beta-thalassaemia
Ⓔ Target cells are associated with hyposplenism and liver disease

7.

Iron

Ⓐ content of blood is about 500 mg per litre

Ⓑ losses in the healthy male are about 3 mg per day

Ⓒ content of the adult body is about 5 g

Ⓓ is usually stored in hepatocytes as haemosiderin

Ⓔ in the healthy diet amounts to 10–15 mg per day

8.

Peripheral blood findings in dietary iron deficiency include

Ⓐ microcytosis preceding the development of hypochromia

Ⓑ ovalocytosis and elliptocytosis

Ⓒ mean corpuscular haemoglobin concentration < 50% of normal

Ⓓ numerous target cells and Howell–Jolly bodies

Ⓔ neutrophil leucocyte hypersegmentation and thrombocytosis

9.

In the treatment of iron deficiency anaemia with iron

Ⓐ folic acid should also be given if the anaemia is severe

Ⓑ treatment is stopped as soon as haemoglobin normalises

Ⓒ haemoglobin should rise by 1 g/L/day

Ⓓ maximal reticulocyte counts usually develop within 7–10 days

Ⓔ parenteral iron is usually more effective than oral iron

10.

Hypochromic microcytic anaemia is a recognised finding in

Ⓐ haemolytic anaemia

Ⓑ primary sideroblastic anaemia

Ⓒ hypothyroidism

Ⓓ beta-thalassaemia

Ⓔ rheumatoid arthritis

11.

Normocytic normochromic anaemia is an expected feature of

Ⓐ alcoholic liver disease

Ⓑ chronic renal failure

Ⓒ hypothyroidism

Ⓓ kwashiorkor

Ⓔ strict vegetarianism

12.

Macrocytic anaemia is a typical finding in

Ⓐ folic acid deficiency

Ⓑ haemolytic anaemia

Ⓒ alcohol abuse

Ⓓ primary sideroblastic anaemia

Ⓔ myelodysplastic syndrome

13.

Typical haematological findings in megaloblastic anaemia include

Ⓐ pancytopenia and oval macrocytosis

Ⓑ neutrophil leucocyte hypersegmentation

Ⓒ anisocytosis and poikilocytosis

Ⓓ reticulocytosis and polychromasia

Ⓔ excess urinary urobilinogen and bilirubinuria

14.

Folate and vitamin B$_{12}$ deficiency both typically produce

Ⓐ subacute combined degeneration of the spinal cord

Ⓑ intermittent glossitis and diarrhoea

Ⓒ mild jaundice and splenomegaly

Ⓓ dementia and peripheral neuropathy

Ⓔ marked weight loss

15.

Characteristic features of Addisonian pernicious anaemia include

Ⓐ onset before the age of 30 years

Ⓑ gastric parietal cell and intrinsic factor antibodies in the serum

Ⓒ increased serum bilirubin and lactate dehydrogenase concentrations

Ⓓ fourfold increase in the risk of developing gastric carcinoma

Ⓔ Schilling test usually reverts to normal with intrinsic factor

16.
Typical features of the myelodysplastic syndromes include

Ⓐ presentation before the age of 40 years
Ⓑ macrocytic anaemia and pancytopenia
Ⓒ ring sideroblasts present on bone marrow cytology
Ⓓ clonal chromosomal abnormalities in 50% of patients
Ⓔ risk of progression to an acute leukaemia

17.
Recognised causes of pancytopenia include

Ⓐ systemic lupus erythematosus
Ⓑ indomethacin and sulphonamide therapy
Ⓒ hepatitis A infection
Ⓓ megaloblastic anaemia
Ⓔ myelodysplastic syndromes

18.
Characteristic features of primary aplastic anaemia include

Ⓐ peak incidence about the age of 60 years
Ⓑ normocytic normochromic anaemia with thrombocytosis
Ⓒ bone marrow trephine is required to confirm the diagnosis
Ⓓ splenomegaly indicating extramedullary erythropoiesis
Ⓔ paroxysmal nocturnal haemoglobinuria

19.
Typical features suggesting intravascular haemolysis include

Ⓐ bilirubinuria and haemoglobinuria
Ⓑ methaemalbuminaemia and haemosiderinuria
Ⓒ increased serum haptoglobin concentration
Ⓓ increased plasma haemoglobin concentration
Ⓔ rigors and splenomegaly

20.
Laboratory features suggesting haemolytic anaemia include

Ⓐ increased serum lactate dehydrogenase concentration
Ⓑ unconjugated hyperbilirubinaemia and excess urobilinogenuria
Ⓒ peripheral blood neutrophil leucocytosis and reticulocytosis
Ⓓ peripheral blood polychromasia and macrocytosis
Ⓔ bone marrow erythroid hyperplasia

21.
Haemolytic anaemia is a recognised complication of

Ⓐ prosthetic heart valves
Ⓑ mycoplasma pneumonia
Ⓒ megaloblastic anaemia
Ⓓ malarial infection
Ⓔ sulphonamide therapy

22.
Splenectomy for patients with hereditary spherocytosis

Ⓐ Should be followed by daily oral penicillin
Ⓑ Should be performed at as young an age as possible
Ⓒ is contraindicated in the presence of gallstones
Ⓓ predisposes to subsequent pneumococcal infection
Ⓔ is reserved for only those patients with massive splenomegaly

23.
Typical features of hereditary spherocytosis include

Ⓐ splenomegaly and gallstones
Ⓑ intravascular haemolysis
Ⓒ decreased RBC osmotic fragility
Ⓓ transient aplastic anaemia
Ⓔ positive Coomb's antiglobulin test

24.
The typical clinical features of sickle-cell anaemia include
- Ⓐ haemolytic and aplastic crises
- Ⓑ neonatal spherocytic haemolytic anaemia
- Ⓒ renal papillary, pulmonary and mesenteric infarction
- Ⓓ splenomegaly with hypersplenism
- Ⓔ bone necrosis and Salmonella osteomyelitis

25.
Recognised hazards in sickle-cell disease include
- Ⓐ high altitude
- Ⓑ pregnancy
- Ⓒ dehydration
- Ⓓ Bier's anaesthetic block
- Ⓔ hypothermia and infection

26.
The typical features of the beta-thalassemias include
- Ⓐ peripheral blood macrocytosis and anaemia
- Ⓑ hepatosplenomegaly and growth retardation
- Ⓒ mongoloid facies with frontal bossing
- Ⓓ neonatal haemolytic anaemia
- Ⓔ leg ulceration and gallstones

27.
The typical features of autoimmune haemolytic anaemia include
- Ⓐ peripheral blood spherocytosis and polychromasia
- Ⓑ fever with haemoglobinuria and haemosiderinuria
- Ⓒ association with systemic lupus erythematosus
- Ⓓ positive Coomb's antiglobulin test and splenomegaly
- Ⓔ association with lymphoproliferative disease

28.
In isoimmune haemolytic disease of the newborn
- Ⓐ ABO rather than Rhesus incompatibility is usually the more severe
- Ⓑ neonatal jaundice is usually present at birth
- Ⓒ hepatosplenomegaly and peripheral blood normoblasts are common
- Ⓓ the disease decreases in severity with successive pregnancies
- Ⓔ anti-D immunoglobulin prevents the development of maternal antibodies

29.
The typical features of polycythaemia rubra vera include
- Ⓐ predominance in females aged < 40 years
- Ⓑ splenomegaly, leucocytosis and thrombocytosis
- Ⓒ headaches, pruritus and peptic ulcer dyspepsia
- Ⓓ decreased leucocyte alkaline phosphatase score
- Ⓔ increased blood viscosity associated with vascular disease

30.
Recognised causes of neutropenia and agranulocytosis include
- Ⓐ folic acid deficiency
- Ⓑ sulphasalazine therapy
- Ⓒ sickle-cell anaemia
- Ⓓ infectious mononucleosis
- Ⓔ carbimazole therapy

31.
Peripheral blood lymphocytosis is an expected finding in
- Ⓐ brucellosis
- Ⓑ pneumococcal pneumonia
- Ⓒ measles and rubella
- Ⓓ Hodgkin's disease
- Ⓔ chronic lymphatic leukaemia

32.
Peripheral blood neutrophil leucocytosis is an expected finding in
Ⓐ connective tissue disease
Ⓑ corticosteroid therapy
Ⓒ pregnancy
Ⓓ whooping cough
Ⓔ mesenteric infarction

33.
Recognised causes of leuco-erythroblastic anaemia include
Ⓐ carcinomatosis
Ⓑ miliary tuberculosis
Ⓒ myelofibrosis
Ⓓ whooping cough
Ⓔ severe bleeding or haemolysis

34.
Characteristic features of acute leukaemia include
Ⓐ rapid onset of fever and anaemia
Ⓑ mouth ulceration and gingival hypertrophy
Ⓒ myalgia, arthralgia and skin rashes
Ⓓ microcytic anaemia and leucopenia
Ⓔ hypocellular bone marrow cytology

35.
Acute lymphoblastic leukaemia
Ⓐ usually develops in patients > 20 years old
Ⓑ typically produces blast cell cytoplasmic Auer rods
Ⓒ responds better to chemotherapy than other acute leukaemias
Ⓓ is the most common of all acute leukaemias
Ⓔ is a typical complication of multiple myeloma

36.
Clinical features of chronic myeloid leukaemia (CML) include
Ⓐ painful splenomegaly and priapism
Ⓑ sternal tenderness, gout and arthralgia
Ⓒ generalised lymphadenopathy
Ⓓ tendency to bleeding and bruising
Ⓔ median survival of 10 years with chemotherapy

37.
The typical laboratory findings in chronic myeloid leukaemia include
Ⓐ leucoerythroblastic anaemia and thrombocytosis
Ⓑ peripheral blood neutrophilia, eosinophilia and basophilia
Ⓒ chromosomal translocation $22q^-/9q^+$ in 90% of patients
Ⓓ increased neutrophil leucocyte alkaline phosphatase score
Ⓔ transformation to acute lymphoblastic leukaemia

38.
Typical features of chronic lymphatic leukaemia include
Ⓐ onset in younger patients than in CML
Ⓑ development of autoimmune haemolytic anaemia
Ⓒ presentation with massive hepatosplenomegaly and anaemia
Ⓓ lymphadenopathy associated with recurrent infections
Ⓔ median survival of 10 years following chemotherapy

39.
The typical laboratory features in chronic lymphatic leukaemia include
Ⓐ hyperuricaemia and thrombocytosis
Ⓑ hypogammaglobulinaemia
Ⓒ peripheral blood lymphocytosis in the absence of lymphoblasts
Ⓓ positive Coomb's test and Bence–Jones proteinuria
Ⓔ transformation to acute leukaemia is more common than in CML

40.
The presence of lymphadenopathy and splenomegaly is typical in
Ⓐ multiple myeloma
Ⓑ chronic lymphatic leukaemia
Ⓒ chronic myeloid leukaemia
Ⓓ infectious mononucleosis
Ⓔ myelofibrosis

41.
The typical features of myelofibrosis include

Ⓐ absence of splenomegaly or lymphadenopathy

Ⓑ leucoerythroblastic blood film with tear-drop poikilocytes

Ⓒ increased leucocyte neutrophil alkaline phosphatase score

Ⓓ folic acid deficiency and hyperuricaemia

Ⓔ absent bone marrow megakaryocytes and thrombocytopenia

42.
Recognised clinical features of multiple myeloma include

Ⓐ peak incidence between the ages 60 and 70 years

Ⓑ amyloidosis with Bence–Jones proteinuria

Ⓒ median survival of 2 years despite chemotherapy

Ⓓ recurrent infections and pancytopenia

Ⓔ increased serum calcium, urate and blood viscosity

43.
In differentiating multiple myeloma from a benign monoclonal gammopathy, the following findings would favour the diagnosis of multiple myeloma

Ⓐ monoclonal gammopathy with normal serum immunoglobulin levels

Ⓑ bone marrow plasmacytosis of > 20%

Ⓒ carpal tunnel syndrome and cardiac failure

Ⓓ Bence–Jones proteinuria

Ⓔ multiple osteolytic lesions on X-ray

44.
A poor prognosis in multiple myeloma is suggested by the presence of

Ⓐ blood urea > 10 mmol/L after rehydration

Ⓑ decreased serum beta$_2$-microglobulin concentration

Ⓒ blood haemoglobin < 80 g/L

Ⓓ Bence–Jones proteinuria

Ⓔ restriction of the activities of daily living

45.
Typical histopathological features of Hodgkin's disease include

Ⓐ Reed–Sternberg binucleate giant cells and lymphocytes

Ⓑ increased tissue eosinophils, neutrophils and plasma cells

Ⓒ increased fibrous stroma in the nodular sclerosing type

Ⓓ frequent involvement of the central nervous system

Ⓔ splenic involvement is rare in the absence of splenomegaly

46.
The clinical features of Hodgkin's disease include

Ⓐ painless cervical lymphadenopathy

Ⓑ anaemia typically indicating bone marrow involvement

Ⓒ impaired T cell function in the absence of lymphopenia

Ⓓ pruritus and alcohol-induced abdominal pain

Ⓔ overall 10 year survival > 60% following treatment

47.
Typical characteristics of non-Hodgkin's lymphoma include

Ⓐ follicular cell histology indicating a low-grade lymphoma

Ⓑ bone marrow and splenic involvement are present from the onset

Ⓒ involvement of the stomach and thyroid gland is common

Ⓓ the majority are T cell rather than B cell in origin

Ⓔ better prognosis in high-grade rather than low-grade lymphomas

48.
Prolongation of the prothrombin time is typical in

Ⓐ fibrinogen deficiency

Ⓑ factor 10 deficiency

Ⓒ factor 7 deficiency

Ⓓ factor 5 deficiency

Ⓔ factor 2 deficiency

49.
Prolongation of the partial thromboplastin time is typical in
Ⓐ factor 1 or 2 deficiency
Ⓑ factor 7 deficiency
Ⓒ factor 8 or 10 deficiency
Ⓓ factor 13 deficiency
Ⓔ factor 9, 11 or 12 deficiency

50.
Disseminated intravascular coagulation is a complication of
Ⓐ amniotic fluid embolism
Ⓑ incompatible blood transfusion
Ⓒ hypovolaemic and anaphylactic shock
Ⓓ septicaemic shock
Ⓔ carcinomatosis

51.
Features of disseminated intravascular coagulation include
Ⓐ thrombocytopenia
Ⓑ burr cells and schistocytes in the peripheral blood
Ⓒ decreased serum fibrin degradation products
Ⓓ normal prothrombin time and normal thrombin time
Ⓔ prolongation of the partial thromboplastin time

52.
The bleeding time is characteristically prolonged in
Ⓐ ascorbic acid deficiency
Ⓑ thrombocytopenia
Ⓒ haemophilia
Ⓓ warfarin therapy
Ⓔ von Willebrand's disease

53.
Haemorrhagic disorders due to decreased clotting factors include
Ⓐ hereditary haemorrhagic telangiectasia
Ⓑ Christmas disease
Ⓒ senile purpura
Ⓓ Henoch–Schönlein purpura
Ⓔ haemophilia

54.
The following statements about severe haemophilia A are true
Ⓐ The disorder is inherited in an X-linked recessive mode
Ⓑ Recurrent haemarthroses and haematuria are typical
Ⓒ Both partial thromboplastin and prothrombin times are prolonged
Ⓓ Factor 8 has a biological half-life of about 12 days
Ⓔ Desmopressin therapy increases factor 8 levels

55.
Haemorrhagic disorders due to defective blood vessels include
Ⓐ von Willebrand's disease
Ⓑ Ehlers–Danlos disease
Ⓒ septicaemia
Ⓓ Christmas disease
Ⓔ uraemia

56.
Recognised causes of thrombocytosis include
Ⓐ myeloproliferative disorders
Ⓑ iron deficiency anaemia
Ⓒ hypersplenism
Ⓓ carcinomatosis
Ⓔ connective tissue disorders

57.
Recognised causes of thrombocytopenia include
Ⓐ megaloblastic anaemia
Ⓑ acquired immunodeficiency syndrome
Ⓒ disseminated intravascular coagulation
Ⓓ von Willebrand's disease
Ⓔ aspirin, thiazide and sulphonamide therapy

58.
Typical features of idiopathic thrombocytopenic purpura include
Ⓐ IgG-mediated thrombocytopenia
Ⓑ predominantly affects patients > 40 years old
Ⓒ prolongation of the bleeding time
Ⓓ palpable splenomegaly
Ⓔ response to corticosteroid therapy

59.
Hypercoagulation abnormalities are a recognised feature of
Ⓐ the lupus anticoagulant (cardiolipin antibody) in SLE
Ⓑ congenital deficiency of antithrombin III
Ⓒ acute myocardial infarction
Ⓓ polycythaemia rubra vera
Ⓔ chronic myeloid leukaemia

14 ONCOLOGY
ANSWERS BEGIN ON P. 221

1.

The following factors are associated aetiologically with the carcinomas listed below

- Ⓐ malignant melanoma — coffee
- Ⓑ cervical carcinoma — chlamydial infection
- Ⓒ hepatocellular carcinoma — hepatitis B infection
- Ⓓ thyroid carcinoma — environmental radiation
- Ⓔ oesophageal carcinoma — tobacco consumption

2.

Tumour markers associated with the following diseases include

- Ⓐ human chorionic gonadotrophin — testicular seminoma
- Ⓑ alpha-fetoprotein — primary hepatocellular carcinoma
- Ⓒ carcinoembryonic antigen — bronchial adenoma
- Ⓓ placental alkaline phosphatase — cervical carcinoma
- Ⓔ CA-125 — breast carcinoma

3.

The following statements about the predictive value of screening tests are true

- Ⓐ The positive predictive value is dependent on the prevalence of the disease
- Ⓑ The negative predictive value is dependent on the specificity of the test
- Ⓒ The sensitivity is inversely related to specificity
- Ⓓ Specificity = % patients with a positive test in patients with the disease
- Ⓔ Sensitivity = % patients with a negative test in subjects without the disease

4.

The paraneoplastic syndromes listed below are typical of the following tumours

- Ⓐ inappropriate ADH activity — adenocarcinoma of lung
- Ⓑ parathyroid hormone activity — squamous cell carcinoma of lung
- Ⓒ polymyositis — gastric carcinoma
- Ⓓ myasthenia-like syndrome — small cell anaplastic lung carcinoma
- Ⓔ acanthosis nigricans — gastric carcinoma

5.

The following statements about tumour staging and response to therapy are correct

- Ⓐ The TNM system defines only tumour size and the number of metastases
- Ⓑ T0 indicates undetectable tumour proven only by aspirate cytology
- Ⓒ Functional status at diagnosis partly predicts prognosis
- Ⓓ A partial response to therapy = > 50% reduction in tumour size
- Ⓔ In the Ann Arbor classification, stage IIb non-Hodgkin gastric lymphoma indicates disease on both sides of the diaphragm

6.

In the Ann Arbor staging of lymphomas

- Ⓐ intra-thoracic and intra-abdominal lymphadenopathy = stage III
- Ⓑ splenomegaly and intra-abdominal lymphadenopathy = stage IIIS
- Ⓒ diffuse hepatic or bone marrow involvement = stage IV
- Ⓓ gastric and splenic involvement = stage IIS
- Ⓔ pulmonary hilar lymphadenopathy with fever = stage IB

7.

In the TNM staging of bronchial carcinoma

- Ⓐ TX indicates positive cytology
- Ⓑ T2 indicates tumour size > 3 cm and/or extension to hilar nodes
- Ⓒ malignant pleural effusion would be staged as T4
- Ⓓ N1 indicates extension to the ipsilateral mediastinum
- Ⓔ M0 indicates the absence of metastases

8.

The following statements about radiotherapy are true

- Ⓐ Ionising radiation damages cell nuclear DNA
- Ⓑ 1 Gray of absorbed radiation = 10 Joule per kilogram of tissue
- Ⓒ Brachytherapy is radiotherapy delivered by an external beam
- Ⓓ Megavoltage teletherapy is used for skin tumours
- Ⓔ Hypoxia enhances tissue sensitivity to irradiation

9.

The following statements about chemotherapy are true

- Ⓐ Methotrexate is an anti-folate blocking nucleotide synthesis
- Ⓑ Vincristine is an alkylating agent blocking DNA transcription
- Ⓒ Adriamycin is a plant alkaloid which disrupts mitotic spindles
- Ⓓ Streptozotocin is a nitrosourea which blocks pyrimidine synthesis
- Ⓔ Melphalan is an alkylating agent which blocks DNA replication

10.

The general principles governing the use of combination chemotherapy include

- Ⓐ the toxic effects of each drug should be closely similar
- Ⓑ each drug should have a similar mode of action
- Ⓒ each drug should be of proven efficacy individually
- Ⓓ drugs used in combination should not have adverse interactions
- Ⓔ the minimum effective dose of each drug should be used

11.

Malignant diseases that are potentially curable using combination chemotherapy include

- Ⓐ malignant melanoma
- Ⓑ myelomatosis
- Ⓒ choriocarcinoma
- Ⓓ anaplastic thyroid carcinoma
- Ⓔ Hodgkin's lymphoma

12.

Malignant diseases refractory to current chemotherapeutic agents include

- Ⓐ squamous cell bronchial carcinoma
- Ⓑ oesophageal carcinoma
- Ⓒ colorectal carcinoma
- Ⓓ ovarian carcinoma
- Ⓔ malignant melanoma

13.

The following adverse effects are associated with the chemotherapy drugs listed below

- Ⓐ alopecia — cyclophosphamide
- Ⓑ acute leukaemia — methotrexate
- Ⓒ cardiomyopathy — adriamycin
- Ⓓ pulmonary fibrosis — cisplatin
- Ⓔ neuropathy — vincristine

14.

Endocrinological therapies useful in the treatment of the malignant disorders include

Ⓐ gonadotrophin releasing hormone for prostatic carcinoma

Ⓑ thyroxine for papillary thyroid carcinoma

Ⓒ progesterone for endometrial carcinoma

Ⓓ aminoglutethamide for testicular teratoma

Ⓔ tamoxifen for breast carcinoma

15.

In the management of pain in patients with malignant diseases

Ⓐ analgesia is best used on an 'as required' basis

Ⓑ NSAID therapy is particularly valuable in bone pain

Ⓒ morphine is more highly soluble than diamorphine

Ⓓ dextropropoxyphene and dihydrocodeine are equipotent

Ⓔ opiate and phenothiazine combinations should be used routinely

16.

The following drugs have clinically useful anti-emetic properties

Ⓐ lorazepam

Ⓑ domperidone

Ⓒ ondansetron

Ⓓ dexamethasone

Ⓔ etoposide

17.

The tumour lysis syndrome is

Ⓐ commoner in children

Ⓑ commoner in the presence of renal impairment

Ⓒ complicated by progressive hypokalaemia

Ⓓ an indication for allopurinol

Ⓔ a cause of hyperphosphataemia

DISEASES OF CONNECTIVE TISSUES, JOINTS AND BONES

15

ANSWERS BEGIN ON P. 223

1.
The following features suggest a functional origin to low back pain
- Ⓐ radiation of pain down the back of one leg to the ankle
- Ⓑ an elevated C reactive protein
- Ⓒ tenderness to superficial touch
- Ⓓ absence of any abnormal physical sign
- Ⓔ stiffness on resting

2.
In a patient with low back pain
- Ⓐ the X-ray finding of spina bifida occulta would explain the symptom
- Ⓑ loss of lumbar lordosis would suggest neoplastic vertebral infiltration
- Ⓒ exacerbation of pain with exercise suggests sacroiliitis
- Ⓓ previous myelography suggests the possibility of arachnoiditis
- Ⓔ spontaneous resolution within 1 month is the commonest outcome

3.
The following statements are true :
- Ⓐ Pes planus is usually painful
- Ⓑ In genu varus the knee deviates towards the midline
- Ⓒ Cubitus valgus is typical of the normal female elbow
- Ⓓ Pes cavus is common in patients with poliomyelitis
- Ⓔ Hallux valgus is usually secondary to crystal arthropathy

4.
The typical findings in fibromyalgia include
- Ⓐ elevation of the ESR
- Ⓑ symptoms of fatigue and an irritable bowel
- Ⓒ coexistent anxiety and depression
- Ⓓ rapid, spontaneous resolution
- Ⓔ musculoskeletal pain without local tenderness

5.
The following statements about musculoskeletal pains are true
- Ⓐ In inflammatory arthritis, pain is typically worse by day
- Ⓑ Ligamentous strain produces pain which is usually only felt on movement
- Ⓒ The pain of impacted fractures is invariably worse on movement
- Ⓓ Muscle pain is typically unaffected by isometric contraction
- Ⓔ In osteoarthrosis, pain is usually worse on resting

6.
In a patient with neck pain
- Ⓐ aggravation by sneezing suggests cervical disc prolapse
- Ⓑ radiation to the occiput suggests disease affecting the upper cervical vertebrae
- Ⓒ associated bilateral arm paraesthesiae suggest angina pectoris as the most likely diagnosis
- Ⓓ otherwise normal joints exclude rheumatoid arthritis as a possible diagnosis
- Ⓔ associated drop attacks suggest vertebral artery compression due to cervical spondylosis

7.
Shoulder pain is a recognised feature of
- **A** myocardial ischaemia
- **B** supraspinatus tendonitis
- **C** bronchial carcinoma
- **D** pneumococcal pneumonia
- **E** cervical spondylosis

8.
In a patient with shoulder pain
- **A** supraspinatus tendonitis is associated with a 'painful arc'
- **B** bicipital tendonitis is associated with a painful arc
- **C** shoulder pain developing beyond 90 degrees abduction suggests infraspinatus tendonitis
- **D** shoulder pain in all directions of movement suggests capsulitis
- **E** subscapularis tendonitis is suggested by pain worsening on resisted abduction

9.
Dupuytren's contracture is
- **A** typically painless
- **B** associated with autosomal dominant pattern of inheritance
- **C** commoner in men
- **D** associated with epilepsy
- **E** surgically irremediable

10.
The thoracic spine is
- **A** the commonest site of symptomatic disc protrusion
- **B** more mobile in rotation than flexion and extension
- **C** normally lordotic
- **D** typically straight in spinal osteoporosis
- **E** usually scoliotic if affected in poliomyelitis

11.
The typical features of rheumatoid arthritis include
- **A** onset usually before the age of 30 years
- **B** a female-male ratio of 3:1
- **C** association with HLA DR4
- **D** progression to bone and cartilage destruction
- **E** sparing of joints of the pelvic and shoulder girdle

12.
Characteristic pathological changes in rheumatoid arthritis include
- **A** diffuse necrotising vasculitis
- **B** increased synovial fluid complement concentration
- **C** subcutaneous nodules with numerous giant cells
- **D** generalised lymphadenopathy
- **E** progression to amyloidosis

13.
Typical features of active rheumatoid arthritis include
- **A** fever and weight loss
- **B** macrocytic anaemia
- **C** anterior uveitis
- **D** thrombocytopenia
- **E** generalised lymphadenopathy

14.
The typical pattern of synovial disease in rheumatoid arthritis includes
- **A** early involvement of the sacro-iliac joints
- **B** symmetrical peripheral joint involvement
- **C** spindling of the fingers and broadening of the forefeet
- **D** distal interphalangeal joint involvement of fingers and toes
- **E** atlanto-axial joint involvement

15.
Extra-articular manifestations of rheumatoid arthritis include
- **A** cutaneous ulceration
- **B** pericardial and pleural effusions
- **C** amyloidosis
- **D** peripheral neuropathy
- **E** hypersplenism

16.

The following statements about rheumatoid arthritis are true

Ⓐ joint pain and stiffness is typically aggravated by rest

Ⓑ the Rose–Waaler test is positive in about 70% of patients

Ⓒ joint involvement is additive rather than flitting

Ⓓ associated scleromalacia typically produces painful red eyes

Ⓔ Raynaud's and sicca syndromes suggest an alternative diagnosis

17.

In the treatment of rheumatoid arthritis

Ⓐ bed rest should be avoided because of bony ankylosis

Ⓑ splinting of the affected joints reduces pain and swelling

Ⓒ associated anaemia responds promptly to oral iron therapy

Ⓓ systemic corticosteroids are contraindicated

Ⓔ non-steroidal anti-inflammatory drugs retard disease progression

18.

Drugs which retard disease progression in RA include

Ⓐ sulphasalazine

Ⓑ phenylbutazone

Ⓒ D-penicillamine

Ⓓ sodium aurothiomalate

Ⓔ azathioprine

19.

A poorer prognosis in rheumatoid arthritis is associated with

Ⓐ insidious onset of rheumatoid arthritis

Ⓑ high titres of rheumatoid factor early in the course of the disease

Ⓒ early development of subcutaneous nodules and erosive arthritis

Ⓓ extra-articular manifestations of the disease

Ⓔ onset with palindromic rheumatism

20.

Recognised features of primary Sjögren's syndrome include

Ⓐ an increased incidence of lymphoma

Ⓑ dryness of the eyes, mouth and vagina

Ⓒ reduced lacrimal secretion rate

Ⓓ a predominance of males amongst affected patients

Ⓔ a positive IgM rheumatoid factor in over 80% of patients

21.

Typical features of seronegative spondyloarthritis include

Ⓐ asymmetrical oligoarthritis

Ⓑ involvement of cartilaginous joints

Ⓒ enthesitis of tendinous insertions

Ⓓ scleritis and episcleritis

Ⓔ mitral valve disease

22.

Features associated with ankylosing spondylitis include

Ⓐ peak onset in the second and third decades

Ⓑ subcutaneous nodules

Ⓒ HLA B27 in > 90% of affected patients

Ⓓ faecal carriage of specific Klebsiella species

Ⓔ family history of psoriatic arthritis and Reiter's syndrome

23.

In osteomalacia

Ⓐ a proximal myopathy may be the presenting feature

Ⓑ bone involvement is characteristically painless

Ⓒ Chvostek's sign may be positive

Ⓓ due to renal disease, 25-hydroxycholecalciferol therapy is advisable

Ⓔ pseudofractures on X-ray are pathognomonic

24.
Features suggesting ankylosing spondylitis include
Ⓐ early morning low back pain radiating to the buttocks
Ⓑ persistence of lumbar lordosis on spinal flexion
Ⓒ chest pain aggravated by breathing
Ⓓ 'squaring' of the lumbar vertebrae on X-ray
Ⓔ erosions of the symphysis pubis on X-ray

25.
In the treatment of ankylosing spondylitis
Ⓐ systemic corticosteroid therapy is contraindicated
Ⓑ prolonged bed rest accelerates functional recovery
Ⓒ spinal radiotherapy modifies the course of the disease
Ⓓ spinal deformity is minimised with physiotherapy
Ⓔ hip joint involvement augurs a poorer prognosis

26.
The typical features of Reiter's disease include
Ⓐ anterior uveitis develops more often than conjunctivitis
Ⓑ non-specific urethritis and prostatitis
Ⓒ symmetrical small joint polyarthritis
Ⓓ onset 1–3 weeks following bacterial dysentery
Ⓔ keratoderma blenorrhagica and nail dystrophy

27.
In Reiter's disease
Ⓐ a peripheral blood monocytosis is commonly found
Ⓑ sacroiliitis and spondylitis develop in most patients
Ⓒ salmonella or shigella species can be cultured from joint aspirates
Ⓓ calcaneal spurs are not apparent radiologically
Ⓔ arthritis resolves within 3–6 months of onset

28.
Psoriatic arthritis
Ⓐ is usually preceded by the development of psoriasis
Ⓑ affects 25% of patients with psoriasis
Ⓒ is commoner in patients with psoriatic nail changes
Ⓓ has a poorer prognosis than does rheumatoid arthritis
Ⓔ responds well to hydroxychloroquine

29.
Recognised patterns of psoriatic arthritis include
Ⓐ asymmetrical oligoarthritis of the fingers and toes
Ⓑ distal interphalangeal joint involvement with nail dystrophy
Ⓒ sacroiliitis and spondylitis
Ⓓ rheumatoid-like symmetrical small joint arthritis
Ⓔ arthritis mutilans with telescoping of the digits

30.
Diseases associated with sero-negative spondyloarthritis include
Ⓐ Sjögren's syndrome
Ⓑ Whipple's disease
Ⓒ coeliac disease
Ⓓ ulcerative colitis
Ⓔ Behçet's disease

31.
Recognised causes of childhood arthritis include
Ⓐ rubella virus infection
Ⓑ rheumatic fever
Ⓒ acute leukaemia
Ⓓ Henoch–Schönlein purpura
Ⓔ meningococcal infection

32.
The following statements about juvenile chronic arthritis are true
Ⓐ Still's disease usually presents with an unexplained arthritis alone
Ⓑ Seropositive polyarthritis resembles adult rheumatoid arthritis
Ⓒ Pauciarticular disease in girls is associated with chronic iritis
Ⓓ Pauciarticular disease in boys resembles ankylosing spondylitis
Ⓔ Polyarticular pattern is seen most commonly

33.
Joint involvement is a recognised feature of the following conditions
Ⓐ acromegaly
Ⓑ sarcoidosis
Ⓒ leprosy
Ⓓ infection with *Borrelia burgdorferi*
Ⓔ syringomyelia

34.
Features of vitamin D deficiency in childhood include
Ⓐ normal serum alkaline phosphatase concentration
Ⓑ delayed motor development
Ⓒ development of epilepsy
Ⓓ irreversible X-ray changes in the long bones
Ⓔ decreasing serum calcium levels in response to treatment

35.
The following statements about infective arthritis are true
Ⓐ The onset is typically insidious
Ⓑ Pre-existing arthritis is a recognised predisposing factor
Ⓒ Small peripheral joints are involved more often than larger joints
Ⓓ *Haemophilus influenzae* is the commonest causative organism in adults
Ⓔ Joint aspiration should be avoided given the risk of septicaemia

36.
The typical features of gonococcal arthritis include
Ⓐ a predominance of young males
Ⓑ pustular or vesicular rashes
Ⓒ tenosynovitis and asymmetrical polyarthritis
Ⓓ positive synovial fluid culture in most instances
Ⓔ chronic joint disease in the majority

37.
Tuberculous arthritis is
Ⓐ a common accompaniment of pulmonary tuberculosis in the UK
Ⓑ characterised by early, florid, destructive joint changes on X-ray
Ⓒ typically associated with a strongly positive tuberculin skin test
Ⓓ usually best confirmed by joint aspiration
Ⓔ best managed by intra-articular antituberculous drugs

38.
Typical features of systemic lupus erythematosus include
Ⓐ a higher prevalence in Caucasian than African women
Ⓑ onset usually in the fourth and fifth decades
Ⓒ impaired function of suppressor T lymphocytes
Ⓓ increased prevalence of HLA B8 and HLA DR3
Ⓔ exacerbations occurring during pregnancy and the puerperium

39.
Characteristic clinical features of systemic lupus erythematosus include
Ⓐ Raynaud's phenomenon
Ⓑ alopecia
Ⓒ an erythematous facial rash which is improved by exposure to ulraviolet light or sunlight
Ⓓ absence of renal complications
Ⓔ neuropsychiatric symptoms

40.

Antinuclear antibodies

ⓐ occur in 95% of patients with systemic lupus erythematosus

ⓑ of anti-dsDNA type are highly specific to systemic lupus erythematosus

ⓒ fluctuate in titre in parallel with clinical activity of disease

ⓓ are rarely found in healthy subjects

ⓔ typically occur in patients with polyarteritis nodosa

41.

Typical haematogical findings in systemic lupus erythematosus include

ⓐ leucocytosis and thrombocytosis

ⓑ impaired coagulation

ⓒ circulating anti-DNA and rheumatoid factor antibodies in high titre

ⓓ elevated CH50, C3 and C4 complement levels in peripheral blood

ⓔ elevated C-reactive protein levels

42.

Drug-induced systemic lupus erythematosus is a recognised adverse drug effect following therapy with

ⓐ aspirin

ⓑ hydralazine

ⓒ oestrogens

ⓓ phenytoin

ⓔ ibuprofen

43.

In the management of systemic lupus erythematosus, the following are of proven value

ⓐ NSAIDs for renal involvement

ⓑ corticosteroid therapy for cerebral involvement

ⓒ plasmapheresis for immune complex disease

ⓓ hydroxychloroquine for skin and joint involvement

ⓔ long term corticosteroid therapy during periods of remission to prevent relapse

44.

Typical features of mixed connective tissue disease include

ⓐ proximal muscle weakness and tenderness

ⓑ diffuse interstitial pulmonary fibrosis

ⓒ anti-ribonucleoprotein antibodies in high titre

ⓓ renal and neurological involvement

ⓔ decreased serum creatine kinase concentration

45.

The clinical features of progressive systemic sclerosis include

ⓐ presentation with Raynaud's phenomenon

ⓑ reflux oesophagitis and dysphagia

ⓒ fibrosing alveolitis

ⓓ ulceration, atrophy and subcutaneous calcification of the fingertips

ⓔ anti-DNA antibodies and decreased serum complement levels

46.

In inflammatory polymyositis

ⓐ an association with HLA B8, HLA DR3 is recognised

ⓑ antinuclear antibodies are characteristically absent

ⓒ electromyography is helpful in differentiation from peripheral neuropathy

ⓓ underlying malignancy is usually present if weight loss is marked

ⓔ an erythematous rash on the knuckles, elbows, knees and face is typical

47.

Features of giant cell arteritis include

ⓐ a predominance in females > 60 years of age

ⓑ pain in the jaw during eating

ⓒ confluent involvement of affected arteries

ⓓ difficulty in rising from the seated position

ⓔ weight loss with normochromic anaemia and high ESR

48.

In polymyalgia rheumatica

Ⓐ antinuclear and rheumatoid factor antibodies are often present in high titre

Ⓑ temporal artery biopsy usually confirms the diagnosis

Ⓒ response to oral corticosteroids typically occurs within 7 days

Ⓓ corticosteroid therapy should be withdrawn after 6 months

Ⓔ sudden uniocular blindness suggests steroid-induced cataract

49.

Factors predisposing to hyperuricaemia and gout include

Ⓐ hypothyroidism

Ⓑ severe exfoliative psoriasis

Ⓒ renal failure

Ⓓ polycythaemia rubra vera

Ⓔ therapy with loop diuretics

50.

The clinical features of gout include

Ⓐ precipitation of an acute attack by allopurinol

Ⓑ cellulitis, tenosynovitis and bursitis

Ⓒ the abrupt onset of severe joint pain and tenderness

Ⓓ serum urate levels fall during an acute attack

Ⓔ loin pain and haematuria

51.

In the treatment of gout

Ⓐ indomethacin increases urinary urate excretion

Ⓑ salicylates control symptoms and accelerate resolution of the acute attack

Ⓒ allopurinol inhibits xanthine oxidase and hence urate production

Ⓓ tophi should resolve with control of hyperuricaemia

Ⓔ allopurinol or probenecid should be given within 24 hours of onset of the acute attack

52.

In pyrophosphate arthropathy

Ⓐ calcium pyrophosphate dihydrate crystals are deposited in the synovial cells

Ⓑ haemochromatosis is a recognised predisposing factor

Ⓒ the clinical appearances are similar to acute gout

Ⓓ the findings on synovial aspiration are indistinguishable from acute gout

Ⓔ intra-articular corticosteroid injections are contraindicated

53.

Osteoarthritis is

Ⓐ evident radiologically in at least 80% of patients > 65 years old

Ⓑ more likely to be generalised and severe in males

Ⓒ characterised by degeneration of cartilage and synovial inflammation

Ⓓ associated with increased collagen synthesis in the affected cartilage

Ⓔ best managed with anti-inflammatory doses of NSAIDs

54.

The clinical features of primary (nodal) osteoarthrosis include

Ⓐ joint pain aggravated by rest and relieved by activity

Ⓑ proximal interphalangeal and MCP joint involvement

Ⓒ involvement of the hip, knee and spinal apophyseal joints

Ⓓ a strong family history of Heberden's nodes

Ⓔ microfractures of subchondral bone

55.

The features of polyarteritis nodosa include

Ⓐ a preponderance in males

Ⓑ an association with circulating immune complexes containing Hepatitis B virus

Ⓒ involvement of small arteries and arterioles

Ⓓ multiple peripheral nerve palsies

Ⓔ severe hypertension

56.
Typical features of Paget's disease of bone include
Ⓐ onset before the age of 40 years
Ⓑ increased serum alkaline phosphatase and urinary hydroxyproline
Ⓒ presentation with headache in elderly patients
Ⓓ delayed healing of fractures
Ⓔ risk of development of osteogenic sarcoma

57.
In a male patient with widespread metastatic bone disease
Ⓐ osteolytic deposits are likely to be due to prostatic carcinoma
Ⓑ the plasma calcium is typically elevated
Ⓒ bone pain is invariably present
Ⓓ the alkaline phosphatase is only elevated if pathological fracture occurs
Ⓔ cyproterone acetate retards progress of the disease

58.
Typical features of primary osteosarcomas include
Ⓐ onset before the age of 20 years
Ⓑ predeliction for the vertebrae
Ⓒ absence of haematogenous metastases
Ⓓ 'sun-ray' appearance on X-ray due to new bone formation
Ⓔ 5 year survival rates > 75% with treatment

59.
Generalised osteoporosis is
Ⓐ usually associated with normal serum calcium, phosphate and alkaline phosphatase
Ⓑ more likely to occur if menopause is early
Ⓒ commonly asymptomatic
Ⓓ a typical complication of untreated Addison's disease
Ⓔ radiologically detectable when 10% of bone mineral content is lost

60.
Typical features of Ewing's sarcoma include
Ⓐ onset between the ages 5 and 15 years
Ⓑ origin in the bone marrow endothelium
Ⓒ presentation with features suggesting osteomyelitis
Ⓓ characteristic 'onion skin' appearance on X-ray
Ⓔ 5 year survival rates < 10% despite amputation

61.
Typical features of osteomyelitis include
Ⓐ onset in the sixth and seventh decade
Ⓑ fever, joint effusion and bone pain
Ⓒ X-ray changes preceding abnormalities on the isotope bone scan
Ⓓ association of salmonella infection in haemophilic patients
Ⓔ sparing of the disc space in vertebral osteomyelitis

62.
Typical laboratory findings in systemic necrotising vasculitis include
Ⓐ peripheral blood lymphocytosis
Ⓑ high titres of anti-DNA antibodies
Ⓒ high titres of anti-neutrophil cytoplasmic antibodies
Ⓓ anaemia with an elevated MCV
Ⓔ haematuria on dipstix testing

63.
The typical features of childhood Still's disease include
Ⓐ systemic onset with fever and an evanescent rash
Ⓑ lymphadenopathy and hepatosplenomegaly
Ⓒ high serum titres of rheumatoid factor
Ⓓ pleurisy and pericarditis
Ⓔ progressive arthritis especially of the cervical spine

64.
The typical features of acute rheumatic fever include
Ⓐ fever, abdominal pain, vomiting and pancarditis
Ⓑ additive rather than flitting arthralgia
Ⓒ onset before 4 years of age
Ⓓ onset within 1 week of streptococcal infection
Ⓔ erythema nodosum rather than erythema marginatum

65.
The following disorders produce joint symptoms and signs
Ⓐ Lyme disease
Ⓑ acromegaly
Ⓒ hypothyroidism
Ⓓ chronic sarcoidosis
Ⓔ amyloidosis

66.
The typical features of chondrosarcoma include
Ⓐ onset before the age of 10 years
Ⓑ occurrence in the long bones
Ⓒ presentation with pain and swelling
Ⓓ 'onion skin' appearance radiographically
Ⓔ 5 year survival > 50% with amputation

67.
Disorders associated with avascular necrosis of bone include
Ⓐ radiotherapy damage
Ⓑ sickle-cell disease
Ⓒ corticosteroid therapy
Ⓓ alcoholism
Ⓔ diabetes mellitus

68.
The typical features of relapsing polychondritis include
Ⓐ onset before the age of 30 years
Ⓑ association with autoimmune disorders
Ⓒ presentation with cough and breathlessness
Ⓓ rapid progression to renal failure
Ⓔ association with HLA B6

16 DISEASES OF THE SKIN

ANSWERS BEING ON P. 231

1.
The following statements about the skin are true

ⓐ The surface area of an adult is approximately 2 m²

ⓑ The weight of an adult's skin is approximately 4 kg

ⓒ Keratinocytes comprise one-third of epidermal cell numbers

ⓓ Langerhans cells synthesise vitamin D in the epidermis

ⓔ Sweat is produced by eccrine glands

2.
In the terminology of skin lesions

ⓐ papules are solid skin elevations > 20 mm in diameter

ⓑ nodules are solid skin masses > 5 mm in diameter

ⓒ vesicles are fluid-containing skin elevations > 5 mm in diameter

ⓓ petechiae are pinhead-sized macules of blood within the skin

ⓔ macules are small raised areas of skin of altered colour

3.
Properties of vehicles for topical skin treatments include

ⓐ creams composed of grease to moisturise dry skin

ⓑ ointments composed of water, grease and an emulsifier

ⓒ pastes composed of grease and an alcohol

ⓓ shake lotions composed of water and powder to aid skin cooling

ⓔ lotions composed of water or alcohol for use in hairy areas

4.
Effects of topical corticosteroid therapy include

ⓐ dermal atrophy most marked in the face and body folds

ⓑ striae in the body folds particularly

ⓒ absence of hypothalamo-pituitary-adrenal axis suppression

ⓓ decreased hair growth particularly of the beard

ⓔ spread of skin infection

5.
Characteristic features of eczema include

ⓐ epidermal oedema and intra-epidermal vesicles

ⓑ delayed hypersensitivity reaction in seborrhoeic eczema

ⓒ increased serum IgA concentration in discoid (nummular) eczema

ⓓ eyelid and scrotal oedema in allergic contact eczema

ⓔ persistence of childhood atopic eczema into adulthood

6.
Typical sensitising agents in contact eczema include

ⓐ aluminium

ⓑ colophony

ⓒ lanolin

ⓓ rubber

ⓔ ethanol

7.
Typical features of psoriasis include
ⓐ well-defined erythematous plaques with adherent silvery scales
ⓑ epidermal thickening and nucleated horny layer cells (parakeratosis)
ⓒ induction of plaques by local trauma
ⓓ an association with HLA CW6
ⓔ exacerbation by propranolol and lithium carbonate therapy

8.
The characteristic clinical features of psoriasis include
ⓐ sparing of the skin over the head, face and neck
ⓑ guttate psoriasis predominantly affecting the elderly
ⓒ nail changes with pitting and onycholysis
ⓓ oligoarthritis particularly associated with nail changes occurring in 5%
ⓔ red non-scaly skin areas in the natal cleft and submammary folds

9.
Appropriate therapeutic schedules in psoriasis include
ⓐ dithranol cream for facial, genital and flexural plaques
ⓑ steroid-antifungal combinations for flexural plaques
ⓒ tar-steroid combinations during withdrawal of steroid creams
ⓓ short wave UVA exposure from sunbeds
ⓔ combined psoralen-UVA photochemotherapy and isotretinoin

10.
The typical features of acne vulgaris include
ⓐ involvement of pilosebaceous glands and their ducts
ⓑ distribution over the face and upper torso
ⓒ infection with the skin commensal *Propronobacterium acnes*
ⓓ increased sebum production containing excess free fatty acids
ⓔ open and closed comedones, inflammatory papules, nodules and cysts

11.
Recognised agents inducing acneiform eruptions include
ⓐ chlorinated hydrocarbons
ⓑ corticosteroid therapy
ⓒ androgenic or oestrogenic steroid therapy
ⓓ lithium carbonate therapy
ⓔ anticonvulsants

12.
Therapies of proven value in acne vulgaris include
ⓐ oral tetracycline or erythromycin drug therapy
ⓑ topical preparations of benzoyl peroxide and retinoic acid
ⓒ oral contraceptive pill
ⓓ cyproterone acetate
ⓔ oral isotretinoin

13.
The characteristic features of rosacea include
ⓐ predominantly affects adolescents
ⓑ increased secretion of sebum with comedones
ⓒ facial erythema, telangiectasia, pustules and papules
ⓓ rhinophyma, conjunctivitis and keratitis
ⓔ non-responsive to oral tetracycline therapy

14.
The typical features of lichen planus include
ⓐ involvement of the skin, nails, hair and mucous membranes
ⓑ dense subepidermal lymphocytic infiltration on histology
ⓒ itchy, purplish, polygonal, shiny skin papules
ⓓ hypopigmentation at sites of previous lesions
ⓔ complete resolution following topical steroid therapy

15.
Characteristic features in Henoch–Schönlein vasculitis include
Ⓐ palpable purpuric rash particularly over the buttocks
Ⓑ lymphocytic infiltration of capillary endothelium
Ⓒ leucocytoclastic vasculitis and endothelial IgA deposition
Ⓓ polyarthritis and mononeuritis multiplex
Ⓔ corticosteroid therapy is mandatory

16.
Systemic causes of pruritus include
Ⓐ oral contraceptives and pregnancy
Ⓑ hypothyroidism and hyperthyroidism
Ⓒ lymphoproliferative and myeloproliferative diseases
Ⓓ iron deficiency anaemia
Ⓔ opiate and antidepressant drug therapy

17.
Skin diseases associated with marked pruritus include
Ⓐ cutaneous vasculitis
Ⓑ lichen planus
Ⓒ atopic eczema
Ⓓ seborrhoeic keratosis
Ⓔ dermatitis herpetiformis

18.
Skin diseases associated with blistering eruptions include
Ⓐ erythema multiforme
Ⓑ dermatitis herpetiformis
Ⓒ pemphigoid
Ⓓ pemphigus vulgaris
Ⓔ guttate psoriasis

19.
Skin diseases associated with HIV infection include
Ⓐ seborrhoeic dermatitis
Ⓑ oral candidiasis
Ⓒ hairy leukoplakia
Ⓓ drug-induced eruptions
Ⓔ Kaposi's sarcoma

20.
Skin diseases associated with photosensitivity include
Ⓐ variegate and hepatic porphyrias
Ⓑ atopic eczema
Ⓒ drug reactions to phenothiazine, thiazide and tetracycline
Ⓓ pyoderma gangrenosum
Ⓔ pityriasis rosea

21.
The typical features of erythema multiforme include
Ⓐ target-like skin lesions of the hands and feet
Ⓑ skin eruption lasting 6–12 weeks
Ⓒ absence of vesiculation or blistering
Ⓓ involvement of the eyes, genitalia and mouth
Ⓔ association with underlying systemic malignancy

22.
Recognised causes of erythema multiforme include
Ⓐ herpes simplex infection
Ⓑ mycoplasmal pneumonia
Ⓒ sulphonamide therapy
Ⓓ systemic lupus erythematosus
Ⓔ pregnancy

23.
The typical features of erythema nodosum include
Ⓐ red hot tender nodules over the shins
Ⓑ lesions disappear over 1–2 weeks
Ⓒ fever, malaise and polyarthralgia
Ⓓ oral and genital mucosal ulceration
Ⓔ predominantly affects the elderly

24.
Recognised causes of erythema nodosum include
Ⓐ sarcoidosis
Ⓑ beta-haemolytic streptococcal infection
Ⓒ inflammatory bowel disease
Ⓓ tuberculosis
Ⓔ contraceptive drug therapy

25.
Cutaneous manifestations of systemic malignancy include
Ⓐ generalised pruritus
Ⓑ acanthosis nigricans
Ⓒ late-onset dermatomyositis
Ⓓ generalised hyperpigmentation
Ⓔ seborrhoeic eczema

26.
Typical features of melanocytic naevi include
Ⓐ usually present from birth
Ⓑ development after the age of 40 years
Ⓒ junctional naevi are smooth, papillomatous, hairy nodules
Ⓓ intradermal naevi are circular, brown macules < 10 mm in diameter
Ⓔ 30% lifetime risk of malignant transformation

27.
Typical features of malignant melanoma include
Ⓐ changing appearance of a preceding melanocytic naevus
Ⓑ diameter of the lesion > 5 mm
Ⓒ irregular colour, border and elevation
Ⓓ personal or family history of melanoma
Ⓔ painless, expanding, subungual area of pigmentation

28.
The typical features of seborrhoeic keratosis include
Ⓐ appearance before the age of 30 years
Ⓑ discrete irregular lesions in light-exposed skin areas
Ⓒ yellow-brown, pedunculated lesions on the trunk or face
Ⓓ lesions exhibit greasy scaling and tiny keratin plugs
Ⓔ eventual transition to squamous cell carcinoma

29.
The typical features of basal cell carcinoma include
Ⓐ predominantly affects the elderly
Ⓑ metastatic spread to the lungs if untreated
Ⓒ occurrence in areas exposed to light or X-irradiation
Ⓓ papule with surface telangiectasia or ulcerated nodule
Ⓔ unresponsive to radiotherapy

30.
The typical features of squamous cell carcinoma include
Ⓐ occurrence in areas exposed to light or X-irradiation
Ⓑ arise from malignant transformation of the Langerhans cells
Ⓒ preceded by leukoplakia on the lips, mouth or genitalia
Ⓓ metastatic spread to the liver and lungs
Ⓔ unresponsive to radiotherapy

31.
In disorders of the nail
Ⓐ koilonychia suggests B_{12} or folate deficiency
Ⓑ onycholysis is associated with psoriasis
Ⓒ leuconychia is a feature of severe liver disease
Ⓓ splinter haemorrhages usually indicate the presence of infective endocarditis
Ⓔ Beau's lines disappear faster from fingernails than toenails

17 PSYCHIATRY
ANSWERS BEGIN ON P. 234

1.
Prevalence rates of psychiatric illness in the UK include
Ⓐ 5% of the general adult population
Ⓑ 50% of patients attending their general practitioner
Ⓒ substance abuse in 15%
Ⓓ 30% of patients admitted to general medical wards
Ⓔ schizophrenia in 5% of the population

2.
Aetiological factors in psychiatric illness include
Ⓐ family history of psychiatric illness
Ⓑ parental loss or disharmony in childhood
Ⓒ stressful life events and difficulties
Ⓓ chronic physical ill-health
Ⓔ social isolation

3.
Important factors in the assessment of mental state include
Ⓐ general appearance, behaviour and speech
Ⓑ mood state and thought content
Ⓒ abnormal beliefs and delusions
Ⓓ abnormal perceptions
Ⓔ intellect and cognitive function

4.
Intellectual impairment should be suspected in the presence of
Ⓐ disordered thought content
Ⓑ auditory hallucination
Ⓒ inappropriate optimism and elation
Ⓓ disorientation in time and place
Ⓔ impaired serial 7s test and arithmetic ability

5.
The following psychiatric definitions are true
Ⓐ delusions — unreasonably persistent, firmly held false beliefs
Ⓑ illusions — abnormal perceptions of normal external stimuli
Ⓒ hallucinations — abnormal perceptions without external stimuli
Ⓓ depersonalisation — perception of altered reality
Ⓔ phobia — abnormal fear leading to avoidance behaviour

6.
Cardinal elements in behavioural therapy include
Ⓐ self-awareness of maladaptive patterns of learned behaviour
Ⓑ systematic desensitisation and flooding
Ⓒ operant conditioning
Ⓓ exploration of repressed unpleasant experiences
Ⓔ modification of negative patterns of thinking

7.
Cardinal elements in cognitive therapy include
Ⓐ restructuring psychological conflicts and behaviour
Ⓑ identification of negative patterns of automatic thoughts
Ⓒ awareness of connections between thoughts, mood and behaviour
Ⓓ reorientation of negative views of the past, present and future
Ⓔ personality assessment and transactional analysis

8.
Typical features of acute confusional states include

Ⓐ impaired consciousness particularly in the evening
Ⓑ impaired attention, concentration and speed of thought
Ⓒ impaired memory, registration, recall and retention
Ⓓ illusions, hallucinations and delusions
Ⓔ anxiety, irritability and depression

9.
Typical features of dementia include

Ⓐ loss of intellectual function without impaired consciousness
Ⓑ impairment of judgment, abstract thought and problem-solving
Ⓒ impairment of long-term memory without loss of short-term memory
Ⓓ personality change with disinhibition and loss of social awareness
Ⓔ psychomotor retardation, anxiety and depression

10.
Typical features of schizophrenia include

Ⓐ thought insertion and thought broadcasting
Ⓑ delusions and passivity feelings
Ⓒ visual hallucinations
Ⓓ thought disorder and thought block
Ⓔ poverty of speech, social withdrawal and flat affect

11.
Features indicating a good prognosis in schizophrenia include

Ⓐ abrupt onset of symptoms
Ⓑ absence of affective symptoms
Ⓒ schizoid personality
Ⓓ catatonic symptoms
Ⓔ family history of schizophrenia

12.
The typical features of depression include

Ⓐ depressed mood for most of the day
Ⓑ insomnia or hypersomnia
Ⓒ loss of pleasure, self-esteem and hope
Ⓓ loss of energy, libido and interest
Ⓔ psychomotor retardation and suicidal thoughts

13.
The typical features of mania include

Ⓐ high self-confidence and self-esteem
Ⓑ reduction in sleep and food intake
Ⓒ flight of ideas
Ⓓ grandiose delusions
Ⓔ impaired attention and concentration

14.
Clinical features of generalised anxiety disorders include

Ⓐ feelings of worthlessness and excessive guilt
Ⓑ depersonalisation and derealisation
Ⓒ feelings of apprehension and impending disaster
Ⓓ breathlessness, dizziness, sweating and palpitation
Ⓔ claustrophobia and agoraphobia

15.
Diseases mimicking anxiety disorders include

Ⓐ alcohol withdrawal
Ⓑ hyperthyroidism
Ⓒ hypoglycaemia
Ⓓ temporal lobe epilepsy
Ⓔ phaeochromocytoma

16.
Typical features of panic disorder include

Ⓐ loss of libido, anhedonism and irritability
Ⓑ recurrent unpredictable attacks of intense anxiety
Ⓒ chest pain, palpitation and breathlessness
Ⓓ delusions and auditory hallucinations
Ⓔ association with primary affective disorders

17.
Typical features of phobic disorder include

Ⓐ predominance in young males
Ⓑ history of specific childhood trauma
Ⓒ avoidance of public transport and shopping areas
Ⓓ sudden intense attacks of breathlessness and faintness
Ⓔ good response to benzodiazepine therapy

18.
Typical features of obsessive compulsive disorder include
Ⓐ consciously-resisted unwanted thoughts and impulses
Ⓑ conscientiousness with perfectionistic personality
Ⓒ short-lived disability without relapses
Ⓓ association with schizophrenia and depression
Ⓔ response to clomipramine and behaviour therapy

19.
Typical features of dissociative disorder include
Ⓐ conscious attempt to manipulate and/or malinger
Ⓑ previous history of multiple recurrent somatic complaints
Ⓒ coexistent disease of the nervous system
Ⓓ gait disturbance or sensory or motor disorder in the limbs
Ⓔ pseudo-seizures, blindness or aphonia

20.
Typical features of anorexia nervosa include
Ⓐ only adolescent girls are affected
Ⓑ amenorrhoea or loss of libido > 3 months
Ⓒ weight loss > 25% or weight 25% below normal
Ⓓ normal perception of body weight and image
Ⓔ retardation of physical sexual development

21.
Typical features of bulimia nervosa include
Ⓐ age of onset at puberty
Ⓑ dramatic weight loss
Ⓒ lack of control of binge-eating
Ⓓ self-induced vomiting and purgation
Ⓔ hospital admission required to control the disorder

22.
Criteria for the diagnosis of alcohol dependence include
Ⓐ increasing tolerance of the effects of alcohol
Ⓑ repeated withdrawal symptoms
Ⓒ priority of drinking over other activities
Ⓓ expansion of the drinking repertoire
Ⓔ relief of withdrawal symptoms by further drinking

23.
Alcohol abuse should be suspected in patients presenting with
Ⓐ painless diarrhoea and/or vomiting
Ⓑ atrial fibrillation and/or hypertension
Ⓒ weight gain and/or gout
Ⓓ peripheral neuropathy and/or epilepsy
Ⓔ infertility and/or insomnia

24.
The typical features of alcohol withdrawal include
Ⓐ early-morning waking with anxiety and tremor
Ⓑ visual or auditory hallucinations
Ⓒ amnesia and epileptic seizures
Ⓓ depression and morbid jealousy
Ⓔ ataxia, nystagmus and ophthalmoplegia

25.
Recognised features of benzodiazepine withdrawal include
Ⓐ heightened sensory perception
Ⓑ hallucinations and delusions
Ⓒ epilepsy and ataxia
Ⓓ manic-depressive-like disorder
Ⓔ poverty of ideas and speech

26.
Risk factors for suicide following attempted suicide include
Ⓐ female sex and age < 45 years
Ⓑ self-poisoning rather than more violent methods of self-harm
Ⓒ absence of a suicide note or previous suicide attempts
Ⓓ chronic physical or psychiatric illness
Ⓔ living alone and/or recently separated from partner

27.
Indications for ECT in depressive illness include
Ⓐ severe depression with paranoid delusions
Ⓑ depressive stupor producing nutritional difficulties
Ⓒ major risk of suicide requiring rapid therapeutic response
Ⓓ unresponsive to or intolerant of antidepressant drug therapy
Ⓔ depression associated with panic disorder

28.
In the management of depression
Ⓐ cognitive therapy helps modify negative patterns of thinking in a positive way
Ⓑ previous life events are more often viewed as positive rather than negative
Ⓒ the patient should be discouraged from devaluation of self
Ⓓ monitoring negative automatic thoughts is central to cognitive therapy
Ⓔ the combination of drug therapy and cognitive therapy is synergistic

29.
The following statements about antipsychotic drugs are true
Ⓐ phenothiazines block central nervous dopamine D_2 receptors
Ⓑ akathisia, dystonia and tardive dyskinesia are attributable to cholinergic side-effects
Ⓒ long-term ocular complications include corneal and lenticular opacities
Ⓓ galactorrhoea suggests an alternative explanation rather than an adverse drug effect
Ⓔ clozapine and risperidone have a greater effect on $5-HT_2$ receptors than cholinergic receptors

30.
The following statements about antidepressant drugs are true
Ⓐ tricyclic drugs inhibit the reuptake of noradrenaline and 5-hydroxytryptamine at synaptic clefts
Ⓑ the onset of antidepressant effects is usually clinically apparent within 2 weeks
Ⓒ selective serotonin reuptake inhibitors are more effective than tricyclic drugs
Ⓓ fluoxetine is an alpha-$_2$-adrenoceptor antagonist without any effect on synaptic amine reuptake
Ⓔ monoamine oxidase inhibitors are less effective than tricyclic drugs for severe depression

31.
Psychiatric illness rather than an organic brain disorder is suggested by
Ⓐ onset for the first time at the age of 55
Ⓑ a family history of major psychiatric illness
Ⓒ no previous history of psychiatric illness
Ⓓ recent occurrence of a major adverse life event
Ⓔ episodes of dysphasia and impaired short-term memory

32.
Authorisation for hospital detention of a mentally ill patient under the provisions of the Mental Health Act, 1983 (England and Wales) requires the signature of
Ⓐ one doctor and a relative/social worker under section 4, lasting for 72 hours
Ⓑ two doctors and a relative/social worker under section 2, lasting for 28 days
Ⓒ only the doctor in charge under section 5(2), lasting for 72 hours
Ⓓ one registered staff nurse under section 5(4), lasting 6 hours
Ⓔ one policeman under section 2, lasting 28 days

18 DISEASES OF THE NERVOUS SYSTEM

ANSWERS BEGIN ON P. 237

1.
Dysphonia would be an expected finding in a patient with
Ⓐ myasthenia gravis
Ⓑ supranuclear bulbar palsy
Ⓒ Parkinson's disease
Ⓓ cerebellar disease
Ⓔ lesions of Broca's area

2.
Dysarthria would be an expected finding in a patient with
Ⓐ bilateral recurrent laryngeal nerve palsies
Ⓑ supranuclear bulbar palsy
Ⓒ cerebellar disease
Ⓓ myasthenia gravis
Ⓔ lesion of Wernicke's area

3.
Upper motor neurone involvement is characterised by
Ⓐ extensor plantar responses
Ⓑ absent abdominal reflexes
Ⓒ muscle fasciculation
Ⓓ increased muscle tone and tendon reflexes
Ⓔ plantar flexion of the great toe in response to rapid dorsiflexion of the toes

4.
Lower motor neurone involvement is characterised by
Ⓐ flaccid muscle tone
Ⓑ the rapid onset of muscle wasting
Ⓒ absent or decreased tendon reflexes
Ⓓ clonus
Ⓔ weakness affecting adductors more than abductors of shoulder

5.
Recognised features of extrapyramidal tract disease include
Ⓐ intention tremor
Ⓑ 'clasp-knife' rigidity
Ⓒ choreo-athetosis
Ⓓ delayed relaxation of the tendon reflexes
Ⓔ delayed initiation of movements

6.
The lateral spinothalamic tract of the spinal cord
Ⓐ transmits pain sensation from the same side of the body
Ⓑ crosses to the opposite side in the medial lemniscus
Ⓒ transmits contralateral light touch sensation
Ⓓ stratifies fibres from the lowest spinal segments innermost
Ⓔ crosses from the thalamus to the contralateral parietal lobe

7.
Loss of tendon reflexes is characteristic of
Ⓐ proximal myopathy
Ⓑ peripheral neuropathy
Ⓒ syringomyelia
Ⓓ myasthenia gravis
Ⓔ tabes dorsalis

8.
The segmental innervation of the following tendon reflexes is
Ⓐ biceps jerk — C5–C6
Ⓑ triceps jerk — C6–C7
Ⓒ supinator jerk — C5–C6
Ⓓ knee jerk — L3–L4
Ⓔ ankle jerk — L5–S1

9.
The following statements about bladder innervation are true
Ⓐ sacral cord lesions usually produce urinary retention
Ⓑ thoracic cord lesions produce urinary urge incontinence
Ⓒ pelvic nerve parasympathetic stimulation causes bladder emptying
Ⓓ pudendal nerve lesions produce automatic bladder emptying
Ⓔ the L1–L2 segment sympathetic outflow mediates bladder relaxation

10.
Typical findings in cerebellar disease include
Ⓐ dysmetria
Ⓑ dysarthria
Ⓒ intention tremor
Ⓓ increased muscle tone
Ⓔ pendular nystagmus

11.
Right homonymous hemianopia usually results from damage to
Ⓐ the left optic tract
Ⓑ the left optic radiation
Ⓒ the optic chiasma
Ⓓ the right lateral geniculate body
Ⓔ the left optic nerve

12.
Features suggesting a third cranial nerve palsy include
Ⓐ paralysis of abduction
Ⓑ absence of facial sweating
Ⓒ complete ptosis
Ⓓ pupillary dilatation
Ⓔ absence of the accommodation reflex

13.
Paralysis of the fourth cranial nerve produces
Ⓐ weakness of the inferior oblique muscle
Ⓑ pupillary dilatation
Ⓒ impaired downward gaze in adduction
Ⓓ elevation and abduction of the eye
Ⓔ nystagmus more marked in the abducted eye

14.
Paralysis of the sixth cranial nerve
Ⓐ produces impaired adduction of the eye
Ⓑ produces enophthalmos
Ⓒ is a characteristic feature of Wernicke's encephalopathy
Ⓓ results from disease of the upper pons
Ⓔ is a recognised feature of posterior fossa tumour

15.
Drooping of the upper eyelid results from a lesion of the
Ⓐ levator palpebrae superioris
Ⓑ third cranial nerve
Ⓒ cervical sympathetic outflow
Ⓓ seventh cranial nerve
Ⓔ parabducens nucleus

16.
Absence of pupillary constriction in either eye on shining a light into the right pupil suggests
Ⓐ bilateral Argyll–Robertson pupils
Ⓑ bilateral Holmes–Adie pupils
Ⓒ right optic nerve lesion
Ⓓ right oculomotor nerve lesion
Ⓔ bilateral Horner's syndrome

17.
Recognised causes of impaired facial sensation include
Ⓐ cavernous sinus disease
Ⓑ trigeminal neuralgia
Ⓒ acoustic neuroma
Ⓓ lesion of the posterior limb of the internal capsule
Ⓔ lesion of the upper cervical cord segments

18.
Features of an intracranial lower motor neurone lesion of the facial nerve include
Ⓐ inability to wrinkle the forehead
Ⓑ increased lacrimation on the affected side
Ⓒ upward deviation of the eye on attempted eyelid closure
Ⓓ deafness due to loss of the nerve to the stapedius muscle
Ⓔ loss of taste over the anterior two-thirds of the tongue

19.
Characteristic features of pseudo-bulbar palsy include
Ⓐ dysarthria
Ⓑ dysphagia
Ⓒ emotional lability
Ⓓ wasting and fasciculation of the tongue
Ⓔ absence of the jaw jerk

20.
The following statements about the Glasgow coma scale are true
Ⓐ the best response to an arousal stimulus should be measured
Ⓑ appropriate motor responses to verbal commands = score 6
Ⓒ spontaneous eye opening = score 4
Ⓓ verbal responses with normal speech and orientation = score 5
Ⓔ the minimum total score = 3

21.
The diagnosis of brain death is supported by
Ⓐ pin-point pupils
Ⓑ absent corneal reflexes
Ⓒ absent vestibulo-ocular responses to caloric testing
Ⓓ absence of spontaneous respiration
Ⓔ preservation of the cough and gag reflexes

22.
Typical features of pre-frontal lobe lesions include
Ⓐ positive grasp reflex
Ⓑ astereognosis
Ⓒ sensory dysphasia
Ⓓ olfactory hallucinations
Ⓔ social disinhibition

23.
Typical features of posterior parietal lobe lesions include
Ⓐ lower homonymous quadrantanopia
Ⓑ constructional apraxia
Ⓒ perceptual rivalry
Ⓓ motor dysphasia
Ⓔ agnosia and acalculia

24.
Typical causes of papilloedema include
Ⓐ migraine
Ⓑ central retinal vein thrombosis
Ⓒ cranial arteritis
Ⓓ chronic ventilatory failure
Ⓔ chronic glaucoma

25.
Jerking nystagmus that changes in direction with the direction of gaze is
Ⓐ compatible with cerebellar hemisphere disease
Ⓑ indicative of a brain stem disorder
Ⓒ compatible with a vestibular nerve lesion
Ⓓ typically accompanied by vertigo and tinnitus
Ⓔ likely to continue following closure of the eyes

26.
The characteristic features of trigeminal neuralgia include
Ⓐ pain lasting several hours at a time
Ⓑ pain precipitated by touching the face and/or chewing
Ⓒ absence of the corneal reflex
Ⓓ predominance in young females
Ⓔ response to anticonvulsants

27.
The typical features of Ménière's disease include
Ⓐ sudden onset of vertigo, nausea and vomiting
Ⓑ progressive sensorineural deafness and tinnitus
Ⓒ rotatory jerking nystagmus and ataxic gait
Ⓓ positional nystagmus usually persists between attacks
Ⓔ restoration of hearing following effective treatment

28.
Typical causes of vertigo include
Ⓐ petit mal epilepsy
Ⓑ acoustic neuroma
Ⓒ vestibular neuronitis
Ⓓ gentamicin drug therapy
Ⓔ otitis media

29.
Wasting and fasciculation of the tongue is a feature of
Ⓐ pseudo-bulbar palsy
Ⓑ myasthenia gravis
Ⓒ motor neurone disease
Ⓓ nasopharyngeal carcinoma
Ⓔ Paget's disease of the skull

30.
Typical features of generalised epilepsy include
Ⓐ loss of consciousness accompanied by symmetrical EEG discharge
Ⓑ invariable presence of an aura
Ⓒ lesion demonstrable on CT brain scanning
Ⓓ induction by photic stimulation
Ⓔ induction by hyperventilation

31.
The clinical features of tonic-clonic seizures include
Ⓐ prodromal phase lasting hours or days
Ⓑ onset with an audible cry due to the aura
Ⓒ sustained spasm of all muscles lasting 30 seconds
Ⓓ interrupted jerking movements lasting 1–5 minutes
Ⓔ flaccid post-ictal state with bilateral extensor plantar responses

32.
The typical features of absence (petit mal) seizures include
Ⓐ loss of consciousness lasting up to 10 seconds
Ⓑ onset at the age 25–30 years
Ⓒ synchronous 3 per second spike and wave activity on EEG
Ⓓ later development of tonic-clonic seizures in 50%
Ⓔ sleepiness lasting several hours post-ictally

33.
Characteristic features of temporal lobe epilepsy include
Ⓐ complex partial seizure with loss of awareness
Ⓑ hallucinations of smell, taste, hearing or vision
Ⓒ déjà vu phenomena associated with intense emotion
Ⓓ progression to tonic-clonic seizure
Ⓔ hemiparesis lasting several hours post-ictally

34.
The management of grand mal epilepsy should include
Ⓐ hospital admission following episodes
Ⓑ return to driving after 1 year free of all seizures
Ⓒ irrevocable loss of an HGV driving licence
Ⓓ combined primidone and phenobarbitone therapy
Ⓔ phenytoin, carbamazepine or sodium valproate therapy

35.
Features suggesting epilepsy as the cause of blackouts include
Ⓐ impairment of vision heralding the attack
Ⓑ urinary incontinence during the attack
Ⓒ eye witness account of jerking movements during the attack
Ⓓ attacks aborted by lying supine
Ⓔ attacks confined to the sleeping hours

36.
Clinical features of raised intracranial pressure include
Ⓐ tachycardia and hypotension
Ⓑ dizziness and lightheadedness
Ⓒ headache aggravated by bending and straining
Ⓓ behavioral and personality changes
Ⓔ sixth or third cranial nerve palsies

37.
The following statements about primary brain tumours are true
Ⓐ meningiomas are commonest in the middle aged
Ⓑ gliomas are commonest in childhood
Ⓒ most childhood brain tumours arise within the posterior fossa
Ⓓ presentation with adult-onset partial seizures is typical
Ⓔ acoustic neuromas usually present in the sixth and seventh decades

38.
Papilloedema due to raised intracranial pressure typically produces
Ⓐ severe visual impairment at presentation
Ⓑ an arcuate scotoma progressing to 'tunnel' vision
Ⓒ pain and tenderness in the affected eye
Ⓓ retinal haemorrhages around the optic disc if rapid in onset
Ⓔ contralateral optic atrophy in tumours of the anterior cranial fossa

39.
Recognised features of migraine include
Ⓐ family history of migraine
Ⓑ onset before the age of puberty
Ⓒ headache is always unilateral and throbbing
Ⓓ premonitory symptoms include teichopsia
Ⓔ hemiparaesthesiae or hemiparesis at onset

40.
There is a major risk of cerebral embolism associated with
Ⓐ calf vein thrombosis
Ⓑ atrial fibrillation
Ⓒ atrial myxoma
Ⓓ infective endocarditis
Ⓔ acute rheumatic fever

41.
Typical causes of transient cerebral ischaemic attacks include
Ⓐ carotid artery stenosis
Ⓑ atrial fibrillation
Ⓒ hypotension
Ⓓ intracerebellar haemorrhage
Ⓔ intracerebral tumour

42.
Clinical features suggesting lacunar stroke include
Ⓐ homonymous hemianopia
Ⓑ motor or sensory dysphasia
Ⓒ facial weakness and arm monoparesis
Ⓓ isolated hemiparesis or hemianaesthesia
Ⓔ history of hypertension or diabetes mellitus

43.
Clinical features suggesting intracerebral haemorrhage include
Ⓐ abrupt onset of severe headache followed by coma
Ⓑ third cranial nerve palsy
Ⓒ retinal haemorrhages and/or papilloedema
Ⓓ onset of stroke on waking from sleep
Ⓔ tinnitus, deafness and vertigo

44.
Typical manifestations of brain stem infarction include
Ⓐ pin-point pupils
Ⓑ vertigo and diplopia
Ⓒ sensory dysphasia
Ⓓ severe headache
Ⓔ bi-directional jerking nystagmus

45.
Functional recovery following stroke is more likely to be poor if
Ⓐ coma is prolonged for > three days
Ⓑ the stroke was haemorrhagic rather than embolic in origin
Ⓒ associated hypertension is severe
Ⓓ there is a conjugate gaze palsy
Ⓔ hemiplegia is left-sided rather than right-sided

46.
Typical features of chronic subdural haematoma in adults include
ⓐ recall of a recent head injury
ⓑ urinary incontinence and ataxia
ⓒ epilepsy without previous headaches
ⓓ hemiplegia and hemianopia of sudden onset
ⓔ fluctuating confusional state

47.
Intracerebral abscess is a typical complication of
ⓐ infective endocarditis
ⓑ bronchiectasis
ⓒ frontal sinusitis
ⓓ otitis media
ⓔ head injury

48.
The typical features of chronic intracerebral abscess include
ⓐ high fever, weight loss and peripheral blood leucocytosis
ⓑ epilepsy persisting after successful treatment of the abscess
ⓒ bradycardia and papilloedema
ⓓ headache, vomiting and confusion
ⓔ positive blood and CSF cultures

49.
The typical features of adult tuberculous meningitis include
ⓐ headache and vomiting
ⓑ fever associated with neck stiffness
ⓒ cranial nerve palsies associated with coma
ⓓ miliary tuberculosis is often present
ⓔ CSF cell count > 400 neutrophil leucocytes/ml

50.
In the treatment of adult pyogenic meningitis
ⓐ penicillin therapy should be given intrathecally initially
ⓑ chloramphenicol therapy should be considered for penicillin-allergic patients
ⓒ antibiotic therapy should not be given before CSF analysis has been undertaken
ⓓ parenteral fluid therapy should be instituted immediately
ⓔ the onset of a purpuric rash suggests drug allergy is likely

51.
Recognised causes of viral meningitis include
ⓐ herpes simplex
ⓑ poliomyelitis
ⓒ arenavirus
ⓓ echo and coxsackie viruses
ⓔ measles and mumps viruses

52.
Typical features of adult viral encephalitis include
ⓐ acute onset of headache and fever
ⓑ partial epilepsy and coma rapidly ensue
ⓒ decreased CSF glucose concentration
ⓓ temporal lobe EEG abnormalities are pathognomonic of herpes simplex infection
ⓔ meningism

53.
Typical features of herpes zoster include
ⓐ the rash heals without scarring
ⓑ permanent dermatomal sensory impairment
ⓒ infection is confined to the posterior root ganglia
ⓓ pain is the first symptom before a rash appears
ⓔ treatment with acyclovir prevents post-herpetic neuralgia

54.

Syphilis should be considered in the differential diagnosis of

Ⓐ late-onset epilepsy

Ⓑ progressive dementia

Ⓒ stroke in young patients

Ⓓ truncal or limb ataxia

Ⓔ septic meningitis

55.

Typical features of tabes dorsalis include

Ⓐ paroxysmal abdominal and girdle pains

Ⓑ loss of pain sensation of the nose, perineum and feet

Ⓒ bilateral ptosis and Argyll–Robertson pupils

Ⓓ urinary incontinence with absent ankle and plantar reflexes

Ⓔ high stepping, stamping gait with muscle hypotonia

56.

Epidemiological characteristics of multiple sclerosis include

Ⓐ predominant occurrence in males

Ⓑ association with HLA A3, B7 and Dw2/DRw2

Ⓒ a prevalence of 1 in 2000 of the UK population

Ⓓ more prevalent in the tropics than in temperate climates

Ⓔ lesions within the CNS are confined to the grey matter

57.

The typical features of multiple sclerosis include

Ⓐ invariable progression with relapses and remission

Ⓑ onset often occurs before the age of puberty

Ⓒ choreoathetosis and parkinsonism

Ⓓ urinary urgency, frequency and incontinence

Ⓔ epilepsy, dysphasia or hemiplegia

58.

Useful investigations in diagnosing multiple sclerosis include

Ⓐ visual and somatosensory evoked potentials

Ⓑ CT and magnetic resonance brain scanning

Ⓒ CSF analysis for oligoclonal IgG bands

Ⓓ electroencephalography

Ⓔ electromyography

59.

The typical features of parkinsonism include

Ⓐ hypokinesia

Ⓑ dementia

Ⓒ intention tremor

Ⓓ lead-pipe rigidity

Ⓔ impaired upward gaze

60.

Findings inconsistent with idiopathic Parkinson's disease include

Ⓐ unilateral onset of the disorder

Ⓑ emotional lability

Ⓒ oculogyric crises

Ⓓ extensor plantar responses

Ⓔ impaired pupillary accommodation reflexes

61.

Parkinsonism is a typical feature complicating

Ⓐ encephalitis lethargica

Ⓑ phenothiazine and butyrophenone therapy

Ⓒ Wilson's disease

Ⓓ repetitive head injury in boxers

Ⓔ methyl-phenyl-tetrahydropyridine exposure

62.
In the management of Parkinson's disease
Ⓐ anticholinergics are first choice agents for hypokinesis
Ⓑ L-dopa should be introduced as soon as diagnosis is made
Ⓒ sialorrhoea invariably indicates overuse of L-dopa
Ⓓ dopamine receptor agonists, unlike L-dopa, do not cause confusion
Ⓔ dyskinesia is a frequent dose-limiting side-effect of L-dopa

63.
The characteristic features of Huntington's chorea include
Ⓐ autosomal recessive inheritance
Ⓑ clinical onset before the age of puberty
Ⓒ progress of dementia arrested with tetrabenazine therapy
Ⓓ choreiform movements of the face and arms particularly
Ⓔ cardiomyopathic changes on echocardiography

64.
The clinical features of motor neurone disease include
Ⓐ insidious onset in elderly males
Ⓑ progressive distal muscular atrophy
Ⓒ progressive bulbar palsy
Ⓓ upper motor neurone signs in the lower limbs
Ⓔ lower motor neurone signs in the upper limbs

65.
The differential diagnosis in motor neurone disease includes
Ⓐ syringomyelia
Ⓑ diabetic amyotrophy
Ⓒ cervical myelopathy
Ⓓ paraneoplastic syndrome
Ⓔ meningovascular syphilis

66.
Typical features of cervical radiculopathy include
Ⓐ pathognomonic X-ray abnormalities of the cervical spine
Ⓑ radicular pain in the arm and shoulder
Ⓒ painful limitation of movements of the cervical spine
Ⓓ C8–T1 sensory and/or motor loss in the upper limb
Ⓔ neurosurgical intervention is often required

67.
The following statements about spinal cord compression are true
Ⓐ metastatic disease is a more common cause than primary tumour
Ⓑ the CSF protein concentration is likely to be normal
Ⓒ local spinal pain and tenderness usually precede motor weakness
Ⓓ urinary urgency is commonly the presenting feature
Ⓔ myelography is the best and most appropriate investigation

68.
Recognised causes of paraplegia include
Ⓐ intracranial parasagittal meningioma
Ⓑ vitamin B₁₂ deficiency
Ⓒ tuberculosis of the thoracic spine
Ⓓ anterior spinal artery thrombosis
Ⓔ spinal neurofibromas and gliomas

69.
The clinical features of hemisection of the spinal cord (Brown–Sequard syndrome) include
Ⓐ pain and temperature sensory loss in the contralateral leg
Ⓑ proprioceptive sensory loss in the ipsilateral leg
Ⓒ an extensor plantar response in the ipsilateral leg
Ⓓ hyperreflexia and weakness of the contralateral leg
Ⓔ hyperaesthetic dermatome on the opposite side of the lesion

70.

In the treatment of established paraplegia

Ⓐ prophylactic antibiotics are indicated to prevent urinary sepsis

Ⓑ pressure sores are not likely to occur unless sensation is lost

Ⓒ urinary retention usually requires long-term catheterisation

Ⓓ flexor spasms and contractures are usually unavoidable

Ⓔ constipation requires dietary treatment and regular enemas

71.

The typical features of syringomyelia include

Ⓐ slow insidious progression of the disease

Ⓑ dissociated sensory loss with normal touch and position sense

Ⓒ loss of one or more upper limb tendon reflexes is invariable

Ⓓ wasting of the small muscles of the hands

Ⓔ hyperreflexia of the lower limbs and extensor plantar responses

72.

Recognised features of neurofibromatosis include

Ⓐ autosomal dominant inheritance

Ⓑ cafe-au-lait spots

Ⓒ association with multiple endocrine neoplasias

Ⓓ intraspinal and intracranial neuromas and meningiomas

Ⓔ nerve deafness

73.

The neurological manifestations of severe vitamin B_{12} deficiency include

Ⓐ mononeuritis multiplex

Ⓑ optic atrophy

Ⓒ confusion and dementia

Ⓓ spastic paraparesis

Ⓔ sensory ataxia

74.

Typical features of the carpal tunnel syndrome include

Ⓐ remission during pregnancy

Ⓑ wasting of the dorsal interossei and lumbricals

Ⓒ pain producing night waking

Ⓓ association with acromegaly and hypothyroidism

Ⓔ complication of both rheumatoid arthritis and amyloidosis

75.

Recognised causes of mononeuritis multiplex include

Ⓐ rheumatoid arthritis

Ⓑ sarcoidosis

Ⓒ polyarteritis nodosa

Ⓓ diabetes mellitus

Ⓔ systemic lupus erythematosus

76.

Recognised causes of a generalised polyneuropathy include

Ⓐ bronchial carcinoma

Ⓑ rheumatoid arthritis and systemic lupus erythematosus

Ⓒ vitamin B_1, B_2, B_6 and B_{12} deficiencies

Ⓓ drugs especially co-trimoxazole, phenytoin and mianserin

Ⓔ diabetes mellitus and chronic renal failure

77.

Clinical features typical of the following polyneuropathies include

Ⓐ predominantly motor loss — lead poisoning

Ⓑ predominantly sensory loss — post-inflammatory polyneuropathy

Ⓒ painful sensory impairment — alcohol abuse

Ⓓ sparing of the cranial nerves — sarcoidosis

Ⓔ prominent postural hypotension — diabetes mellitus

78.

The following findings suggest a likely cause of a peripheral neuropathy

Ⓐ peripheral blood punctate basophilia

Ⓑ atrophic glossitis and weight loss

Ⓒ hyponatraemia with urinary osmolality of 300 mosm/kg

Ⓓ recent discovery of Kayser–Fleischer corneal rings

Ⓔ family history of neurofibromatosis

79.

The typical features of Guillain–Barré polyneuropathy include

Ⓐ onset within 4 weeks of an acute infective illness

Ⓑ severe back pain and peripheral paraesthesiae

Ⓒ ascending flaccid paralysis with areflexia

Ⓓ sparing of the respiratory and facial nerves

Ⓔ normal CSF protein concentration and cell count

80.

Non-metastatic neurological complications of malignancy include

Ⓐ meralgia paraesthetica

Ⓑ carpal tunnel syndrome

Ⓒ cerebellar ataxia

Ⓓ progressive dementia

Ⓔ myasthenic syndrome

81.

Characteristic features of myasthenia gravis include

Ⓐ motor dysphasia

Ⓑ circulating anti-acetylcholine receptor antibodies

Ⓒ onset of the disease between the ages 15 and 50 years

Ⓓ muscle wasting

Ⓔ intermittent diplopia and ptosis

82.

In the treatment of myasthenia gravis

Ⓐ pupillary miosis, salivation and sweating typify excessive therapy

Ⓑ pyridostigmine therapy is best given with propantheline once per day

Ⓒ thymectomy is mandatory as soon as the diagnosis is confirmed

Ⓓ corticosteroid therapy produces a transient myasthenic crisis

Ⓔ the prognosis is significantly worse if associated with thymoma

83.

The typical features of Duchenne muscular dystrophy include

Ⓐ presentation in the third year of life

Ⓑ calf muscle hypertrophy

Ⓒ difficulty in rising from the floor

Ⓓ normal serum creatine phosphokinase concentration

Ⓔ death is usually due to cardiac and respiratory failure

84.

Recognised causes of proximal myopathy include

Ⓐ hypothyroidism and hyperthyroidism

Ⓑ type I diabetes mellitus

Ⓒ Cushing's syndrome and acromegaly

Ⓓ Addisonian pernicious anaemia

Ⓔ chronic alcohol abuse

19 GERIATRIC MEDICINE

ANSWERS BEGIN ON P. 245

1.
The following are physiological changes associated with normal ageing
Ⓐ decreased calcium phosphate content per 100 g bone
Ⓑ high tone hearing loss
Ⓒ increased tissue sensitivity to insulin
Ⓓ increased standing postural sway
Ⓔ decreased suppressor T cell function

2.
The following drugs are useful in the management of some patients with urinary incontinence
Ⓐ loperamide
Ⓑ oxybutynin
Ⓒ bisacodyl
Ⓓ oestrogen
Ⓔ indoramin

3.
Pharmacodynamic and pharmacokinetic consequences are attributable to the following changes that occur in the elderly population
Ⓐ increased lean body mass
Ⓑ increased percentage body fat
Ⓒ reduced plasma binding
Ⓓ reduced first pass hepatic metabolism
Ⓔ decrease in number of cell receptors

4.
The following statements regarding elderly citizens of the UK are true
Ⓐ dementia is present in 15% of the population over the age of 75 years
Ⓑ 75% of subjects aged over 85 years can wash unaided
Ⓒ 95% of subjects aged over 85 years can toilet themselves
Ⓓ 50% of subjects over the age of 75 years maintain independent households
Ⓔ the population aged > 65 years increased by 30% during the period 1961–1981

5.
Elderly individuals
Ⓐ have an increased core-skin temperature gradient
Ⓑ have reduced cutaneous temperature discrimination
Ⓒ shiver less efficiently in response to cooling
Ⓓ stop shivering when core temperature falls < 35°C
Ⓔ are more likely to die from stroke during cold weather

6.
When compared to healthy young people, hospitalised elderly patients who fall have
Ⓐ reduced variability of step length
Ⓑ reduced step frequency
Ⓒ increased step width
Ⓓ increased step length
Ⓔ greater antero-posterior sway in women than in men

7.
The following conditions cause urinary incontinence
Ⓐ detrusor instability
Ⓑ faecal impaction
Ⓒ dementia despite normal bladder cystometry
Ⓓ atrophic vaginitis
Ⓔ prostatic carcinoma

8.
Adverse drug reactions in the elderly are
Ⓐ three times more common than in the under 65's
Ⓑ the cause of 50% of all admissions to geriatric units
Ⓒ usually due to drugs used for gastrointestinal disease
Ⓓ more likely to occur with drugs that have a high therapeutic index
Ⓔ usually due to alterations in the pharmacodynamics and pharmacokinetics

20 ACUTE POISONING

ANSWERS BEGIN ON P. 246

1.
The following statements about drug metabolism are true

Ⓐ Apparent volume of distribution = volume of total body water

Ⓑ First order elimination = rate of renal clearance of a drug

Ⓒ Drug clearance = amount of the drug removed from plasma per hour

Ⓓ First-pass elimination = degree of drug excretion in the first hour

Ⓔ Bioavailability = amount of the drug bound to specific receptors

2.
The following statements about pharmacokinetics are true

Ⓐ 50% of steady state concentration is achieved in one half-life

Ⓑ The drug half-life = time taken to eliminate half the dose given

Ⓒ Steady state is achieved after approximately five half-lives

Ⓓ Drug bioavailability is enhanced by intravenous administration

Ⓔ Drug absorption and excretion are increased when drugs are in a non-ionised state

3.
The following statements about drug absorption are true

Ⓐ Oral drug absorption is reduced if nausea or pain are present

Ⓑ Only 10% of drugs given by pressurised aerosols reach the lungs

Ⓒ Buccal and transdermal routes avoid first-pass hepatic metabolism

Ⓓ Rectal administration avoids pre-systemic hepatic elimination

Ⓔ Drug absorption within the stomach is enhanced by food or alcohol

4.
The following examples of pharmacokinetic variability are true

Ⓐ Lipid-soluble drug bioavailability is enhanced by food

Ⓑ Chronic liver disease reduces the bioavailability of propranolol

Ⓒ Hypoalbuminaemia decreases drug concentrations in the free form

Ⓓ Impaired neonatal glucuronidation increases chloramphenicol toxicity

Ⓔ Ampicillin increases plasma concentrations of oral contraceptives

5.
Examples of pharmacokinetic interactions include

Ⓐ allopurinol inhibits the metabolism of azathioprine

Ⓑ amitriptyline delays gastric emptying and the absorption of drugs

Ⓒ digoxin and verapamil compete for renal tubular secretion

Ⓓ effect of methotrexate is inhibited by NSAID therapy

Ⓔ antibiotics alter gut flora disrupting enterohepatic drug cycling

6.
The following drugs inhibit drug metabolism by reducing hepatic enzyme activities

Ⓐ carbamazepine

Ⓑ ciprofloxacin

Ⓒ metronidazole

Ⓓ allopurinol

Ⓔ erythromycin

7.
The following statements about self-poisoning are true
Ⓐ The majority of patients are middle-aged and/or suicidal
Ⓑ 50% of episodes are associated with alcohol intoxication
Ⓒ 66% of patients ingest drugs prescribed for family members
Ⓓ 50% of patients have a previous history of self-poisoning
Ⓔ 75% of patients repeat self-poisoning within 12 months

8.
Clinical features suggestive of self-poisoning include
Ⓐ coma in patients under the age of 40 years
Ⓑ strabismus and nystagmus in young patients
Ⓒ evidence of self-injury e.g. scars on the forearms
Ⓓ evidence of needle tracks suggesting drug abuse
Ⓔ circumoral acneiform rash suggesting solvent abuse

9.
Immediate measures in the management of self-poisoning include
Ⓐ identification of the ingested poison
Ⓑ use of specific antidotes and antagonists
Ⓒ maintenance of the airway and respiratory function
Ⓓ maintenance of blood pressure and circulatory function
Ⓔ induction of vomiting by salt water

10.
The following statements about gastric lavage are true
Ⓐ Lavage is preferable to the use of ipecacuanha in children
Ⓑ The position of the tube should be checked under X-ray control
Ⓒ In comatose patients, endotracheal intubation must precede lavage
Ⓓ Patients should lie on their left side in a feet-down tilt
Ⓔ Activated charcoal should be given following completion of lavage

11.
The use of gastric lavage or ipecacuanha following self-poisoning
Ⓐ should be avoided if petroleum distillates have been ingested
Ⓑ with aspirin is unlikely to be helpful 8 hours after ingestion
Ⓒ with tricyclic antidepressants is indicated 8 hours post-ingestion
Ⓓ should always be undertaken if paraquat has been ingested
Ⓔ should never be undertaken in hypothermic patients

12.
The following treatments are effective in poisoning with the following drugs
Ⓐ Forced alkaline diuresis — salicylates
Ⓑ Dimercaprol — arsenic
Ⓒ Flumazenil — opiates and analogues
Ⓓ N-acetylcysteine — paracetamol
Ⓔ haemoperfusion — medium acting barbiturates

13.
Typical features 12 hours after paracetamol poisoning include
Ⓐ nausea and vomiting
Ⓑ coma and internuclear ophthalmoplegia
Ⓒ prolongation of the prothrombin time
Ⓓ metabolic acidosis and hypoglycaemia
Ⓔ prevention of liver damage with methionine

14.
Typical features 8 hours after salicylate poisoning in an adult include
Ⓐ coma and dilated pupils
Ⓑ deafness, tinnitus and blurred vision
Ⓒ hypokalaemia and respiratory alkalosis
Ⓓ hyperventilation, sweating and restlessness
Ⓔ an empty stomach before gastric lavage

15.
Typical features following benzodiazepine poisoning include
Ⓐ ataxia, dysarthria, nystagmus and drowsiness
Ⓑ severe systemic hypotension and respiratory depression
Ⓒ nausea, vomiting and diarrhoea
Ⓓ convulsions, muscle spasms and papilloedema
Ⓔ resolution of symptoms in < 12 hours in lorazepam poisoning

16.
Typical features following barbiturate poisoning include
Ⓐ hypotension and hypothermia
Ⓑ coma and respiratory depression
Ⓒ skin blisters on dependent areas
Ⓓ sweating, restlessness and hallucinations
Ⓔ nausea, vomiting and abdominal pain

17.
Typical features following amitriptyline poisoning include
Ⓐ coma, hyperreflexia and extensor plantar responses
Ⓑ warm, dry skin and dry mouth
Ⓒ pinpoint pupils
Ⓓ hallucinations and urinary retention
Ⓔ convulsions and cardiac tachyarrhythmias

18.
Poisoning with drugs containing dextropropoxyphene produces
Ⓐ hyperventilation and agitation
Ⓑ coma with pinpoint pupils and hypotonia
Ⓒ hypotension and hypothermia
Ⓓ high plasma paracetamol concentration
Ⓔ absence of a response to naloxone therapy

19.
Typical features of morphine poisoning include
Ⓐ nausea, vomiting and pallor
Ⓑ coma, miotic pupils and hyporeflexia
Ⓒ hypoventilation and hypothermia
Ⓓ hypotension and respiratory arrest
Ⓔ non-cardiac pulmonary oedema

20.
Typical features of elemental iron poisoning include
Ⓐ nausea, vomiting and abdominal pain
Ⓑ tachypnoea and tachycardia
Ⓒ acute gastrointestinal haemorrhage
Ⓓ encephalopathy and circulatory failure
Ⓔ pyloric stricture presenting 6 weeks later

21.
Typical features of lithium carbonate poisoning include
Ⓐ response to forced diuresis
Ⓑ thirst and polyuria
Ⓒ management by haemodialysis if plasma level > 5 mmol/L
Ⓓ hypernatraemia and hypokalaemia
Ⓔ prolongation of the QRS and QT intervals and AV block on ECG

22.
Findings consistent with ethanol poisoning include
Ⓐ drowsiness, dysarthria, ataxia and nystagmus
Ⓑ hyponatraemia and hypoglycaemia
Ⓒ hypothermia
Ⓓ metabolic acidosis
Ⓔ aspiration pneumonia

23.
Methanol poisoning characteristically produces
Ⓐ the features of ethanol intoxication
Ⓑ abdominal pain, vomiting and convulsions
Ⓒ fixed, dilated pupils and papilloedema
Ⓓ severe metabolic acidosis due to lactic acid
Ⓔ severe toxicity only in volumes > 100 ml

24.

In ethylene glycol poisoning

Ⓐ toxicity is primarily due to ethylene glycol itself

Ⓑ papilloedema and ophthalmoplegia are typical features

Ⓒ lactic acidosis and renal failure frequently develop

Ⓓ hypokalaemia and hypercalcaemia are typical

Ⓔ treatment with alcohol may be valuable

25.

Organophosphate poisoning is characteristically associated with

Ⓐ sewage workers

Ⓑ vomiting, abdominal pain and diarrhoea

Ⓒ sweating, hypersalivation and bronchorrhoea

Ⓓ coma, convulsions and muscle twitching

Ⓔ clinical response to obidoxime therapy

1 GENETIC FACTORS IN DISEASE

1.
- **A** T — In addition there are 2 X chromosomes in females and 1 X and 1 Y in males
- **B** T — In contrast to somatic cell nuclei which are diploid
- **C** F — Haploid male cell (sperm) may contain an X or a Y chromosome
- **D** F — Occurs during meiosis
- **E** F — One X chromosome is inactive and appears as the Barr body in the nucleus

2.
- **A** T — The most common form of numerical chromosome aberration
- **B** T
- **C** T — Liveborn frequency is 0.6%
- **D** F — Gene expression can be affected by the parental origin of the abnormal chromosome
- **E** T — No genetic material is lost

3.
- **A** F — Peripheral blood lymphocytes are the most convenient source for chromosome study
- **B** F — 47,XX,+21
- **C** T
- **D** T
- **E** F — 47,XY,+18

4.
- **A** F — Proband is a male
- **B** T — As indicated by the double line
- **C** F — Both are alive and unaffected
- **D** F — Dizygotic twin
- **E** F

5.
- **A** T
- **B** F — Can be of either sex
- **C** F — All female
- **D** F — Male to male transmission is characteristically absent in X-linked inheritance
- **E** T

6.
- **A** F — 75% will carry the gene, 25% will be normal homozygotes
- **B** F — Children of either sex could be affected
- **C** T
- **D** T — 25% chance that a single child will be affected
- **E** F — 25% chance of a grandchild being affected

7.
- **A** T
- **B** F — Parent is almost always affected
- **C** F — An equal chance
- **D** F — Unaffected children are free of the mutant gene
- **E** F — Some affected individuals are clinically normal—'non-penetrance'

8.
- **A** T — The most common human aneuploidy
- **B** F — Only about 5% are translocations
- **C** T
- **D** F — Most siblings will be chromosomally normal
- **E** F — Polyploidy = chromosome number is a multiple of 23, e.g. triploidy = 69 chromosomes

9.
Ⓐ F Cardiac abnormalities are rare
Ⓑ F Intelligence is usually normal, but mild mental retardation may be seen
Ⓒ F Affected individuals are typically tall
Ⓓ F FSH and LH are typically elevated in hypergonadotrophic hypogonadism
Ⓔ T A secondary phenomenon seen in many types of gonadal failure

10.
Ⓐ T Due to gonadal (ovarian) dysgenesis
Ⓑ F Affected individuals are typically short in stature
Ⓒ T May also be a short neck with low hairline
Ⓓ T Producing the so called wide carrying- angle
Ⓔ T Other cardiac abnormalities include aortic stenosis and bicuspid aortic valve

11.
Ⓐ T Absence of male to male transmission is a key feature of all X-linked inheritance
Ⓑ T
Ⓒ T If the X chromosome is inherited from the father
Ⓓ F 50% of his sisters will be carriers and 50% normal
Ⓔ T All the female children of an affected grandfather would carry the gene

12.
Ⓐ F Autosomal recessive
Ⓑ T
Ⓒ T
Ⓓ F Autosomal recessive
Ⓔ T Similarly familial hypercholesterolaemia, adult polycystic disease and Huntington's disease

13.
Ⓐ F X-linked dominant mode of inheritance
Ⓑ T Haemophilia is also an X-linked recessive trait
Ⓒ F Autosomal dominant
Ⓓ F Autosomal recessive
Ⓔ T

14.
Ⓐ T Like other aminoacidopathies such as phenylketonuria
Ⓑ F Only congenital erythropoietic porphyria is not inherited as an autosomal dominant
Ⓒ T Early onset hereditary ataxia associated with cardiac abnormalities
Ⓓ T Abnormal copper metabolism leads to neurological and hepatic damage
Ⓔ T Congenital defect of bilirubin uptake and conjugation

15.
Ⓐ F Multifactorial disorder
Ⓑ T Autosomal recessive
Ⓒ F Multifactorial disorder
Ⓓ T Autosomal recessive
Ⓔ T Autosomal dominant

16.
Ⓐ F 64 possible codons — the code is said to be degenerate
Ⓑ T Introns are non-coding regions in base sequences
Ⓒ F Occurs in the cytoplasm
Ⓓ T
Ⓔ T Sickle-cell anaemia exemplifies such 'point mutation'

17.
Ⓐ F Multifactorial disorder more frequent in males
Ⓑ T Risk is greater for children of affected individuals of the less commonly affected sex
Ⓒ T Presence of additional affected family members increases risk
Ⓓ F In contrast with the chromosomal disorder Down's syndrome
Ⓔ T Risks are higher for relatives of an individual with a more severe malformation

18.
Ⓐ F TSH is measured
Ⓑ T Permitting genetic counselling
Ⓒ T
Ⓓ F Used in sickle-cell anaemia
Ⓔ T Some affected subjects exhibit retinal abnormalities

19.
Ⓐ F Screening is offered to pregnant women in the UK
Ⓑ F Confirmatory evidence is obtained by amniocentesis
Ⓒ F Measured at 16–19 weeks
Ⓓ T Such as spina bifida and anencephaly
Ⓔ F Reduced

20.
Ⓐ T 95% of patients with AS carry this antigen
Ⓑ F Association with blood group O
Ⓒ T
Ⓓ T
Ⓔ T Also associated with ankylosing spondylitis

21.
Ⓐ F Enzymes cleave DNA
Ⓑ T
Ⓒ T Minute quantities can now be detected with PCR techniques
Ⓓ T
Ⓔ T

22.
Ⓐ T
Ⓑ T
Ⓒ T
Ⓓ T
Ⓔ T

23.
Ⓐ T Can be performed as early as 10 weeks
Ⓑ T Safely locates the placenta
Ⓒ F
Ⓓ T
Ⓔ T

IMMUNOLOGICAL FACTORS IN DISEASE

2

1.
- **A T** Particularly bacteria
- **B T** Also capable of phagocytosis
- **C T** Also activated by interferons
- **D T** Opsonisation facilitates phagocytosis
- **E T** Also induces T cell proliferation

2.
- **A F** Large granular lymphocytes
- **B T** And cells which act as mediators of delayed hypersensitivity
- **C T** E.g. via production of IL-4
- **D T** Possess the CD4 marker
- **E F** Amplifies T cell proliferation

3.
- **A F** B lymphocytes
- **B T** And in the respiratory tract and other mucosae
- **C T** Responsible for fetal passive immunity
- **D F** Only 20%, IgG = 70%+
- **E T** Involved in B lymphocyte maturation and regulation

4.
- **A T**
- **B F** A function of IgM predominantly
- **C T** LgG also fixes complement
- **D F** No direct defensive role
- **E F** This is a function of IgD

5.
- **A F** Both pathways activate these enzymes
- **B T** Synthesized in the liver
- **C F** Immune complexes
- **D F** Bacterial products
- **E T** Autosomal dominant inheritance

6.
- **A F** A distinct cell series with basophilic staining properties
- **B T** And immediate hypersensitivity
- **C T** And IgE
- **D F** Activated by opioids
- **E T** Mediators of inflammation and chemotaxis

7.
- **A T** Attracted by T cell eosinophilic chemotactic factor
- **B T** Most severe when antigen injected
- **C T** Many vasoactive products are released
- **D T** Preferably i.m.; used in lower dosage i.v.
- **E F** Can be induced by cold or local skin trauma

8.
- **A T** Specific T_{DTH} lymphocytes are involved
- **B F** Intracellular location e.g. tuberculosis, leprosy, syphilis
- **C T** Granulomatous reactions such as sarcoidosis
- **D T** Jewellery and garment clips
- **E F** Cells are predominantly epidermal

9.
- **A T** Due to recruitment of inflammatory mediators
- **B T** Also on the antigen/antibody ratio and the nature of antigen
- **C F** 6–24 hours after exposure
- **D F** 10 days after exposure
- **E F** IgG antibodies

10.
A T   As in older age
B T   E.g. sperm in vas deferens occlusion
C T   E.g. Group A haemolytic streptococci
D T   E.g. methyldopa
E T   Expression of MHC class 2 surface antigens important

11.
A T   On the short arm
B F   Only two classes
C F   Also occur on platelets
D T   Cells which initiate and control immune responses
E T

12.
A T   Also multiple sclerosis
B T   And many of the reactive arthritides
C T   Also coeliac disease
D F   HLA DR4
E F   HLA B14

13.
A F   H1 receptors only
B T   Useful in asthma
C F   No direct immunosuppressive action
D T   Also suppress macrophage function
E T   A non-cytotoxic effect

14.
A F   Normal
B F   There are no mature lymphocytes
C T   But susceptibility to infection remains
D T   Linked to HLA DR3
E F   Not B cell-dependent

15.
A T   Viral infections are frequently fatal in infants
B T   B cell function is normal
C T   Absent circulating T cells
D T   Causing neonatal hypocalcaemic convulsions
E T   Fetal thymic graft can help

16.
A F   RNA retrovirus
B T   With decreased numbers and abnormal function
C T   Also show reduced responses to some antigens
D T   With subsequent impaired killing and cytokine secretion
E T   Antiplatelet antibodies are detectable

17.
A T   2–6 months
B F   Inactivated toxin is used
C T   Like tetanus
D F   Active immunisation
E F   Contraindicated due to danger of dissemination

18.
A F
B T   Especially in combination with immunosuppressive drugs
C T   Reduces plasma viscosity
D T   Especially in patients with respiratory paralysis
E F   Venesection is usually undertaken

19.
A F   Cell mediated immunity is the more important
B F   HLA antigen groups have the major role
C T   Lymphocytes carry all class I and II MHC antigens
D T   1 in 4 in siblings
E T   Graft versus host disease

20.
A T   Antigen if the most important drive to B and T cell proliferation
B T   Producing a decline in antigen
C T   Comprise 35% of circulating peripheral T cells
D F   Induce suppressor cells
E T   Idiotype is the antigen-specific component of an antibody

21.

A T Glomerular basement membrane antibodies
B T Parietal cell antibodies
C T Acetylcholine receptor antibodies
D T TSH receptor antibodies
E T Anti-mitochondrial antibodies

3 CLIMATE AND ENVIRONMENTAL FACTORS IN DISEASE

1
Ⓐ T   Secondary to fluid retention
Ⓑ T   Facilitating salt retention
Ⓒ F   Decreased
Ⓓ F   Decreased with decreased salt content
Ⓔ F   Increased stroke volume

2.
Ⓐ T   Intracellular and extracellular
Ⓑ T   Lack of thirst means may mislead the unwary
Ⓒ F   Sweating continues unabated
Ⓓ T   Salt and water replacement and a cool environment
Ⓔ F   Salt losses are greater in the unacclimatised

3.
Ⓐ T   Perhaps simply due to inappropriate clothing
Ⓑ T   Above 42° death is likely
Ⓒ F   Absent
Ⓓ F   'Hot dry man'
Ⓔ F   Usually abrupt onset with rapid progression

4.
Ⓐ T   Can occur secondary to use of some drugs
Ⓑ T   Impeding sweating
Ⓒ T   Decreased renal blood flow and rhabdomyolysis
Ⓓ T   May be disseminated intravascular coagulation
Ⓔ T   Or phenothiazines

5.
Ⓐ T   With hypotension and hypoglycaemia
Ⓑ T   Sometimes a presenting feature
Ⓒ T   Or acute hepatic failure
Ⓓ T   Particularly in the elderly
Ⓔ T   Especially barbiturates and phenothiazines

6.
Ⓐ F   Haemoconcentration
Ⓑ T   May be as low as 25 degrees
Ⓒ T   And even loss of consciousness
Ⓓ F   Bradycardia and J waves on the ECG
Ⓔ T   Check amylase and blood gases

7.
Ⓐ F   Unusual below 2500 metres
Ⓑ F   May prevent development
Ⓒ T   Also breathlessness, dizziness and insomnia
Ⓓ T   Even progressing to coma
Ⓔ F   Significant risk of thrombosis due to dehydration and hyperviscosity

8.
Ⓐ T   Death occurs within 2 weeks
Ⓑ F   Lymphocytes are the most sensitive
Ⓒ F   However, above this, death becomes increasingly likely
Ⓓ F   Requires doses > 10 Gy
Ⓔ T   80% of background radiation is attributable to radon

9.
Ⓐ F   Food and drink
Ⓑ T   Abdominal pain, gastrointestinal upset and dysgeusia
Ⓒ F   Adult lead levels = 10–25 μg/100 ml
Ⓓ T   Together with punctate basophilia of the RBCs
Ⓔ F   Chelation therapy is advisable if blood lead > 100 μg/100 ml

10.
Ⓐ T   Early signs
Ⓑ T   Peripheral neuropathies are common
Ⓒ T   In severe poisoning
Ⓓ F   Suggests acute poisoning
Ⓔ F   Suggests acute poisoning

11.

Ⓐ F 1 atmosphere = 760 mmHg
Ⓑ T Also causes hypoxia on surfacing
Ⓒ T Pressure rises by 1 atmosphere for each 10 m of depth
Ⓓ F Occurs in rapid ascent without expiration from shallower depths
Ⓔ F Typically the tympanic membrane

12.

Ⓐ T Rarely reversible 4 hours or more after surfacing
Ⓑ F Due to intra-lymphatic gas
Ⓒ F Affects fatty tissues particularly
Ⓓ T The 'staggers' and the 'chokes'
Ⓔ F Neurological deficits usually persist

4 DISEASES DUE TO INFECTION

1.
- **A** T From rats' or dogs' urine
- **B** F
- **C** T Lice, fleas, ticks, mites
- **D** T Ticks
- **E** F Faecal-oral

2.
- **A** T
- **B** T
- **C** T Like hepatitis A
- **D** F Faecal-oral
- **E** T

3.
- **A** F 3 times during the first 6 months of life
- **B** T
- **C** F At 12–24 months
- **D** T
- **E** T

4.
- **A** F
- **B** T Also in other immunosuppressed states
- **C** T
- **D** F
- **E** T Diminishes the effectiveness of live vaccines

5.
- **A** T Inactivated vaccine also available
- **B** F
- **C** F
- **D** T Do not give to immunosuppressed patients
- **E** F

6.
- **A** T Active immunisation also available
- **B** T In susceptible injured patients
- **C** T Post-exposure protection
- **D** F
- **E** T

7.
- **A** T
- **B** T
- **C** T
- **D** T
- **E** T

8.
- **A** T E.g. malaria
- **B** T E.g. abattoir workers and Q fever
- **C** T E.g. in-land water sports enthusiasts and leptospira
- **D** T E.g. penicillin hypersensitivity
- **E** T E.g. farmers and brucellosis

9.
- **A** T Also includes asymptomatic patients
- **B** F This is classed as group A infection
- **C** F Group C includes conditions meeting CDC/WHO case definition
- **D** T
- **E** F This would be group A

10.
- **A** T Affects the tongue and mouth
- **B** T Especially *pneumocystis* carinii
- **C** T
- **D** T Sometimes with atypical mycobacteria
- **E** T

11.
Ⓐ T
Ⓑ F Male homosexuality is the commonest risk factor in the UK
Ⓒ F Greater affect on T lymphocytes
Ⓓ F CD4 helper T cells are principally involved
Ⓔ F Prognosis is worse

12.
Ⓐ T
Ⓑ T The catarrhal phase
Ⓒ F They precede the rash
Ⓓ T
Ⓔ F Contact should be avoided for 7 days after the onset of the rash

13.
Ⓐ T Especially in the immunocompromised
Ⓑ T Occurs in the convalescent phase due to an immune reaction
Ⓒ F
Ⓓ F
Ⓔ T

14.
Ⓐ T A togavirus
Ⓑ F Constitutional symptoms and polyarthritis are both worse in adults
Ⓒ T
Ⓓ T
Ⓔ T Greatest risk is in the first 4 weeks

15.
Ⓐ T Termination should be offered if infection proven
Ⓑ F
Ⓒ F
Ⓓ T
Ⓔ F

16.
Ⓐ T
Ⓑ F Infectivity is generally low
Ⓒ T
Ⓓ F Pain suggests pancreatitis or oophoritis
Ⓔ F It is usually unilateral and postpubertal

17.
Ⓐ T Especially HS type 2
Ⓑ T HS type 1
Ⓒ T HS type 1
Ⓓ F Varicella zoster virus
Ⓔ T HS type 1 — 'herpetic whitlow'

18.
Ⓐ T
Ⓑ T And malaise and anorexia
Ⓒ F
Ⓓ T
Ⓔ T Especially if there is dysphagia or breathing difficulty

19.
Ⓐ T
Ⓑ T
Ⓒ T
Ⓓ T
Ⓔ F Adults are more severely affected

20.
Ⓐ F Adults or the immunosuppressed
Ⓑ T
Ⓒ F May occur in mumps
Ⓓ T
Ⓔ T

21.
Ⓐ T Especially dogs and foxes
Ⓑ F Average 4–8 weeks
Ⓒ T It is usually fatal
Ⓓ T
Ⓔ T

22.
Ⓐ T
Ⓑ T Highly infectious
Ⓒ T In severe cases
Ⓓ F 7–21 days
Ⓔ T Overall mortality 50%

23.
Ⓐ T Transmitted from monkeys
Ⓑ F 3–6 days
Ⓒ F There is leucopenia
Ⓓ T
Ⓔ F Supportive therapy only

24.
Ⓐ T
Ⓑ T Fever may remit on day 4–5 ('saddleback')
Ⓒ T But non-specific
Ⓓ T Rash starts peripherally
Ⓔ F There is no vaccine

25.
Ⓐ T *Chlamydia psittaci*
Ⓑ F *Rickettsia prowazeki*
Ⓒ T *Chlamydia trachomatis*
Ⓓ T *Chlamydia trachomatis*
Ⓔ F *Coxiella burnetii*

26.
Ⓐ F No symptoms may occur before vision fails
Ⓑ T With entropion and trichiasis
Ⓒ T
Ⓓ T Oral tetracycline is also effective
Ⓔ F It is due to corneal scarring

27.
Ⓐ T 4–14 days
Ⓑ T But non-specific
Ⓒ T As in other 'atypical' pneumonia
Ⓓ F
Ⓔ F Tetracycline is effective

28.
Ⓐ T Due to cold agglutinins
Ⓑ T
Ⓒ T The commonest clinical problem
Ⓓ T Rare, complicating pneumonia
Ⓔ T

29.
Ⓐ T Lice and fleas
Ⓑ T with widespread clinical manifestations
Ⓒ T
Ⓓ F Under 40%
Ⓔ T

30.
Ⓐ T Especially butchers and abattoir workers
Ⓑ T
Ⓒ F Acute Q fever is a flu-like illness
Ⓓ T
Ⓔ F Tetracyclines, rifampicin or chloramphenicol

31.
Ⓐ T Ixodes species of tick
Ⓑ T An annular red lesion
Ⓒ T Or meningitis or radiculopathy
Ⓓ T Not in acute stages
Ⓔ T And cephalosporins

32.
Ⓐ T Louse- or tick-borne
Ⓑ F Typically under 3 weeks
Ⓒ T
Ⓓ T
Ⓔ T

33.
Ⓐ F 4–21 days
Ⓑ T
Ⓒ T With abrupt onset
Ⓓ F Aseptic meningitis characterises *L. canicola* infection
Ⓔ T Mortality is 15–20%

34.
Ⓐ T
Ⓑ T
Ⓒ T Warts
Ⓓ T Anogenital lesions
Ⓔ T Wart-like lesions

35.
Ⓐ F *T. pallidum*
Ⓑ F Infectivity persists if untreated
Ⓒ T
Ⓓ T But may be 90 days
Ⓔ F

36.
- **A** T Perhaps with lymphadenopathy
- **B** T Differentiate from viral warts
- **C** T 'Snail-track' ulcers
- **D** F Meningeal involvement is rare
- **E** F Cardiac involvement is a feature of late disease

37.
- **A** F They are typically positive
- **B** T
- **C** T Due to dorsal column spinal disease
- **D** T Typically with calcification
- **E** F

38.
- **A** F 2–10 days
- **B** T Dysuria, discharge or no symptoms
- **C** T
- **D** T With septicaemia
- **E** T Or cefotaxime or spectinomycin

39.
- **A** T In around 50% of cases
- **B** T Less common than *C. trachomatis*
- **C** T Suggesting Reiter's disease
- **D** F
- **E** F Tetracycline or erythromycin

40.
- **A** F Granuloma inguinale due to *Donovania granulomatis*
- **B** T
- **C** T Tender lymph nodes
- **D** T
- **E** T

41.
- **A** T More often Herpes simplex
- **B** T *Haemophilus ducreyii* infection
- **C** T
- **D** T With oral ulcers, iritis and arthropathy
- **E** F

42.
- **A** F Type 2 more than type 1
- **B** T Healing is more rapid in recurrent attacks
- **C** T
- **D** T
- **E** F It shortens first attacks and may prevent recurrence

43.
- **A** T Most commonly in children
- **B** T The face is spared
- **C** F *Streptococcus pyogenes*
- **D** F Suggests an alternative diagnosis
- **E** F Suggests diphtheria

44.
- **A** T *Streptococcus pyogenes*
- **B** F Systemic upset is common
- **C** T The rash has a palpably raised edge
- **D** F
- **E** T

45.
- **A** T In 90% of cases
- **B** T
- **C** T Often secondary to viral infection
- **D** T Often complicating vaginal infection
- **E** T

46.
- **A** F It does not follow ingestion of infected foodstuffs
- **B** T There is severe systemic upset
- **C** T Perhaps with renal failure
- **D** F
- **E** T Similar to scarlet fever

47.
- **A** T
- **B** T Due to vasodilatation
- **C** F Due to peripheral vasodilatation and capillary damage
- **D** F Leucopenia may suggest a poor prognosis
- **E** F Urgent antibiotic therapy after taking the appropriate cultures

48.
Ⓐ F May occur in either
Ⓑ T Suggests anterior nasal infection and myocarditis
Ⓒ T Streptococcal exudate is easily removed
Ⓓ T Occasionally with peripheral polyneuritis
Ⓔ F There is rarely a marked fever at onset

49.
Ⓐ F Tissue fixed toxin cannot be neutralised
Ⓑ F This requires adrenaline, fluid and antihistamine
Ⓒ F Causes fever, urticaria and joint pains
Ⓓ F Vital
Ⓔ F Recovery is complete in survivors

50.
Ⓐ T
Ⓑ T A highly infectious stage
Ⓒ T Lasting 1 or more weeks
Ⓓ F Swabs from the posterior nasopharyngeal wall are better
Ⓔ F

51.
Ⓐ T
Ⓑ T With rapid progression
Ⓒ T Septicaemia usually precedes meningitis
Ⓓ F
Ⓔ F Chemoprophylactic treatment of close contacts is preferred

52.
Ⓐ F As long as several weeks
Ⓑ T Causing trismus
Ⓒ F They are painful
Ⓓ T
Ⓔ F Not often achieved

53.
Ⓐ F Antitoxin is given intravenously
Ⓑ F Antitoxin should be given as soon as possible
Ⓒ T
Ⓓ F Necessary to control spasms
Ⓔ T Metronidazole if penicillin allergic

54.
Ⓐ F 12–72 hours after ingestion
Ⓑ T
Ⓒ T
Ⓓ T Diplopia may be the earliest symptom
Ⓔ F Bound toxin cannot be neutralised

55.
Ⓐ T Farmers, butchers and dealers in hides, hair, wool
Ⓑ F 1–3 days
Ⓒ T Painless but itchy
Ⓓ T
Ⓔ F The organism is widely sensitive

56.
Ⓐ F 3 weeks
Ⓑ T Joint pains and anorexia also
Ⓒ T But rarely
Ⓓ T Due to localised granulomatous disease
Ⓔ F Neutropenia and lymphocytosis

57.
Ⓐ T 3–6 days or less
Ⓑ F Transmitted in rodents by fleas
Ⓒ F Bubonic plague is commoner
Ⓓ T The bubo is the affected lymph node mass
Ⓔ T

58.
Ⓐ T Usually asymptomatic carriers
Ⓑ F 10–14 days
Ⓒ T And relative bradycardia
Ⓓ T
Ⓔ T

59.
Ⓐ T May remain infectious for years
Ⓑ T Septicaemia is characteristic during the first week
Ⓒ T
Ⓓ T Especially in patients with sickle-cell disease
Ⓔ T

60.
- **A** T — Abrupt onset
- **B** T
- **C** F — The rash may be more pronounced
- **D** F
- **E** F — Intestinal complications are less frequent

61.
- **A** F — Bacteraemia in the first week
- **B** F — More likely in second or third week
- **C** F — Leucopenia is typical
- **D** F — There are frequent false negatives
- **E** F — It may suggest a septicaemic focus

62.
- **A** T — Salmonella has similar incubation
- **B** T — A toxin mediated food poisoning
- **C** T — Or chemical poisoning
- **D** T — Typically *E. coli* 0157
- **E** T

63.
- **A** F — *Shigella sonnei*
- **B** T
- **C** F — Faecal contamination of food and milk is most important
- **D** F — Bloodstained purulent stools with abdominal pain
- **E** F — Antibiotics are often unnecessary — trimethoprim or ciprofloxacin

64.
- **A** T
- **B** F — Hours rather than days
- **C** T — Typically without abdominal pain
- **D** T — Fluid replacement must be prompt
- **E** F — Typically a metabolic acidosis

65.
- **A** T — Interfere with cell wall synthesis
- **B** T — Resistance by beta-lactamase-producing organisms is common
- **C** T — Used in combination with amoxycillin as co-amoxyclav
- **D** F — Hypersensitivity may be shared
- **E** F — Never give intrathecally

66.
- **A** F — Tetracyclines are bacteriostatic
- **B** T — Causes tooth discolouration in the fetus and child
- **C** T — As can minocycline
- **D** T — Calcium chelates tetracycline
- **E** T — Also coxiellae and brucella

67.
- **A** T — Especially in the elderly
- **B** T — Loop diuretics increase the ototoxic risk
- **C** T — Plasma levels and duration of therapy correlate with risk of toxicity
- **D** F — No anti-anaerobic activity
- **E** T — If they must be used, levels must be carefully measured

68.
- **A** T
- **B** F — Hence less likely to disrupt bowel flora
- **C** T
- **D** T — In appropriate dosage
- **E** F

69.
- **A** T — Especially useful in *H. influenzae* meningitis
- **B** T — Although ciprofloxacin is the drug of choice
- **C** T — Gentamicin, ceftazidime or ciprofloxacin are preferred
- **D** F — Azlocillin plus gentamicin
- **E** F — Tetracycline plus rifampicin for 4 weeks

70.
- **A** T
- **B** F — Tetracycline plus rifampicin is better
- **C** T — Active against most of the enterobacteria
- **D** F — Only moderate activity
- **E** F

71.
Ⓐ T 'Grey baby' syndrome due to poor hepatic conjugation
Ⓑ T
Ⓒ T Typically in patients with AIDS
Ⓓ T
Ⓔ F Also inactive against *Ureaplasma urealyticum*, a cause of urethritis

72.
Ⓐ T
Ⓑ T Or ciprofloxacin for meningococcal or *H. influenzae* infections
Ⓒ T
Ⓓ F Avoid except in combination with other drugs
Ⓔ T To prevent endocarditis

73.
Ⓐ T
Ⓑ T Used in prophylaxis of influenza A
Ⓒ T Also active in Lassa fever
Ⓓ T Used in AIDS
Ⓔ T Like acyclovir, useful orally or parenterally

74.
Ⓐ T
Ⓑ F The organism cannot be grown in artificial media
Ⓒ F There is no risk of infection in tuberculoid leprosy
Ⓓ T
Ⓔ F Characteristic of the tuberculoid form

75.
Ⓐ T Sweat glands are also affected
Ⓑ T Infective risk is non-existent
Ⓒ T Perhaps with anaesthetic cutaneous macules
Ⓓ F This is a type 2 lepra reaction seen in lepromatous patients
Ⓔ F This would suggest lepromatous disease

76.
Ⓐ F Infectivity is high
Ⓑ F Is multi-bacillary disease
Ⓒ T No cell-mediated immune response
Ⓓ F Suggests tuberculoid disease
Ⓔ F Macules occur, but sensation is retained

77.
Ⓐ T To prevent the emergence of drug resistance
Ⓑ T Rifampicin renders patients non-infective in days
Ⓒ T Because of the long generation time of *M. leprae*
Ⓓ T
Ⓔ T Then 5 years follow-up

78.
Ⓐ T Sporozoites enter the liver within 30 minutes
Ⓑ T
Ⓒ T Duration of the pre-patent period varies
Ⓓ F Only vivax and ovale persist in this form
Ⓔ F Fertilisation occurs in the mosquito

79.
Ⓐ F It may be transmitted by blood transfusion
Ⓑ F Only vivax and ovale
Ⓒ F Release of RBC schizonts produces symptoms
Ⓓ F They only parasitise these cells at certain stages
Ⓔ F P. falciparum may parasitise capillary endothelium in some sites

80.
Ⓐ F Onset is insidious, fever without pattern and often low
Ⓑ F Haemolysis is predominant
Ⓒ T Especially in brain, kidney, liver, lungs and gut
Ⓓ T Severe infection is rare
Ⓔ T

81.
A T
B T
C T *P. malariae* may persist but clinical recrudescence is rare
D T Especially in vivax and ovale
E T

82.
A T Due to cerebral anoxia
B T Severe haemolysis and haemoglobinuria
C T Acute tubular necrosis
D T
E T

83.
A T May develop many months after exposure
B F Subacute course with intermittent loose stools
C F Lesions are often most marked in the caecum
D T Flask-shaped ulcers
E F One-third of individuals in endemic areas are symptomless carriers

84.
A T Due to mucosal ulceration
B T Rarely due to transdiaphragmatic rupture
C T Very rare
D T May mimic carcinoma
E T Especially in homosexuals

85.
A F Free amoebae or cysts are rarely found
B F Exudate in the stool should be examined for trophozoites
C T Ultrasound-guided aspiration is useful
D T Or tinidazole
E T

86.
A F 1–3 weeks
B F Ingestion of contaminated water
C T
D T Mimics other malabsorptive conditions such as coeliac disease
E T Tinidazole is even more effective

87.
A T Immunocompromised patients are most at risk
B T Most infections are asymptomatic
C T Termination is suggested in seronegative mothers with first trimester infection
D T Can also cause thrombocytopenia
E T

88.
A T
B T Occasionally longer in *gambiense* infections
C T At the site of the bite
D T
E T Unless cerebral infection has developed

89.
A T Also spread by infected blood transfusions
B T Cutaneous lesion with regional nodes
C T
D T Megaoesophagus and megacolon
E T Established tissue damage cannot be reversed

90.
A T Also spread from infected blood transfusions
B F 1 month to 10 years
C F Splenomegaly is characteristic
D F Diagnosis by examination of stained smears of bone marrow, spleen or liver
E T Pentamidine is alternative

91.
A T Secondary to initial cutaneous ulceration
B F Typically painless and not involving nodes
C F Occurs in visceral leishmaniasis
D F
E F Typically positive except in diffuse cutaneous leishmaniasis

92.
A T *Schistosoma haematobium, japonicum* and *mansoni*
B F Eggs are passed in urine and/or stool
C T With local papular dermatitis
D F Portal hypertension not seen in *S. haematobium*
E T Or oxamniquine or metrifonate

93.
A F Pulmonary disease also occurs
B T Due to early egg deposition in the bladder mucosa
C F Adult worms can live for 20 years
D T
E F *S. japonicum*

94.
A T Also endemic in regions of S. America
B T Due to deposition of eggs in colonic mucosa
C F Portal hypertension is seen, but liver failure is rare
D T
E F The small bowel is unaffected

95.
A T Endemic in the Yellow River basin
B F Infection is by cutaneous penetration
C T Both the small and large bowel may be affected
D T In about 5% of infections
E F *S. japonicum* produces more eggs — infective consequences are worse

96.
A F *T. saginata* is the beef tapeworm
B F Asymptomatic usually
C F But worms may be seen in faeces
D F
E T Prevention by thorough cooking

97.
A F The pork tapeworm
B F Liberated in the stomach
C T Commonly deposited in muscle, brain, or subcutaneous tissue
D T Once deposited they do not migrate
E F

98.
A T May be many years before clinical manifestations appear
B T Usually an asymptomatic event
C T Right lobe of the liver is the commonest site
D F Care must also be taken during excision
E F But further enlargement may be prevented

99.
A F Seen in the colon
B T Worms may be visible
C T
D F The small bowel is unaffected
E T Cross-infection and autoinfection are common

100.
A F Food contaminated by mature ova
B T Pneumonitis with peripheral eosinophilia
C T Due to large masses of worms
D F Abdominal discomfort
E T

101.
A T Producing itchy cutaneous rash
B T With pain, diarrhoea, steatorrhoea and weight loss
C T
D T Intensely itchy
E T Seen in HIV

102.
A T
B F Clinical manifestations are due to dead or dying larvae
C T Visceral larva migrans and ocular granulomas
D T Tissue and blood eosinophilia
E T Or albendazole

103.
Ⓐ F Ingestion of partially cooked pork or ham
Ⓑ T With local symptoms and systemic upset
Ⓒ T During larval invasion
Ⓓ T
Ⓔ T Severe infections can be fatal

104.
Ⓐ F Vector is a fly, *Chrysops* species
Ⓑ F 3 months minimum
Ⓒ T Following the movement of adult worms
Ⓓ T Occasionally
Ⓔ T

105.
Ⓐ T A painful bite
Ⓑ F Worms can live for over 15 years
Ⓒ T Nodules contain adult worms
Ⓓ T
Ⓔ T

106.
Ⓐ F Commonly 14–28 days
Ⓑ T
Ⓒ F 2–4 weeks
Ⓓ T
Ⓔ T

107.
Ⓐ T
Ⓑ F Most are non-infectious within 24 hours of antibiotic therapy
Ⓒ T
Ⓓ F Infectious for 1 week after swellings appear
Ⓔ T

108.
Ⓐ F Urease levels in the gastric mucosa are increased due to the presence of HP (CLO test)
Ⓑ F HP eradication has no clinically significant effect on oesophagitis
Ⓒ T Hence concomitant acid-lowering drug therapy in eradication regimes
Ⓓ T Eradication rates are increased from 65% to > 85%
Ⓔ T Recurrence rates are > 80% without HP eradication

109.
Ⓐ T
Ⓑ F DNA virus causing an acute polyarthritis
Ⓒ F DNA poxvirus producing wart-like skin lesions
Ⓓ T Enteroviruses like coxsackie, hepatitis A and polio viruses
Ⓔ T

110.
Ⓐ F Zoonoses endemic in pigs, domestic animals and birds
Ⓑ T
Ⓒ T Especially with *Y. seudotuberculosis*
Ⓓ T Especially with *Y. enterocolitica*
Ⓔ F Tetracycline or gentamicin are more useful

5 DISEASES OF THE CARDIOVASCULAR SYSTEM

1.

A T Typical chest pain occurring at rest does not exclude myocardial ischaemia

B F May also radiate to the shoulders, arms or back

C F Rapid resolution is atypical — pain usually lasts for minutes

D F Oesophageal pain may mimic angina — precipitation by swallowing may be useful

E T Can disappear as exercise continues — 'second wind' effect ('walk through' angina)

2.

A F Suggests episodic bradycardia — Adams–Stokes attacks

B F Nausea and lightheadedness typically precede vasovagal attacks

C F Exertional syncope is a feature of severe aortic stenosis

D F Elderly patients do not usually lose consciousness during a fall

E T Circulatory collapse or arryhthmia in massive embolism

3.

A T Due to severe reduction in cardiac output

B T 'Cardiac cachexia' — weight gain due to oedema is more common

C T Due to hepatic and gastrointestinal congestion

D T Diuresis is induced by adopting the supine position

E T A manifestation of pulmonary congestion

4.

A F Supplied by the right coronary artery in 90%

B T These receptors also mediate inotropic responses

C F Varies between 15 and 30 mmHg in health

D F Restricts electrical connections between the atria and ventricles to the AV node

E F The product of heart rate and ventricular stroke volume

5.

A F Measured from the start of the P wave to the start of the R wave

B T

C T Heart rate = 1500/R–R interval (mm) (or 300/R-R interval (cm))

D T Reflecting the electrical dominance of the left ventricle

E F Represents atrial depolarisation

6.

A F 'Double peak' pulse is found in mixed aortic stenosis and regurgitiation

B F Found in severe airways obstruction or pericardial tamponade

C T Also typical of aortic regurgitation, pregnancy and therapy with nitrates et al

D F Pulsus alternans is beat-to-beat variation in pulse volume with a regular rate

E F Suggests severe aortic stenosis

7.

Ⓐ F The right internal jugular vein is the best manometer

Ⓑ F Measured from the manubriosternal junction (Angle of Louis)

Ⓒ F Venous tone increases with anxiety

Ⓓ F The rise may be more obvious in patients with cardiac failure

Ⓔ T On inspiration, heart rate rises, JVP falls and systemic arterial BP falls

8.

Ⓐ F Indicate atrial systole against a closed tricuspid valve and are seen in AV dissociation

Ⓑ T Also seen in pulmonary hypertension

Ⓒ T Better termed 'cv' waves are synchronous with right ventricular systole

Ⓓ T 'Kussmaul's sign' is associated with pulsus paradoxus

Ⓔ F There can be no 'a' waves in atrial fibrillation

9.

Ⓐ F Due to a palpably loud first heart sound and typical in mitral stenosis

Ⓑ T

Ⓒ F Such a thrill suggests a VSD — a mitral thrill is typically apical

Ⓓ T Also a feature of obesity or pericardial effusion

Ⓔ T Best appreciated as a supra–apical, rocking sensation

10.

Ⓐ F Occurs in mid–diastole due to rapid ventricular filling

Ⓑ T Due to variations in stroke volume

Ⓒ F Typically loud in mitral stenosis

Ⓓ T Due to delayed closure of the aortic valve compared with the pulmonary valve

Ⓔ F Coincides with atrial contraction and hence cannot occur in atrial fibrillation

11.

Ⓐ F Rapid left ventricular filling cannot occur if the mitral valve is stenosed

Ⓑ T Found in healthy hearts with a large stroke volume e.g. pregnancy

Ⓒ T Typically loud and occurs early in diastole

Ⓓ T Also in right ventricular failure

Ⓔ F Lone AF indicates normal ventricular function

12.

Ⓐ F Diastolic murmurs should always be regarded as pathological

Ⓑ T Typically at the left sternal edge

Ⓒ F Suggests aortic or pulmonary regurgitation

Ⓓ T Or hypertrophic cardiomyopathy

Ⓔ F Best heard at the apex with the patients lying on their left side

13.

Ⓐ F The heart rate is unreliable in making this distinction

Ⓑ F Suggests an SVT

Ⓒ T Suggests atrioventricular dissociation

Ⓓ F Occurs with both especially if left ventricular function is abnormal

Ⓔ F ECG complexes in VT are typically broader than 0.14 s

14.

Ⓐ F The CTR should be not greater than 0.5

Ⓑ F 'False negative' tests occur in 15–20%

Ⓒ T

Ⓓ T Pressure gradients can be extrapolated from measuring intracardiac flow velocities

Ⓔ T Ejection fraction is usually measured using this technique

15.
Ⓐ F Typically, the R–R interval variability decreases
Ⓑ T The commonest cause of supraventricular tachyarrhythmias
Ⓒ T Important to remember when assessing 24 hour ECG recordings
Ⓓ F This suggests complete heart block; sinus arrest is characterised by missing P waves
Ⓔ T Characteristic and predisposes to systemic emboli from intracardiac clot

16.
Ⓐ F Adenosine therapy can terminate an attack but has no role in prophylaxis
Ⓑ T
Ⓒ T Thought to be due to atrial natriuretic peptide release
Ⓓ F
Ⓔ F Bundle branch block can occur during rapid ventricular rates — 'rate-dependent aberrance'

17.
Ⓐ T Re-entrant circuit includes AV node and the accessory bundle
Ⓑ T
Ⓒ T Consider WPW in young patients with episodes of atrial fibrillation
Ⓓ F PR interval is shortened and a delta wave is seen in the QRS complex
Ⓔ F Differential effects on the normal and anomalous pathways can increase cardiac rate

18.
Ⓐ F A regular tachycardia
Ⓑ F Carotid sinus massage slows conduction in the AV node and may slow ventricular rate
Ⓒ F An ectopic atrial focus with abnormal P waves
Ⓓ T
Ⓔ F QRS complexes are usually narrow

19.
Ⓐ T
Ⓑ F Underlying structural heart disease is common and promotes the recurrence of AF
Ⓒ T Warfarin therapy reduces the annual risk to about 1.5%
Ⓓ T Episodes of sinus bradycardia or sinus arrest may coexist making drug therapy difficult
Ⓔ T Indicating concomitant AV nodal disease, a common finding in elderly patients

20.
Ⓐ F A greater risk reduction is achieved with warfarin therapy
Ⓑ T
Ⓒ T The onset of AF may precipitate heart failure
Ⓓ F Cardioversion should only be avoided if the patient is not taking anticoagulant therapy
Ⓔ T A common cause and left ventricular function is usually normal

21.
Ⓐ T The pulse is irregular with weak or missed beats
Ⓑ F Often occur in and are noticed by individuals with structurally normal hearts
Ⓒ F Usually become more frequent during exertion
Ⓓ T
Ⓔ F No beneficial effect on subsequent mortality

22.
Ⓐ T Often ischaemic heart disease
Ⓑ T A class III agent
Ⓒ F A prolonged QT interval predisposes to recurrent VT
Ⓓ F No effect on cardiac rate
Ⓔ F The treatment of choice in acute heart failure with VT

23.
- **A** F Arterial pulses are absent
- **B** T Also consider hypomagnesaemia
- **C** F Don't delay — it's easier to treat early than late
- **D** F
- **E** F Cardioversion is vital — prior lignocaine may diminish responsiveness to DC shock

24.
- **A** T Strange but true
- **B** F Ventricular fibrillation is the commonest underlying arrhythmia
- **C** T A cause of 'electro-mechanical' dissociation
- **D** F Adrenaline should be given intravenously
- **E** T

25.
- **A** T Also advise stopping smoking and excessive consumption of tea or coffee
- **B** F Ambulatory or stress ECG monitoring or electrophysiological testing may be needed
- **C** T More often used however in bradycardias
- **D** F Single drug therapy is preferable to avoid adverse effects
- **E** F Control of ischaemia or heart failure can avert the need for antiarrhythmic therapy

26.
- **A** F Prolongs the refractory period of conducting tissue; shortens it in cardiac muscle
- **B** F Often converts atrial flutter to atrial fibrillation
- **C** T
- **D** F Potentiated by hypokalaemia
- **E** T Increases myocardial excitability

27.
- **A** T Also lignocaine therapy
- **B** T Calcium channel blocking effect on smooth muscle
- **C** T
- **D** F An adverse effect of amiodarone therapy
- **E** T

28.
- **A** T E.g. lignocaine-like drugs
- **B** T
- **C** T E.g. amiodarone
- **D** T E.g. verapamil, nifedipine
- **E** T E.g. sotalol and amiodarone

29.
- **A** F Also exhibits class III activity
- **B** T
- **C** F
- **D** T
- **E** F

30.
- **A** T In common with other class III drugs
- **B** T
- **C** F Effective in both
- **D** F
- **E** F Can be safely used in heart failure

31.
- **A** T Conversely, a short PR interval produces a loud first heart sound
- **B** F Fixed PR = Mobitz type II; variable PR (Wenckebach phenomenon) = Mobitz type I
- **C** F PR intervals gradually increase
- **D** T Due to AV dissociation
- **E** F Can be narrow if the escape rhythm arises from within the bundle of His

32.
- **A** F Pacing has no effect on symptoms or prognosis
- **B** F Mobitz type II with symptoms is usually paced
- **C** T Mortality is reduced only if AV block is the underlying problem
- **D** T
- **E** F May respond to atropine and is often transient unlike in anterior infarcts

33.
Ⓐ F May result from right ventricular hypertrophy
Ⓑ F No axis shift unless associated with left bundle hemiblock
Ⓒ F Causes enhanced physiological splitting; fixed splitting suggests an ASD
Ⓓ T Causes reversed splitting
Ⓔ F Left Anterior hemiblock produces Left Axis deviation

34.
Ⓐ F Suggests cardiogenic shock
Ⓑ F Suggests septic shock
Ⓒ T
Ⓓ T Due to cerebral hypoperfusion
Ⓔ F Causes oliguria

35.
Ⓐ F Hypovolaemic shock occurs
Ⓑ T Acute right ventricular failure
Ⓒ F
Ⓓ T
Ⓔ T

36.
Ⓐ T Higher filling pressures are necessary to maintain cardiac output
Ⓑ F Pulmonary artery wedge pressure measurements are much better
Ⓒ T Heart rate and contractility are increased by high dose dopamine
Ⓓ T
Ⓔ F Occasionally used when either hypovolaemia or RV infarction is suspected

37.
Ⓐ F High flow oxygen in concentrations > 35% should be administered
Ⓑ T Also has a vasodilating effect
Ⓒ T
Ⓓ F Can safely be used with systolic pressures > 90 mmHg
Ⓔ F Both preload and afterload are reduced

38.
Ⓐ F Right atrium dilates
Ⓑ F No chamber enlargement
Ⓒ T Secondary to pulmonary hypertension
Ⓓ T Secondary to pulmonary hypertension
Ⓔ T Secondary to pulmonary hypertension

39.
Ⓐ F RV hypertrophy usually develops
Ⓑ T Due to outflow obstruction
Ⓒ F
Ⓓ F An intracardiac tumour
Ⓔ T

40.
Ⓐ T Via direct renal effects and aldosterone release
Ⓑ F Angiotensin II is more important
Ⓒ F Usually suggests free water excess
Ⓓ F Marked increase in sympathetic neural activity
Ⓔ T Occurs in response to atrial distension

41.
Ⓐ T Also reduces mortality
Ⓑ F Other factors favouring thromboembolism outweigh this effect
Ⓒ F Prognosis is unchanged
Ⓓ F Due to afterload reduction from a direct smooth muscle effect
Ⓔ F Has a modest positive inotropic effect in sinus rhythm

42.
Ⓐ F Both minor, non-specific manifestations
Ⓑ F Both minor
Ⓒ T Suggest CNS involvement and carditis
Ⓓ F Erythema marginatum is the classical rash
Ⓔ T Both are major manifestations

43.

A T First symptoms appear at valve areas of around 2 cm²

B F Occurs in only 50%

C F Produces a double right heart border and a enlarged left atrial appendage

D F Embolic risk over 10 years is 10% compared with 35% if atrial fibrillation is present

E T Mitral regurgitation is a contraindication

44.

A F Early diastolic murmurs suggest aortic or pulmonary regurgitation

B F Present only if there is severe calcification and immobility of the valve

C T Due to right ventricular hypertrophy

D F Tapping but undisplaced apex beat; displacement suggests mitral regurgitation

E F Occurs just after the second heart sound

45.

A T

B T Due to pulmonary hypertension

C F Reduced by afterload reduction e.g. ACE inhibitor therapy

D T

E T

46.

A F Typically causes aortic regurgitation

B T Due to papillary muscle or chordal damage

C T

D T Classical triad of changing murmur, fever and emboli

E T Rare cause of an acute myocarditis

47.

A F Early systolic click implies the stenosis is valvular

B F Suggests coexistent aortic regurgitation

C T Implying left ventricular hypertrophy

D T

E F Quiet S2 if the valve is heavily calcified and immobile

48.

A T Also Reiter's disease and psoriatic arthritis

B T Due to cystic medial necrosis

C T Typically affects the ascending aorta

D F Produces the 'machinery murmur'

E T Rare granulomatous arteritis of the aorta

49.

A F Austin Flint murmur due to turbulence around the anterior mitral cusp

B F Flow murmur due to an increased stroke volume

C F A left parasternal heave suggests right ventricular hypertrophy

D T Hence the increase in pulse pressure

E F Suggests severe acute regurgitation with rapid equalisation of aortic/LV pressures

50.

A F Best heard in inspiration

B F Both may cause ascites

C F A prominent 'a' wave and slow 'y' descent

D F Stenosis may produce a presystolic hepatic pulsation

E T The pulmonary valve may also be affected

51.

A F Acyanotic unless associated with a VSD and right to left shunt

B T

C F Pulmonary component of S2 is usually soft

D T Due to right ventricular hypertrophy and stenosis

E T Post-stenotic dilatation of the pulmonary artery

52.
Ⓐ T *Streptococcus viridans* alone accounts for 30–40% of cases
Ⓑ T
Ⓒ F About 30% have no identifiable predisposing cardiac lesion
Ⓓ T
Ⓔ F Vegetations may be too small to be detected

53.
Ⓐ F Sensitivity of blood cultures does not correlate well with peaks of fever
Ⓑ F Onset of therapy is best judged by illness severity
Ⓒ F Total duration of therapy should be not less than 4 weeks
Ⓓ T Also suggest abscess or drug resistance
Ⓔ T The embolic risk is high in such patients

54.
Ⓐ F Risk is decreased by oestrogen therapy
Ⓑ T Effect is measurable within 6 months of stopping
Ⓒ T Not more than 2–4 units per day
Ⓓ T
Ⓔ F Both confer increased risk

55.
Ⓐ F Usually normal
Ⓑ F Fall in BP suggests significant ischaemia
Ⓒ F False negatives may occur
Ⓓ F Useful in patients with convincing history but normal ETT
Ⓔ F Important to exclude anaemia and valvular stenosis

56.
Ⓐ F But it improves the prognosis
Ⓑ F Extensive first pass hepatic metabolism
Ⓒ T Beta blockers potentiate alpha adrenoceptor-mediated spasm
Ⓓ F A nitrate free period should be achieved
Ⓔ F All three main classes are equally efficacious

57.
Ⓐ F No effect on mortality
Ⓑ F Used to dilate graft stenoses
Ⓒ F About 55% are asymptomatic
Ⓓ T Also useful in triple vessel coronary artery disease
Ⓔ F Spontaneous improvement is common due to the growth of a collateral circulation

58.
Ⓐ F Frequently occurs de novo
Ⓑ T Should therefore be actively managed
Ⓒ T
Ⓓ F Exercise testing must be deferred until symptoms have settled
Ⓔ F Usually resolves with therapy but angioplasty and surgery may become necessary

59.
Ⓐ T Due to activation of the autonomic nervous system
Ⓑ T
Ⓒ T Suggests a large infarct
Ⓓ T
Ⓔ T 15% of infarcts are believed to be clinically 'silent'

60.
Ⓐ T Both could occur in response to pain and anxiety
Ⓑ F Pericarditis is unusual in the first 12 hours
Ⓒ F Suggests an inferior myocardial infarction
Ⓓ T Suggests left ventricular impairment
Ⓔ F Suggests infarction occurred more than 12 hours ago

61.
Ⓐ T Vascular events are reduced by 25%
Ⓑ F
Ⓒ F
Ⓓ T Limits infarct expansion
Ⓔ T Reduces mortality by 25%

62.
Ⓐ F The risk-benefit ratio of thrombolytic therapy patients > 80 years is unknown
Ⓑ F More beneficial if ST elevation is present
Ⓒ T
Ⓓ F Should be administered on basis of ECG and clinical impression
Ⓔ T Much more antigenic than genetically-engineered thrombolytic agents

63.
Ⓐ T 30% reduction in short-term mortality
Ⓑ T The earlier thrombolysis is given the better the results
Ⓒ T Intramuscular injections predispose to haematoma
Ⓓ F Similarly, nitrate therapy has no effect on the early mortality rate
Ⓔ F Mobilisation should begin on day 2 in the absence of cardiac failure

64.
Ⓐ F Only if symptoms are associated
Ⓑ F Suppressing ectopic beats has no effect on subsequent VF rate or survival
Ⓒ F May respond to thrombolysis, atropine or resolve spontaneously
Ⓓ F Cardioversion should immediately follow a praecordial thump
Ⓔ T More likely to be successful than drug treatment

65.
Ⓐ T 50% occur within 2 hours
Ⓑ F Late VF has a poorer prognosis
Ⓒ T Rehabilitation programmes can be helpful
Ⓓ T
Ⓔ T Limiting infarct size improves prognosis

66.
Ⓐ F Early studies established a link between mortality and a single BP reading
Ⓑ F Elevated systolic BP is associated with increased cardiovascular mortality
Ⓒ T
Ⓓ T
Ⓔ F Only 5% have secondary hypertension

67.
Ⓐ F In contrast to coarctation of the aorta
Ⓑ T Conn's syndrome
Ⓒ T
Ⓓ T Also pregnancy
Ⓔ F In contrast to hypothyroidism

68.
Ⓐ F Suggests connective tissue disease
Ⓑ F Suggests coarctation of the aorta
Ⓒ F A non-specific finding in hypertension
Ⓓ F Suggests renal artery stenosis
Ⓔ F Suggests polycystic kidney disease

69.
Ⓐ F Arteriolar thickening, irregularity and tortuosity are detectable
Ⓑ T
Ⓒ T Hypertension predisposes to atheroma formation
Ⓓ T
Ⓔ F Also intracerebral and subarachnoid haemorrhage

70.
Ⓐ F Hypokalaemic alkalosis suggests this diagnosis
Ⓑ F Exclusion requires renal arteriography or radionuclide renography
Ⓒ F Urinary VMA is measured in suspected phaeochromocytoma
Ⓓ T To detect renal disease or coexistent diabetes
Ⓔ T Other causes are rare

71.
A F Occurs in many hypertensives
B F Indicates LVH
C T
D T Papilloedema may occur
E T Mortality is 80% untreated

72.
A F Rapid reduction is more dangerous than beneficial
B F If used, the dose must be carefully titrated to response
C F Sublingual nifedipine may be effective
D T Such as frusemide, nifedipine or sodium nitroprusside
E F Impair renal function given bilateral disease

73.
A T
B F Smoking is the most important remediable risk factor
C F
D F Good evidence of efficacy in the elderly
E T Excessive consumption is a significant factor in 10–15% of hypertensives

74.
A T
B T Common particularly in asymptomatic patients
C T But rare
D T Conn's syndrome is suggested by a hyperkalaemic alkalosis
E T May also develop during follow-up

75.
A T Chronically elevated left atrial pressure
B T Increased pulmonary flow
C T Increased pulmonary vascular resistance
D T Increased pulmonary vascular resistance
E T Increased pulmonary flow

76.
A F Commoner in females
B T Symptoms appear late
C F
D T Also found in other types of pulmonary hypertension
E T The Graham Steell murmur of pulmonary regurgitation

77.
A T With profound hypoxaemia
B F Suggests pulmonary infarction
C T Non-specific
D T Non-specific
E F Classical ECG pattern is S_1, Q_3, T_3

78.
A T Sometimes difficult to differentiate from pneumonia
B T May be evanescent
C T
D T Cavitation of necrotic lung tissue
E T Detectable clinically or on chest X-ray

79.
A F Unhelpful except in acute massive embolism
B F High flow, high concentration oxygen is indicated
C F May further lower the blood pressure
D T Continue heparin until the prothrombin ratio (INR) is stable
E F Continue for 3 months

80.
A T
B F ECG changes are non-specific
C T Especially adriamycin and daunorubicin
D T
E T Also influenza, HIV and others

81.
A T Heart failure and a small heart
B T Systolic function is well preserved
C T Amyloid can also cause a dilated cardiomyopathy
D T Hypereosinophilic syndrome — Loeffler's endocarditis
E F Heart is usually of normal size

82.

A T   But previous ischaemic heart disease may all be silent

B F   Suggests a previous anterior myocardial infarct as the cause

C T

D F   Regional dyskinesis suggests underlying coronary artery disease

E T   Non-specific

83.

A T   50% of cases are autosomal dominant

B T   Mimicking aortic stenosis

C T

D T   LV outflow obstruction and secondary mitral regurgitation

E F   Suggests calcific aortic stenosis

84.

A F   Sharp pain worsened by posture and movement

B F   Localisation and character vary greatly

C T   In contrast to ischaemia — convex upwards

D F   May occur if in pericarditis complicating acute myocardial infarction

E F   Widespread ECG changes

85.

A T   Also other malignant diseases

B T   Also other connective tissue diseases

C F   coxsackie B

D T   Rare in the UK

E F   Causes fetal cardiac disease in pregnant females

86.

A F   Left heart failure is unusual

B T   But pericardial calcification may be seen

C F   Often no relevant previous history of disease

D T   Classical features

E T   With 'systolic collapse' of the JVP

87.

A F   With a left to right shunt

B T   Usually due to a shunt through a VSD

C F   No shunt

D T   Right to left shunt through a VSD

E F   Left to right shunt

88.

A F   Only happens if the shunt reverses

B F   Typically presents with a murmur in an otherwise healthy infant

C F   Continuous 'machinery' murmur is typical (systolic and diastolic)

D T   A rare sign

E T

89.

A T   Frequently coexists

B F   Cardiac failure is more likely to develop in infancy

C T   A useful but unusual finding

D T   Rib notching is due to enlarged collateral vessels

E F   Left not right ventricular hypertrophy develops

90.

A T   Due to a patent fossa ovalis

B F   Occurs late, and rarely

C F   Splitting is fixed and wide

D T   In primum defect there may be left axis deviation

E F   Surgery is indicated when the pulmonary/systolic flow ratio is > 3/2

91.

A F   Pansystolic

B F   No cardiomegaly

C T   Prophylaxis is indicated

D F   Surgery only indicated if right sided pressures rise

E T   Symptomless murmur is a frequent presentation

92.
A T Right-sided pressures exceed left-sided pressures
B F Pulmonary changes are irreversible
C F CXR shows enlarged central pulmonary arteries
D T Classical
E F May change dramatically or disappear

93.
A F No aortic stenosis
B T Cyanosis may be absent; clubbing develops later
C F A single component to the second heart sound
D F ECG shows RVH; CXR shows small pulmonary arteries and a 'boot-shaped heart'
E F Due to adrenergically mediated increase in RV outflow obstruction

94.
A F Increase of 30–50%
B T Masking or mimicking underlying heart disease
C T Vascular resistance declines
D T 'Flow' murmur
E T

95.
A T Increased coagulability
B T Increased coagulability
C T Due to venous stasis
D T Low cardiac output and immobility
E T Increased coagulability

96.
A F Suggests acute arterial insufficiency
B T Clinical signs are frequently absent
C T Marked erythema might suggest cellulitis
D T
E T Suggesting pulmonary embolism

97.
A F Rest relieves but elevation worsens pain
B F Painless ulcers suggest underlying diabetes
C F Anaemia or diabetes may produce claudication without loss of the pulses
D F Exercise promotes growth of the collateral circulation
E F Anticoagulation is unhelpful

98.
A T Unopposed alpha-adrenoceptor mediated vasospasm
B T Immune complexes form in peripheral vessels
C T And other connective tissue diseases
D T
E F

99.
A T Causing cerebral, limb or mesenteric ischaemia
B T If there is shunt reversal
C T Due to mural thrombus
D T May produce mycotic aneurysms
E T Only if there is LV dilatation and failure

100.
A F Suggests deep venous thrombosis
B F Suggests pulmonary embolism
C T
D T Suggesting ischaemic colitis
E T Suggesting stroke

101.
A T Tissue collagen is abnormal
B T Hypertension predisposes
C T
D F No association
E T

102.
A T Type A aneurysms
B T Due to infarction of the spinal cord
C T The pain is often described as 'tearing'
D T Type A aneurysms
E T Haemothorax

103.
Ⓐ T
Ⓑ F   Describes Grade 2
Ⓒ F   Describes Grade 3
Ⓓ T
Ⓔ T

10.4
Ⓐ F   'Artifact' due to transmission of carotid artery pulsation
Ⓑ T   Absent in atrial fibrillation
Ⓒ F   Peak pressure prior to opening of the tricuspid valve
Ⓓ T
Ⓔ T   Onset of ventricular filling

105.
Ⓐ F   Records falsely higher BP measurements
Ⓑ T
Ⓒ F   Disappearance of the sound marks phase V diastolic pressure
Ⓓ F   Hence the need to record and use phase V as the diastolic pressure
Ⓔ F   Random BP measurements correlate well with cardiovascular risk

106.
Ⓐ F   Proceeds from endocardium to epicardium
Ⓑ F   Produces a negative deflection
Ⓒ T   Absent in left BBB
Ⓓ T   Hence the predominant S wave as depolarisation moves away from AVR
Ⓔ T   An aid to the diagnosis of left ventricular hypertrophy

6 DISEASES OF THE RESPIRATORY SYSTEM

1.
Ⓐ F   Peripheral cyanosis
Ⓑ T   Often with crepitations
Ⓒ T   Usually without hypoxaemia
Ⓓ F   Peripheral cyanosis
Ⓔ T   If there is respiratory failure

2.
Ⓐ F   Never causes finger clubbing
Ⓑ T   Also chronic suppurative pulmonary infections
Ⓒ T   Also chronic malabsorptive diseases
Ⓓ T   Unlike extrinsic allergic alveolitis
Ⓔ F   Can occur in cyanotic congenital heart disease

3.
Ⓐ F   A congenital skeletal deformity
Ⓑ T   AP diameter is normally less than the lateral diameter
Ⓒ F   Cricosternal distance is reduced
Ⓓ T   Also use of other accessory muscles
Ⓔ T   The normal angle is acute

4.
Ⓐ F   Expansion is reduced on the affected side
Ⓑ F   Stony dull
Ⓒ T   Often an area of bronchial breath sounds
Ⓓ T   As is vocal fremitus
Ⓔ F   Sometimes heard above the effusion

5.
Ⓐ T   Particularly if there is associated pleuritic pain
Ⓑ T   But not stony dull
Ⓒ F   Bronchial breath sounds
Ⓓ T   With whispering pectoriloquy
Ⓔ F   There may be crepitations alone

6.
Ⓐ T   On the affected side
Ⓑ F   Implies effusion
Ⓒ F   Diminished or absent
Ⓓ T   As for vocal fremitus
Ⓔ F   No specific added sounds

7.
Ⓐ T   But often normal in small pneumothorax
Ⓑ F   Or hyperresonant
Ⓒ F   Typically diminished or absent
Ⓓ F   Reduced or absent
Ⓔ T

8.
Ⓐ F   Due to arterial hypoxaemia
Ⓑ F   Chest wall compliance is reduced
Ⓒ T   Increased resistance to airflow
Ⓓ T   Lung volume is reduced
Ⓔ T   Ventilatory capacity is reduced

9.
Ⓐ F   Separates middle from upper
Ⓑ F   Aspiration is commoner on the right
Ⓒ T
Ⓓ T   To around the 6th costal cartilage
Ⓔ F   By type II pneumocytes

10.
Ⓐ F   About 7.5 L/min
Ⓑ T   Dead space ventilation is about 2.5 L/min
Ⓒ F   About 5 L/min
Ⓓ T
Ⓔ T   Ventilation/perfusion ratio varies from the base to apex

11.
Ⓐ T Chest wall compliance is reduced
Ⓑ F Non-elastic resistance is increased
Ⓒ F Non-elastic resistance is increased
Ⓓ T Pulmonary compliance is reduced
Ⓔ F Non-elastic resistance is increased

12.
Ⓐ F Sensitivity is increased
Ⓑ F Also peripheral chemoreceptors
Ⓒ F Also sensitive to arterial PCO_2
Ⓓ F Such patients are dependent on 'hypoxic drive'
Ⓔ T

13.
Ⓐ F Hyperventilation unless embolism is massive
Ⓑ T With type II respiratory failure
Ⓒ F Hyperventilation
Ⓓ F Hyperventilation and type I failure
Ⓔ T Type II respiratory failure may ensue

14.
Ⓐ F More than 70% is normal
Ⓑ F Carbon monoxide is used
Ⓒ T The lungs are hyperinflated
Ⓓ T A restrictive disorder may develop
Ⓔ F They measure obstructive ventilatory defects

15.
Ⓐ T Also cutaneous venodilatation
Ⓑ T Progressing to coma
Ⓒ F Skin is warm
Ⓓ T Due to vasodilatation
Ⓔ T And flapping tremor are probably due to hypoxia

16.
Ⓐ F Typically type II failure
Ⓑ F Respiratory muscle paralysis causes type II failure
Ⓒ T Arterial PCO_2 is typically normal
Ⓓ T Ventilatory drive is usually maintained
Ⓔ F Causes acute type II failure — asphyxia

17.
Ⓐ T Causes alveolar hypoventilation
Ⓑ T Paralysis of respiratory muscles
Ⓒ F Causes hypoxaemia alone
Ⓓ F Type I respiratory failure
Ⓔ F Arterial PCO_2 rises in the later stages of severe attacks

18.
Ⓐ T kPa of oxygen declines with altitude
Ⓑ F Indicated when PO_2 < 7.3 breathing air
Ⓒ T Also in other situations when Hb is maximally saturated
Ⓓ F Occurs only in neonates
Ⓔ T Such shunts may be extra- or intrapulmonary

19.
Ⓐ F High concentrations of oxygen are contraindicated
Ⓑ T Aids controlled delivery of oxygen concentrations < 30%
Ⓒ T Useful for controlled oxygen therapy
Ⓓ F Humidification is only required with high concentration masks
Ⓔ F Can occur after > 24 hours of > 40% oxygen

20.
Ⓐ F Cardiac output often falls
Ⓑ T Improves oxygenation in atelectatic areas
Ⓒ F A tightly fitting face or nasal mask can be used
Ⓓ F Can occur with all forms of mechanical ventilation
Ⓔ T

21.
Ⓐ F Controlled oxygen therapy is best given by Ventimask or nasal cannulae
Ⓑ F A central respiratory stimulant
Ⓒ F Depresses respiration and can impair expectoration
Ⓓ F May help relieve bronchospasm
Ⓔ T In patients with cor pulmonale and chronic bronchitis

22.
A F There is a protein rich pulmonary exudate
B T A systemic upset and multi-organ failure
C F Crepitations are typical
D T 'Ground glass' appearance on CXR due to alveolar oedema
E T But not in all cases

23.
A F Parainfluenza 1,2,3
B F Typically *H. Influenzae*
C T May also cause pneumonia
D F Influenza A, B, RSV and parainfluenza
E T

24.
A T Immunisation offers limited protection therefore
B F 1–3 days
C T Occasionally
D T Also bronchiolitis, bronchopneumonia and secondary bacterial infection
E T May be rapidly progressive and fatal

25.
A T May mimic coryza
B T Or *haemophilus influenzae*
C T With stridor or dyspnoea
D T
E F Crepitations suggest a lower respiratory tract disease

26.
A T With headache, anorexia and myalgia
B F Early and middle adult life
C F Signs of consolidation e.g. bronchial breath sounds dominate
D T Bacteraemia and WCC > 20 000 are associated with a poorer prognosis
E T May accompany other acute febrile illnesses

27.
A F
B T Myocarditis is rare
C T Septicaemic shock has a poor prognosis
D T Consider the possibility if stony dullness develops
E F Subphrenic abscess may cause pleural effusion or empyema

28.
A T Sputum and blood cultures are therefore mandatory
B T A form of suppurative pneumonia
C T May be rapidly progressive in this situation
D T Lung infection may be a secondary phenomenon
E T Flucloxacillin or erythromycin are indicated

29.
A F Consolidation and sometimes cavitation
B T
C T May be blood-stained
D F Ceftazidime and ciprofloxacin are also valuable
E F More often associated with pre-existing ill health e.g. alcoholics

30.
A T Classically barracks
B T Anaemia is rarely severe, but may suggest diagnosis
C T In contrast to pneumococcal pneumonia
D T In contrast to bacterial pneumonias
E T Drugs of choice

31.
A F Transmitted in inhaled water droplets
B T Gastrointestinal symptoms should suggest the diagnosis
C T More frequently than in other pneumonic illnesses
D T In contrast to 'typical' bacterial pneumonia
E T Continue for at least 14 days

32.
Ⓐ T
Ⓑ T Chest X-ray is mandatory in a febrile patient
Ⓒ F More common in pneumococcal infection
Ⓓ T Leucopenia can occur in severe pneumococcal infection
Ⓔ T Rare in pneumococcal disease

33.
Ⓐ T Used in higher dosage 120 mg/kg/day
Ⓑ T
Ⓒ T Useful but not always curative
Ⓓ T Or famciclovir
Ⓔ T

34.
Ⓐ F Occurs at the extremes of life
Ⓑ T Often with *Staph. aureus*
Ⓒ F Leucocytosis is typical
Ⓓ F Suggests lobar pneumonia
Ⓔ T Particularly in severe childhood infection

35.
Ⓐ T Suggested by chronic purulent sputum and localised crackles
Ⓑ F Typically lobar or segmental
Ⓒ T As does persisting partial bronchial occlusion without collapse
Ⓓ T But it may be mimimal or absent
Ⓔ T Particularly in aspiration of gastric contents

36.
Ⓐ T Bacteria secondarily infect the damaged pulmonary tissue
Ⓑ T Producing lobar collapse or impaired secretion clearance
Ⓒ T Systemic upset is marked
Ⓓ F Obstruction typically produces signs of collapse
Ⓔ T An air-fluid level may be apparent

37.
Ⓐ F Older ages predominate
Ⓑ T Also other immunocompromised patients
Ⓒ T *Mycobacterium bovis* is now rare
Ⓓ T Due to immunosuppression
Ⓔ F Reactivation of dormant infection is more common

38.
Ⓐ F Typically symptomless
Ⓑ T Mediastinal, cervical or mesenteric nodes are most frequently involved
Ⓒ F Suggests sarcoidosis
Ⓓ T Can also accompany pulmonary sarcoid
Ⓔ F A hypersensitivity phenomenon typically associated with positive tuberculin test

39.
Ⓐ T Onset may be sudden or insidious
Ⓑ T Pancytopenia or a leukaemoid reaction
Ⓒ T But chest X-ray is usually abnormal
Ⓓ T Respiratory symptoms may also be minimal
Ⓔ T Positive urine, sputum or marrow cultures may be obtained

40.
Ⓐ F Sputum is typically smear-positive
Ⓑ T But any lobe may be affected
Ⓒ T In contrast to primary disease
Ⓓ F Unusual
Ⓔ T Pathognomonic

41.
Ⓐ T Superinfection of a cavity
Ⓑ T Associated with chronic immune stimulation
Ⓒ T Due to haematogenous dissemination
Ⓓ T Suggested by chronic productive cough
Ⓔ T Due to vertebral or paraspinal abscess formation

42.
A F False negatives may occur
B T Between 2 and 4 days
C T Implies active or previous infection
D F Diffuse skin induration and perhaps necrosis
E F False positives may occur

43.
A T Minimises resistance and reduces duration of treatment
B F Patients can be regarded as non-infectious after 1 week of therapy
C F 6 and 9 month regimes are of proven efficacy
D F Hence their great value in the treatment of TB meningitis
E F More often due to non-compliance

44.
A F Causes vestibular disturbance and deafness
B F Polyneuropathy
C F Ethambutol causes optic neuritis
D T As may rifampicin
E F Streptomycin causes this

45.
A F Unless there is a recent contact history without previous immunisation
B T Isoniazid for 12 months
C T Pre-emptive therapy prevents the onset of refractory active TB in AIDS
D T Reduces the risk of miliary TB or TB meningitis
E T Providing there has been no previous TB immunisation

46.
A F No association
B T Usually in a tuberculous cavity
C T A severe, rapidly progressive illness
D T Typically with wheeze, pulmonary infiltrates and peripheral eosinophilia
E F Type III and IV immune responses

47.
A F Immediate hypersensitivity reaction
B T With rhinorrhea and nasal obstruction
C F The discharge is watery
D T Permitting precise allergen identification
E T Oral antihistamines and topical steroids may also help

48.
A T Allergic rhinitis or eczema may coexist
B F Unusual but skin tests may usefully establish atopy
C T Sometimes without obvious precipitant
D T Such as asthma, allergic rhinitis or eczema
E F Its presence might suggest allergic bronchopulmonary aspergillosis

49.
A F Occurs in non-smokers also
B F Atopy is absent
C T As can infection
D T Contrast to early-onset disease
E T Keeping with the absence of atopy

50.
A T But bradycardia may occur in life-threatening attacks
B F Usually < 50% of expected PEFR
C T But may diminish in severe attacks
D F $PaO_2 < 8kPa$
E T $PaCO_2$ may remain normal until the late stages

51.
A F High concentration, high flow should be used
B T Intravenous beta$_2$-adrenoceptor agonists can also be used
C F Of no proven value in acute attacks
D T Maintain corticosteroid therapy for at least 7 days in severe attacks
E T Exclude pneumothorax and ventilatory failure

52.
- **Ⓐ T**
- **Ⓑ T** And elevated total serum IgE
- **Ⓒ F** *Aspergillus fumigatus*
- **Ⓓ T** Transient pulmonary infiltrates may also be seen
- **Ⓔ T** Chronic low-dose steroid therapy may be necessary

53.
- **Ⓐ T** May be associated with myasthenia gravis
- **Ⓑ T** Anterior superior mediastinum
- **Ⓒ F** Pulmonary apical mass
- **Ⓓ T** Retrocardiac opacity
- **Ⓔ T** Can be multiple

54.
- **Ⓐ F** Suggests vocal cord paralysis
- **Ⓑ T** Obstruction may supervene
- **Ⓒ F** A cause of hoarseness
- **Ⓓ T** Due to left recurrent laryngeal palsy
- **Ⓔ T** Voice may remain impaired

55.
- **Ⓐ T** And toxocara infestation
- **Ⓑ F** Eosinophilia is necessary for the diagnosis
- **Ⓒ F** Wheeze may be absent
- **Ⓓ T** Or imipramine or phenylbutazone
- **Ⓔ T** Pulmonary infiltrates and eosinophilia (PIE)

56.
- **Ⓐ F** Acute dyspnoea without wheeze is characteristic
- **Ⓑ T** Flu-like symptoms may exist
- **Ⓒ T** Typically bilateral
- **Ⓓ F** Airway obstruction is absent
- **Ⓔ T** Also may be positive in healthy subjects

57.
- **Ⓐ F** Residual volume increases
- **Ⓑ F** Decreased TCO suggests coexistent emphysema
- **Ⓒ F** Mucus secretion is increased
- **Ⓓ F** Reduced FEV/FVC ratio
- **Ⓔ F** Symptoms for at least 3 consecutive months for at least 2 successive years

58.
- **Ⓐ F** Usually associated with chronic bronchitis
- **Ⓑ F** Respiratory failure is usually a late complication
- **Ⓒ T** In contrast with uncomplicated chronic bronchitis
- **Ⓓ T** Cough predominates in chronic bronchitis
- **Ⓔ T** But very rare

59.
- **Ⓐ F** Most obvious in expiration
- **Ⓑ T** Tracheal 'tug' due to mediastinal descent
- **Ⓒ T** A sign of hyperinflation
- **Ⓓ T** And other accessory respiratory muscles
- **Ⓔ F** Often no added sounds

60.
- **Ⓐ T** Suggesting pulmonary hypertension
- **Ⓑ T** A sign of hyperinflation
- **Ⓒ F** Peripheral vessels may be attenuated
- **Ⓓ F** Sign of left ventricular failure
- **Ⓔ F** Signs of left ventricular failure

61.
- **Ⓐ T** Predisposes to recurrent infection
- **Ⓑ T** Infected secretions accumulate distal to obstruction
- **Ⓒ T** Ciliary dysfunction and recurrent infection
- **Ⓓ T** Mucus plugging of airways
- **Ⓔ F**

62.
- **Ⓐ F** Copious sputum production
- **Ⓑ T** Recurrent pneumonia
- **Ⓒ T** Secondary to inflammatory bronchial change
- **Ⓓ T** Complicating pneumonia
- **Ⓔ T** In the presence of large amounts of secretions

63.
Ⓐ T At least
Ⓑ F Occasionally used if the affected area is confined to one lobe
Ⓒ F Only if accompanied by increased volume and signs of infection
Ⓓ T Or bronchography to demonstrate the extent of disease
Ⓔ T Respiratory reserve will be impaired

64.
Ⓐ T Often termed 'obstructive emphysema'
Ⓑ F Not if there is obstructive emphysema
Ⓒ T Infection occurs with variable frequency
Ⓓ T Clinical signs may be subtle
Ⓔ F Right main bronchus is more vertically aligned

65.
Ⓐ F Young males or females
Ⓑ T Extremely rare
Ⓒ T Tumours are vascular
Ⓓ T Due to bronchial obstruction
Ⓔ T Due to bronchial obstruction

66.
Ⓐ F 50% of all male cancer deaths
Ⓑ F Streaking of sputum with blood in a smoker is more typical
Ⓒ F Squamous 50%, adenocarcinoma 15%
Ⓓ T As is mesothelioma
Ⓔ T The major aetiological factor

67.
Ⓐ F 10% are surgically treatable
Ⓑ F Endobronchial lesions may be clinically silent
Ⓒ F Only applies to resected squamous carcinoma
Ⓓ F Cytology may be obtained from sputum or metastatic tissue
Ⓔ F More often absent with small cell type

68.
Ⓐ T With ataxia and nystagmus
Ⓑ T 'Eaton–Lambert' syndrome
Ⓒ T Usually bilateral
Ⓓ T Usually distal sensorimotor
Ⓔ T Skin rash and proximal myopathy

69.
Ⓐ T Also seen in CLL and Hodgkin's lymphoma
Ⓑ T Hyponatraemia is often the clue
Ⓒ T Hypokalaemia, pigmentation and proximal myopathy
Ⓓ F Malignant hypercalcaemia is usually caused by bony metastases not PTH
Ⓔ F Typically peripheral squamous cell tumours

70.
Ⓐ F Typically Type I respiratory failure
Ⓑ T With or without evidence of connective tissue disease
Ⓒ T But not in extrinsic allergic alveolitis
Ⓓ F Dyspnoea, dry cough and crackles
Ⓔ T But this is not completely specific

71.
Ⓐ F Does not progress in the absence of PMF
Ⓑ F Depends on radiological features
Ⓒ T May cavitate
Ⓓ T Usually due to smoking
Ⓔ F Frequently no specific signs

72.
Ⓐ T Typically upper zone changes
Ⓑ T Specific but not highly sensitive
Ⓒ F Continues to progress despite reduced exposure
Ⓓ T Caplan's syndrome
Ⓔ T But now rare

73.
Ⓐ F Often calcify
Ⓑ F But do raise the suspicion of malignancy
Ⓒ T Although cryptogenic fibrosing alveolitis is possible
Ⓓ F A restrictive not an obstructive ventilatory defect
Ⓔ F Seldom necessary

74.
Ⓐ F Cotton dust produces byssinosis, mouldy sugar cane produces bagassosis
Ⓑ T Fungal antigens *Micropolyspora faeni*
Ⓒ F Tin produces stannosis, siderosis results from iron oxide
Ⓓ T Usually pigeons or budgies
Ⓔ F Produces malt worker's lung

75.
Ⓐ F Caseating granulomata e.g. TB are associated with cavitation
Ⓑ F Typically negative
Ⓒ F Erythema nodosum is the typical skin lesion
Ⓓ F The normal course in Stage 1 and 2 disease
Ⓔ F Due to increased vitamin D sensitivity

76.
Ⓐ T Usually bilateral
Ⓑ T Typically the seventh nerve
Ⓒ T Or uveitis
Ⓓ F Non-erosive arthropathy or bone cysts
Ⓔ T Or lacrimal or other salivary glands

77.
Ⓐ F Transudate in CCF
Ⓑ T Sometimes bloodstained or with eosinophils
Ⓒ T Most frequently on the right
Ⓓ T With polymorphonuclear leucocytes
Ⓔ F Severe hypoalbuminaemia produces transudates

78.
Ⓐ T Stony dull percussion and impaired voice transmission
Ⓑ F An exudate is more likely to be associated with malignancy
Ⓒ F An effusion may be the sole X-ray finding
Ⓓ F May be seen in rheumatoid disease and SLE
Ⓔ T Fluid is rich in chylomicrons

79.
Ⓐ F Typically unilateral
Ⓑ T Or a recent diagnostic aspiration
Ⓒ T Suggests lung abscess, antibiotic resistance or hypersensitivity
Ⓓ T Perhaps complicating subphrenic infection
Ⓔ F Frequently sterile post-antibiotic therapy

80.
Ⓐ T A small pneumothorax may be asymptomatic
Ⓑ F Diminished or absent breath sounds
Ⓒ F Mediastinal shift suggests tension
Ⓓ T Pleurectomy may also be necessary
Ⓔ T Particularly if bilateral

7 DISEASES OF THE ALIMENTARY TRACT AND PANCREAS

1.

Ⓐ F Gastrointestinal peptides also play a role

Ⓑ T Cricopharyngeus muscle is tonically contracted

Ⓒ T Via the enteric plexuses

Ⓓ T Drugs, acute systemic illness or mechanical obstruction may cause delayed transit

Ⓔ F Liquid emptying is only slightly impaired

2.

Ⓐ T E.g. vasoactive intestinal peptide and substance P

Ⓑ F Anticipatory centrally mediated secretory phase

Ⓒ T And thence to the myenteric and submucous plexuses

Ⓓ F Generally stimulatory

Ⓔ F Autonomic nervous system is also involved

3.

Ⓐ T An important defence mechanism

Ⓑ T Synthesized by B lymphocytes

Ⓒ T With chylomicrons and lipoproteins

Ⓓ F Actively absorbed throughout the entire small intestine

Ⓔ T Most of the water ingested is absorbed in the small bowel

4.

Ⓐ T And other skin disorders such as pemphigus

Ⓑ F The tongue and buccal mucosa are spared

Ⓒ T The Stevens–Johnson syndrome when mucosal involvement is predominant

Ⓓ T Herpes simplex type 1 infection can be severe in the immunocompromised

Ⓔ T Oral thrush can be severe in AIDS or in patients on corticosteroid therapy

5.

Ⓐ T Via formation of an oesophageal web — 'sideropenic dysphagia'

Ⓑ T May also be associated with regurgitation and recurrent aspiration

Ⓒ F Asymptomatic unless complicated by malignancy

Ⓓ T But stroke and Parkinsonism are more common neurological causes

Ⓔ F South American trypanosomiasis — Chagas' disease

6.

Ⓐ F May be hazardous, particularly if a pouch is not suspected

Ⓑ T Due to aspiration and/or airway compression

Ⓒ F Typically presents in later life

Ⓓ T Due to aspiration

Ⓔ F Dysphagia only progresses very slowly

7.
Ⓐ T A feature of iron deficiency
Ⓑ F Hypochlorhydria may be associated with impaired iron absorption
Ⓒ T A rare association of iron deficiency
Ⓓ F but dysphagia is occasionally functional
Ⓔ F Post-cricoid web

8.
Ⓐ T Due to regurgitation and aspiration
Ⓑ F Failure to relax the LOS with loss of ganglion cells in Auerbach's plexus on histology
Ⓒ F Acid reflux is prevented by the non-relaxing lower oesophageal sphincter
Ⓓ T Even if the obstruction is treated
Ⓔ T If this fails cardiomyotomy may be indicated

9.
Ⓐ F Oesophagogastric hiatus hernia is more common
Ⓑ F Tends not to occur given the normal position of the LOS
Ⓒ F Epigastric pain and postprandial fullness are typical
Ⓓ F The lower oesophageal sphincter is normal
Ⓔ F But can be complicated by volvulus of the stomach

10.
Ⓐ T
Ⓑ F Typical symptoms are those of acid reflux
Ⓒ F Most are asymptomatic and do not have reflux oesophagitis
Ⓓ F May occur with reflux oesophagitis alone
Ⓔ F Surgery is rarely required given the efficacy of medical therapy

11.
Ⓐ T There is oesophageal muscular hypertrophy and degenerative change in the vagus nerves
Ⓑ T But presentation can be at any age
Ⓒ T Emotion may precipitate contraction
Ⓓ F Uncoordinated contractions per se may cause dysphagia
Ⓔ F Only if the contractions are associated with acid reflux

12.
Ⓐ T
Ⓑ F 80–90% are squamous cell
Ⓒ F Dysphagia is typically well localised
Ⓓ F 90% are in the lower two thirds
Ⓔ T And betel nut chewing in the East

13.
Ⓐ F More suggestive of reflux with oesophagitis and stricture formation
Ⓑ T Usually slowly progressive
Ⓒ F Early weight loss relates to poor intake
Ⓓ T To lymph nodes, liver and mediastinum
Ⓔ F 5 year survival is about 5%

14.
Ⓐ F
Ⓑ F May play a role in benign gastric ulcer
Ⓒ F Associated with hypochlorhydria — 'no acid, no ulcer'
Ⓓ T Implicated in > 90% of cases
Ⓔ T Associated with both gastric and duodenal ulcer recurrence rates

15.
Ⓐ T Hunger pain
Ⓑ T Perhaps with the 'pointing sign'
Ⓒ T Pain is characteristically periodic
Ⓓ F More suggestive of gastro-oesophageal reflux disease
Ⓔ T Relieved by antacid or food

16.
ⓐ F Symptoms correlate poorly with disease activity
ⓑ T Tobacco also has an aetiological role
ⓒ F No specific dietary advice is required
ⓓ T Biopsy helps exclude or confirm malignancy
ⓔ F Suggests either reflux dyspepsia or persistent peptic ulceration due to *H. pylori* infection

17.
ⓐ F Only about 20%; most have reflux dyspepsia or functional dyspepsia
ⓑ F 85% relapse if HP has not been eradicated
ⓒ F Cause diarrhoea; aluminium-containing antacids cause constipation
ⓓ T Due to potential accumulation of bismuth, acid-lowering drugs are preferable
ⓔ T 35% of all gastric ulcers are **not** associated with HP, most of which are NSAID-induced

18.
ⓐ T Gastric ulcer 20%, varices 10%
ⓑ T Higher mortality in the elderly and especially in patients who re-bleed
ⓒ T Cushing's stress ulcers
ⓓ T Diagnostic yield reduces with time post admission
ⓔ T 75% of patients with GI bleed have recently taken NSAIDs cf. 50% of 'control' patients

19.
ⓐ F Typically pain-free
ⓑ T Sympathetic nervous activation
ⓒ T Particularly in older patients
ⓓ F Blood urea may rise due to digestion of the blood in the gut
ⓔ F Only present if preceding iron deficiency

20.
ⓐ F A sign of hypovolaemia
ⓑ F Bradycardia may occur in profound blood loss
ⓒ F Haemoglobin level is normal until haemodilution occurs
ⓓ F May be useful in patients with GI bleeding without haematemesis
ⓔ T Patients should first be haemodynamically stable if possible

21.
ⓐ F Sometimes necessary but can be hazardous in patients with liver disease
ⓑ F Colloid infusion and packed red cells are adequate for volume replacement
ⓒ T Crystalloids rapidly redistribute to the extravascular space
ⓓ T Facilitates restoration and monitoring of optimal circulating volume
ⓔ F Consider surgical options in all patients with continuing major bleeding

22.
ⓐ F 25% occur in acute ulcers
ⓑ T Especially anterior wall ulcers
ⓒ F Symptoms depend on peritoneal soiling
ⓓ F Vomiting is common
ⓔ T But abdominal rigidity typically persists

23.
ⓐ F Hypokalaemic metabolic alkalosis
ⓑ F Suggests more distal obstruction
ⓒ T Paradoxical aciduria due to renal tubular mechanisms
ⓓ T Unusually, patients may feel like eating immediately after vomiting
ⓔ F Often prominent peristaltic waves from left to right across the epigastrium

24.
Ⓐ F Tumour is usually in the pancreas or duodenum
Ⓑ T 50% of tumours have metastasised at presentation
Ⓒ T Occur in one third of patients
Ⓓ F 40% have diarrhoea not constipation
Ⓔ T Acid secretion is already maximally stimulated

25.
Ⓐ F 10–20 years or longer post surgery
Ⓑ T Perhaps due to small stomach syndrome
Ⓒ F Iron absorption is partly dependent on gastric acidity
Ⓓ T Vitamin B_{12} deficiency may also occur
Ⓔ F Only in the stagnant loop syndrome

26.
Ⓐ F Symptoms develop within 30 minutes
Ⓑ F Liquid emptying is more rapid
Ⓒ F Due to the release of GI hormones and neurotransmitters not hypoglycaemia
Ⓓ T Avoidance of fluids at meals may help
Ⓔ F Suggests hypoglycaemia characterising late dumping

27.
Ⓐ T May also cause peptic ulceration
Ⓑ F Barium meal is unhelpful
Ⓒ T Acute mucosal injury
Ⓓ T And therapeutic use of iron preparations
Ⓔ T Prophylaxis with H_2 antagonist may help

28.
Ⓐ F Typically asymptomatic
Ⓑ T Atrophic gastritis with absence of intrinsic factor
Ⓒ T Chronic superficial and atrophic gastritis, and gastric atrophy
Ⓓ T Partially relating to reflux of duodenal contents
Ⓔ T Particularly if gastric atrophy or metaplasia present

29.
Ⓐ F Japan has highest incidence
Ⓑ F 5 times more common
Ⓒ F Association with blood group A
Ⓓ T Especially the infiltrating form
Ⓔ T Either gastroenterostomy or partial gastrectomy

30.
Ⓐ F
Ⓑ F But may present as a malignant ulcer
Ⓒ F 5% survival
Ⓓ F Iron deficiency anaemia is typical
Ⓔ T Virchow's node

31.
Ⓐ T Haematogenous metastases also occur
Ⓑ F None available
Ⓒ F May present later, be more difficult to resect
Ⓓ T The commonest cause of this rare skin disorder
Ⓔ T Stomach appears rigid with rapid barium transit

32.
Ⓐ F Only 1%
Ⓑ F 2 L
Ⓒ F Trypsin release mediated by cholecystokinin
Ⓓ T Secreted by D cells
Ⓔ T Bicarbonate is also secreted in the pancreatic fluid

33.
Ⓐ F Typically impaired GTT
Ⓑ F May be seen in acute pancreatitis
Ⓒ F Pancreatic visualisation is superior with CT
Ⓓ F Surgery may be necessary
Ⓔ T Biliary tract disease is a rare aetiologic factor

34.
A T   But rare in childhood mumps
B T   Rare causes
C T   50% are associated with biliary tract disease
D T   Also thiazides and corticosteroids
E T   Common cause in the UK

35.
A F   Guarding occurs relatively late
B F   Serum amylase rises rapidly
C T   Or pancreatic abscess or non-pancreatic cause
D F   Hypocalcaemia
E F   May be absent or diminished due to paralytic ileus

36.
A F   Diagnostic laparotomy is rarely required
B F   Effective pain relief is important
C F   Heart rate alone is a poor guide to volume losses
D T   Shock and respiratory failure are serious complications
E T   Continue until peristalsis returns

37.
A T   Sometimes relieved by crouching or leaning forward
B T   Pancreatic proteases assist vitamin B_{12} absorption
C F   Occasionally in cystic fibrosis
D T   May persist for days or weeks
E T   But insensitive diagnostic tests

38.
A F   Increasing in incidence in Western countries
B T   Most often in the seventh decade
C T   And high dietary fat
D F   5 year survival is rare
E F   Majority have metastatic spread at presentation

39.
A T   The vast majority
B F   Head of pancreas in 60%
C F   Obstructive jaundice
D T   Even in the absence of metastatic spread
E T   Usually tumour in the head of pancreas

40.
A T   Solubilised by bile acids
B F   Active absorptive process
C T   Unabsorbed lactose is metabolised to hydrogen in the colon
D F   A marker of protein-losing enteropathy
E T   A test for fat malabsorption

41.
A T   Chyme traverses the small bowel too rapidly
B F   Bile acid deconjugation increases
C T   6 g protein produces 1 g nitrogen
D T   But produces steatorrhoea
E T   But much more marked in pancreatic insufficiency

42.
A F   Peak incidence ages 1–5 years and 20–39 years
B T   Symptoms return without dietary indiscretion
C T   A component of the gluten protein
D F   Villous atrophy should resolve
E T   Also anti-gliadin IgA antibody titres

43.
A T   Reduced small intestinal motility
B F   Vitamin B_{12} deficiency
C F   Suggests progressive systemic sclerosis
D F   Oral tetracycline
E F   Encourages small bowel bacterial overgrowth

44.

Ⓐ T And vice versa

Ⓑ F Early adult life most commonly

Ⓒ F Affects any part of the alimentary tract

Ⓓ T Bile acid malabsorption predisposes

Ⓔ F Crohn's granulomata are non-caseating

45.

Ⓐ T In contrast to ulcerative colitis

Ⓑ F Diarrhoea is the principal symptom in colonic disease

Ⓒ T With episodes of colicky pain

Ⓓ T In contrast to ulcerative colitis

Ⓔ F Inflammation is transmural

46.

Ⓐ F B_{12} deficiency occurs but not due to IF deficiency

Ⓑ T Pyoderma gangrenosum is another rare cutaneous association

Ⓒ T Seronegative spondyloarthritis

Ⓓ T Stomatitis may be severe

Ⓔ F But colonic cancer may occur

47.

Ⓐ F Unless there is severe generalised colitis

Ⓑ F Use if infection, abscess or bacteraemia suspected

Ⓒ F Intravenous hydrocortisone in severe active disease

Ⓓ T Binds bile salts and impairs fat absorption

Ⓔ F Major role is in colonic disease

48.

Ⓐ T Also femoral hernia

Ⓑ T Diffuse mesenteric ischaemia

Ⓒ F Paralytic ileus occurs

Ⓓ F Strangulation impairs blood supply and leads to paralytic obstruction

Ⓔ F But the converse may occur

49.

Ⓐ F Late or absent in colonic obstruction

Ⓑ T

Ⓒ T Absent bowel sounds suggest paralytic ileus

Ⓓ F Fluid stools can occur — 'spurious' diarrhoea

Ⓔ T Usually with constant severe pain

50.

Ⓐ T Often a mixed growth of organisms

Ⓑ F Mortality is about 10%

Ⓒ F Usually local spread from mesenteric lymph node

Ⓓ F Chemical inflammation due to bile, pancreatic or small bowel contents

Ⓔ F Rigidity typically lessens as the disease progresses

51.

Ⓐ F Urinary frequency, diarrhoea or tenesmus

Ⓑ F Diarrhoea not constipation

Ⓒ T With dull percussion note at the lung base

Ⓓ T Also useful as a guide to aspirate and drain abscesses

Ⓔ F Treatment is by drainage

52.

Ⓐ F Vague central abdominal pain

Ⓑ T Mural lymphoid swelling, stricture or faecolith

Ⓒ T Classical features occur in < 50%

Ⓓ F Both are notably uncommon

Ⓔ F Suggests another diagnosis

53.

Ⓐ T Proctitis is a typical finding

Ⓑ F Suggests Crohn's disease

Ⓒ T Due to oedema and hyperplasia

Ⓓ F Affects mucosa and submucosa only

Ⓔ F Suggests Crohn's disease

54.
- **A F** Both have a peak incidence at about age 20 but can occur at any age
- **B T** Smoking is associated with Crohn's disease not UC
- **C F** Also occurs in severe Crohn's colitis
- **D F** Not useful in distinguishing the two disorders
- **E F** But less common than in Crohn's disease

55.
- **A T** Also occurs in Crohn's disease and rheumatoid arthritis
- **B T** Suggested by abnormal liver function tests
- **C T** Any acute colitis
- **D T** Long-standing disease (> 10 years)
- **E T** Large joints especially or spondyloarthritis

56.
- **A F** Pyrexia may occur without infection
- **B T** As may loperamide
- **C T** Minority require surgery
- **D F** Improves as the disease improves; indication for nutritional support
- **E T** Or if there is progressive colonic dilatation or perforation

57.
- **A F** Oral steroids are reserved for more active disease
- **B F** Reduces the rate of relapse
- **C T** 'Steroid-sparing' effect helps minimise adverse effects
- **D T** Also erythema multiforme
- **E F** All sulphapyridines may cause headaches

58.
- **A F** Pelvic colon is most commonly involved
- **B F** No causative association
- **C F** Colonoscopy may be required to exclude malignancy
- **D F** But symptoms may be improved
- **E T** Such as acute diverticulitis

59.
- **A T** Exclusion of malignancy may be necessary
- **B F** But this may be a feature of chronic diverticulosis
- **C T** With or without perforation
- **D F** Left iliac fossa or hypogastric pain is typical
- **E T** Or coloenteric or colovaginal

60.
- **A F** Most occur in the left hemicolon
- **B T** And tubulo-villous and villous adenomata
- **C T** > 50% are malignant > 2 cm in size
- **D T** Causing mechanical bowel obstruction
- **E F** Bleeding or mucous discharge are common

61.
- **A F** Autosomal dominant with an incidence of 1 in 24 000
- **B F** Typically presents in mid-30s
- **C T** Carcinoma is usually present when symptoms commence
- **D T** Also associated with sebaceous cysts and osteomas of the jaw (Gardner's syndrome)
- **E F** Immunosuppressives have no role; prophylactic colectomy is warranted

62.
- **A T** In Western communities
- **B F** 75% occur in the left hemicolon
- **C T** Particularly in the presence of colonic polyps
- **D F** Spread not beyond muscularis
- **E F** Majority are palpable hence the need to do a PR examination

63.
- **A T** Non-specific presentation leads to diagnostic delay
- **B T** Late event in right sided tumours
- **C F** Portal venous dissemination to the liver is typical
- **D F** Synchronous tumours occur in 2%
- **E T** But too insensitive for initial routine diagnostic purposes

64.
A F Family history in 30%
B F Symptoms usually date from birth
C T In the pelvic colon and rectum
D F Rectum is empty
E F Excision of the abnormal segment with colorectal anastomosis

65.
A F Superior mesenteric artery supplies the midgut
B T Predisposing to cardiogenic embolism
C T May be bloody diarrhoea
D T Progression may be rapid
E F Usually fluid-filled loops with little air seen

66.
A F Diarrhoea without rigors would be typical
B F Occlusion of the inferior mesenteric artery, usually with a diseased SMA
C T May be a history of intermittent abdominal pain previously
D T May be visible on a plain abdominal film
E T But 10% progress to gangrene and peritonitis

67.
A F Such symptoms suggest organic pathology
B F Typically affects females aged 16–45 years
C T Many also have dyspeptic and urinary symptoms
D T Pain may be relieved by defecation
E T May be tenesmus, mucous PR and diarrhoea

68.
A T Probably the most important therapeutic tools
B F Investigations are important in older patients
C T Anxiety and/or depression is often associated with refractory symptoms
D F Although occasionally psychiatric intervention may be necessary
E F Use loperamide, a safer opioid that does not cross the blood-brain barrier

8 DISEASES OF THE LIVER & BILIARY SYSTEM

1.
Ⓐ T Accessed via fenestrations in the endothelium
Ⓑ T Only 25% of hepatic blood flow
Ⓒ F At its maximum postprandially
Ⓓ T Activity may be determined by their location in the acinus
Ⓔ F Comprise 10–15%

2.
Ⓐ F Last for up to 1 day before gluconeogenesis becomes the major source of glucose
Ⓑ T And inhibits gluconeogenesis
Ⓒ T Insulin levels fall during a fast, permitting these metabolic activities
Ⓓ T And lactate
Ⓔ F Only in fulminant hepatic failure

3.
Ⓐ F Also from catabolism of other haem-containing proteins e.g. myoglobin
Ⓑ F Bound to albumin
Ⓒ T By enzymes of the smooth endoplasmic reticulum
Ⓓ F Only reabsorbed after metabolism to stercobilinogen
Ⓔ T And as the oxidation products stercobilin and urobilin

4.
Ⓐ F Unconjugated hyperbilirubinaemia
Ⓑ T As almost all bilirubin is unconjugated and albumin bound
Ⓒ F Most of the serum bilirubin is unconjugated
Ⓓ F Unconjugated bilirubin is increased
Ⓔ F Urobilinogen is an unreliable indicator of hepatobiliary disease

5.
Ⓐ F Neither ALT nor AST is specific to the liver
Ⓑ F Typically less than fivefold
Ⓒ F May be elevated in either
Ⓓ F Changes in serum ALT precede changes in the serum bilirubin
Ⓔ F Only the gamma glutamyl transferase levels increase

6.
Ⓐ T Therefore not specific to liver disease
Ⓑ F Not usually more than doubled
Ⓒ T Excess synthesis in cholestasis
Ⓓ F No prognostic value
Ⓔ F No site-specific pattern

7.
Ⓐ F The half-life of serum albumin is about 20–26 days
Ⓑ F May reflect bypass of hepatic immune mechanisms
Ⓒ T But not completely specific
Ⓓ T Half-lives of clotting factors 2, 7, 9 and 10 are short (5–72 hours)
Ⓔ F Typically an increased IgM level

8.
Ⓐ T Provided lesions are > 2 cm in diameter
Ⓑ F May be normal in disease
Ⓒ F Supero-anterior surfaces are seen best
Ⓓ F Approximately 0.05%
Ⓔ T Also TB and hepatic vein obstruction; protein concentration < 30 g/L = transudate

9.
Ⓐ T Hepatocytic (canalicular) cholestasis
Ⓑ T Secretion of polypeptide tumour products
Ⓒ T Malabsorption of fat-soluble vitamin D
Ⓓ F Suggest pancreatic carcinoma (Courvoisier's law)
Ⓔ T Hepatocyte bilirubin transport is variably disturbed

10.
Ⓐ F Usually less than 100 µol/L
Ⓑ T In skin and sclerae
Ⓒ F Urobilin discolours the urine
Ⓓ T Due to excess reticuloendothelial activity
Ⓔ F Suggests cholestatic jaundice

11.
Ⓐ F Typically autosomal dominant
Ⓑ T Causing failure of bilirubin conjugation
Ⓒ T And no abnormality of other liver function tests
Ⓓ T Sometimes used as a diagnostic test
Ⓔ F Unconjugated hyperbilirubinaemia is the sole abnormality

12.
Ⓐ F An oral hypoglycaemic
Ⓑ F May cause acute hepatitis
Ⓒ T A phenothiazine antipsychotic
Ⓓ T Often dose/duration dependent
Ⓔ T And also pregnancy

13.
Ⓐ F May be a mononuclear infiltrate
Ⓑ F These areas tend to be more affected
Ⓒ T Leading to 'bridging' necrosis
Ⓓ T 'Councilman bodies'
Ⓔ F Seen in alcoholic and other toxic liver disease

14.
Ⓐ T Faecal-oral spread of a picornavirus
Ⓑ F 2–4 weeks
Ⓒ F But children are more frequently infected
Ⓓ T Non-specific findings
Ⓔ F Chronic hepatitis does not occur

15.
Ⓐ F Viraemia is only transient in hepatitis A
Ⓑ F Spontaneous recovery is the typical outcome
Ⓒ T But a recognised rarity
Ⓓ T Serological investigations should distinguish
Ⓔ T Some will have natural endogenous protection

16.
Ⓐ T E.g. pancreatic carcinoma
Ⓑ F Not a useful distinguishing feature
Ⓒ T Less than doubled in viral hepatitis
Ⓓ T Suggests obstruction with cholangitis
Ⓔ T Sometimes relative lymphocytosis in viral hepatitis

17.
Ⓐ T A reliable marker of hepatitis B infection
Ⓑ T A DNA hepadna virus
Ⓒ F Occurs in 1–10% of adults
Ⓓ T Alternative serological evidence of infection should be sought
Ⓔ F Carriage rates are highest in the middle and far East

18.
Ⓐ F Average incubation 3 months
Ⓑ T Or other exposure to blood or blood products
Ⓒ T May cause serum sickness
Ⓓ T Hepatitis A is usually a mild illness
Ⓔ F And hepatic cirrhosis also occurs

19.
Ⓐ T With varying degrees of severity
Ⓑ T Hepatitis E rarely progresses to chronic disease
Ⓒ F Hepatitis C type may progress to chronic disease
Ⓓ T But incubation may be longer
Ⓔ T Although serological screening methods have greatly reduced this

20.

Ⓐ T An incomplete virus

Ⓑ T Alone or with hepatitis B

Ⓒ T Incapable of replication alone

Ⓓ T Often limited by resolution of hepatitis B

Ⓔ T Hepatitis B may then resolve

21.

Ⓐ T Without evidence of pre-existing liver disease

Ⓑ F Suggest chronic liver disease

Ⓒ T With confusion and asterixis (liver flap)

Ⓓ T Renal failure is an ominous development

Ⓔ T Occurs late, if at all

22.

Ⓐ F Serum albumin has a long half life

Ⓑ T Impaired hepatic gluconeogenesis

Ⓒ T Useful in determining prognosis

Ⓓ F Typically not so elevated unlike the serum transaminases

Ⓔ F May be a polymorphonuclear leucocytosis

23.

Ⓐ T To minimise encephalopathy

Ⓑ T

Ⓒ T Disseminated intravascular coagulation may also be present

Ⓓ T Frequent blood glucose monitoring is vital

Ⓔ T Thiopentone is used if there is renal failure

24.

Ⓐ T Portal tracts may be expanded

Ⓑ F Hepatocytes are spared

Ⓒ F A feature of aggressive hepatitis

Ⓓ F A feature of aggressive hepatitis

Ⓔ F Correlates with chronic persistent hepatitis, although overlap occurs

25.

Ⓐ F Symptoms are mild or absent

Ⓑ F No evidence of chronic liver disease

Ⓒ T Serum ALT is modestly elevated

Ⓓ F

Ⓔ F Persistent hepatitis only without change in hepatocytes

26.

Ⓐ F Due to autoimmune liver disease

Ⓑ F But symptoms persist

Ⓒ F Also fatigue, anorexia and jaundice

Ⓓ F And other signs of chronic liver disease

Ⓔ F Altered steroid hormone metabolism

27.

Ⓐ T In contrast to autoimmune hepatitis

Ⓑ F A chronically progressive course is more typical

Ⓒ F Signs are sparse; hepatomegaly is commonest

Ⓓ T Particularly if HBsAg present

Ⓔ F Hepatoma is more common

28.

Ⓐ T Coomb's positive

Ⓑ T Perhaps with thyrotoxicosis

Ⓒ T Less commonly

Ⓓ T Also seen in primary biliary cirrhosis

Ⓔ T More commonly transient arthralgia

29.

Ⓐ T Found in 50–66% of patients with autoimmune hepatitis

Ⓑ T But confirmatory biopsy is necessary

Ⓒ T In presence of elevated serum ALT levels

Ⓓ F Suggests Wilson's disease

Ⓔ F Suggests primary biliary cirrhosis

30.

Ⓐ F Biopsy is often better delayed for 6 months

Ⓑ T Most ultimately develop cirrhosis

Ⓒ F About 10% die within 5 years despite treatment

Ⓓ T Azathioprine also enables smaller steroid doses to be used

Ⓔ F And hepatitis C infection

31.
Ⓐ F Liver size reduces as disease progresses
Ⓑ F Mild splenomegaly due to portal hypertension
Ⓒ T Particularly in alcoholic liver disease
Ⓓ T Particularly in alcoholic cirrhosis
Ⓔ T Abdominal distension may also be due to ascites

32.
Ⓐ F The majority of cases in the UK are alcohol related
Ⓑ T Or a later complication of chronic infection
Ⓒ F May cause acute massive hepatic necrosis
Ⓓ T More than 5–10 years of steady drinking
Ⓔ F Produces a fatty liver (steatosis)

33.
Ⓐ T Multiple small right-to-left shunts
Ⓑ T As does falling serum albumin and rising prothrombin time
Ⓒ F Peripheral vasodilatation occurs
Ⓓ T Visceral blood flow is generally reduced
Ⓔ T As may splenomegaly and ascites

34.
Ⓐ T And a flapping tremor
Ⓑ F Highly atypical — suggests other pathology
Ⓒ T Sometimes sleep reversal
Ⓓ F Transaminase level does not correlate with severity
Ⓔ T And other neuropsychiatric problems

35.
Ⓐ T Spontaneous bacterial peritonitis should not be overlooked
Ⓑ T Often aggravated by diuretic use
Ⓒ T Or trauma
Ⓓ T Increased protein load in gut
Ⓔ F Reduces colonic ammonia absorption

36.
Ⓐ F Restriction to 20–40 mmol/day is usually required
Ⓑ F A palliative, symptomatic measure with no prognostic impact
Ⓒ F Calorie restriction is not required
Ⓓ F Weight loss > 1 kg/day may precipitate renal impairment
Ⓔ T Restriction may be necessary to control encephalopathy

37.
Ⓐ T Or reduced below 20 g/day
Ⓑ F May worsen or precipitate encephalopathy
Ⓒ T Avoid in uraemia
Ⓓ F May be required for coexistent ascites but may worsen encephalopathy
Ⓔ T Hypoglycaemia may coexist

38.
Ⓐ F No intrinsic renal damage
Ⓑ F Suggest glomerulotubular disease
Ⓒ T Normal renal response to secondary hyperaldosteronism
Ⓓ F Ratio > 1.5
Ⓔ F Hypovolaemia is more common

39.
Ⓐ T May be higher in presence of encephalopathy and ascites
Ⓑ F Stops bleeding in 80%
Ⓒ T Constricts splanchnic arterioles
Ⓓ T Unless exsanguinating, 20% are bleeding from non-variceal source
Ⓔ F TIPSS (portasystemic stent shunting) or surgery may be needed

40.
Ⓐ F Somatostatin may be useful in acute bleeds
Ⓑ T Also used in acute bleeds
Ⓒ T Beta blockers reduce portal pressure
Ⓓ T Considered to be better than sclerotherapy
Ⓔ T

41.
Ⓐ F Middle-aged females
Ⓑ F May precede jaundice by months or years
Ⓒ T Vitamin D malabsorption and hepatic osteodystrophy
Ⓓ F Suggests obstruction of large bile duct
Ⓔ F High titres of anti-mitochondrial antibody

42
Ⓐ T And on elbows, knees and buttocks
Ⓑ F Prognosis excellent in the absence of symptoms or signs
Ⓒ T Splenomegaly occurs as portal hypertension develops
Ⓓ F Suggests biliary obstruction
Ⓔ F None proven to be effective

43.
Ⓐ T Inherited as an autosomal recessive
Ⓑ T Typically over 40 years
Ⓒ T 'Bronzed diabetes'
Ⓓ F May be a congestive cardiomyopathy
Ⓔ F Melanin not iron deposition

44.
Ⓐ T Sometimes accompanying an acute hepatitis in children
Ⓑ T Or fulminant hepatic failure or cirrhosis
Ⓒ T A variety of extrapyramidal syndromes may be seen
Ⓓ F Serum copper falls, hepatic copper is increased
Ⓔ T K–F rings are an important diagnostic clue

45.
Ⓐ T Intrahepatic parenchymal
Ⓑ T Intrahepatic presinusoidal
Ⓒ T Commonest cause worldwide
Ⓓ T Leading to portal vein thrombosis
Ⓔ T Intrahepatic parenchymal

46.
Ⓐ T Most commonly alcoholic cirrhosis
Ⓑ T A fungal poison
Ⓒ T Occurs in 30% of those with cirrhosis
Ⓓ F No chronic hepatic sequelae
Ⓔ T And anabolic steroids

47.
Ⓐ T Pain in a cirrhotic should be suggestive
Ⓑ T Tumours are vascular and spread locally
Ⓒ F May be a hepatic bruit
Ⓓ T Rises in 90% of cases
Ⓔ F 10% are suitable for surgery

48.
Ⓐ T Secondary to biliary obstruction
Ⓑ T Secondary to portal pyaemia
Ⓒ T Acute pancreatitis
Ⓓ T Infection via hepatic artery
Ⓔ T Direct local spread

49.
Ⓐ F Jaundice is usually mild and uncommonly obstructive
Ⓑ T Splenomegaly suggests coexistent pathology
Ⓒ T May be right shoulder tip pain
Ⓓ T Single lesions are more common in the right liver
Ⓔ T Multiple organisms in one third

50.
Ⓐ F Common hepatic duct
Ⓑ F Normal CBD < 8 mm in diameter
Ⓒ F Distal common bile duct usually joins pancreatic duct
Ⓓ F Principally vagal tone controls the gallbladder muscle wall
Ⓔ T

51.
Ⓐ F The converse applies
Ⓑ F 40% of patients > 60 years old
Ⓒ T But pigment stones are the more common in the developing countries
Ⓓ T Usually calcium bilirubinate
Ⓔ F Hepatic hypersecretion of cholesterol more important

52.

Ⓐ T Increased hepatic cholesterol secretion

Ⓑ T Multiple factors including impaired gallbladder motility

Ⓒ T Pigment stones

Ⓓ T Pigment stones

Ⓔ T Impaired gallbladder function

53.

Ⓐ F Cystic duct or gallbladder neck are obstructed in 90%

Ⓑ F 50% are infected

Ⓒ F May be acalculous

Ⓓ F Atropine may reduce choledochal sphincter spasm

Ⓔ F Most gallstones are radiolucent

54.

Ⓐ F Jaundice occurs in only 20%

Ⓑ F Pain typically continuous

Ⓒ T Murphy's sign

Ⓓ F May follow passage of a gallstone into intestine or biliary surgery

Ⓔ T May be absent in the elderly

55.

Ⓐ F Associated with gallstones and ulcerative colitis

Ⓑ T Often with weight loss

Ⓒ F Suggests hepatocellular carcinoma

Ⓓ T But not a specific finding

Ⓔ F Commonest treatment is palliative stenting

56.

Ⓐ F Female preponderance — most aged > 70 years

Ⓑ F Adenocarcinoma

Ⓒ T Can also be suspected by the findings on ultrasound scanning

Ⓓ T Usually diagnosed at routine cholecystectomy for gallstones

Ⓔ F Often advanced at diagnosis since presentation is usually late

9 NUTRITIONAL FACTORS IN DISEASE

1.
- **A** F 2–10μg per day
- **B** T And riboflavin
- **C** T Optimally 10% of total calories
- **D** T Highest level for a specific vitamin
- **E** F Approximately 1 g

2.
- **A** T Or 16 kJ/g
- **B** F About 9 kcal (36 kJ)/g
- **C** F All disaccharides
- **D** T And arachidonic acid
- **E** T Arginine is an additional essential amino acid in infants

3.
- **A** F About 2700 kcal (11.3 MJ)
- **B** F Ketosis occurs below 100 g a day
- **C** T And niacin and vitamin E
- **D** T Minimum around 40 g
- **E** F 200 μg of folate per day

4.
- **A** T About 7000 kJ (1750 kcal) per day
- **B** F Declines with age
- **C** F Greater in males
- **D** T But dependent on activity
- **E** T Overweight 25–30, obese > 30

5.
- **A** F BMI < 16
- **B** T 'Famine oedema'
- **C** T And weakness, amenorrhoea or impotence
- **D** T Adolescents may maintain hair growth
- **E** F Brain weight is preserved; bradycardia is the rule

6.
- **A** F Increased FFA levels
- **B** T Plasma glucagon also rises
- **C** T False-negative Mantoux may occur
- **D** T And occasionally a metabolic acidosis
- **E** T Also pancytopenia

7.
- **A** F Predominantly protein deficiency with a normal total energy intake
- **B** F Protein and energy malnutrition in infancy
- **C** F BMI is normal or low normal
- **D** T Compromised humoral and cell mediated immunity
- **E** T Exacerbated by diarrhoeal illness

8.
- **A** T And absence of oedema
- **B** T Weight < 60% standard for age
- **C** T With low plasma lipids
- **D** F Features of kwashiorkor
- **E** T Contributing to dermatosis

9.
- **A** T Dehydration and infection
- **B** T Especially hypokalaemia and hypomagnesaemia
- **C** F Isolated calorie replacement may do so
- **D** F And resolves on re-feeding
- **E** T And growth monitoring (mnemonic **GOBI**)

10.
- **A** T Chiefly as calcium hydroxyapatite
- **B** T 350–550 mg daily for children
- **C** T
- **D** F Impair absorption e.g. whole grain cereals and spinach
- **E** F Correlates poorly

11.
- **A T** 8 mg/day for men
- **B F** 15% is absorbed
- **C T** E.g. red muscle meat or organ meat
- **D F** Average loss 2 mg/day due to menstruation
- **E F** Contains 250 mg of iron

12.
- **A F** Goitre alone or with hypothyroidism
- **B F** Hard water contains more fluoride
- **C T** Acrodermatitis enteropathica
- **D T** And skeletal rarefaction
- **E F** More likely in breast-fed infants

13.
- **A T** A, D, E, K are the fat-soluble vitamins
- **B F** Occurs as retinol in animal produce and as carotene in plants
- **C T** Both conditions are the result of vitamin A deficiency and lead to blindness
- **D F** Minimum recommended daily intake = 1–2 mg
- **E T** Present as retinol

14.
- **A F** Some margarines are fortified
- **B T** But less efficiently produced in old age
- **C F** But metabolism partly occurs in the liver
- **D T** 1-alpha hydroxylation occurs in the kidney and 25-hydroxylation in the liver
- **E T** And stimulates osteoclast proliferation

15.
- **A T** Osteomalacia occurs after fusion
- **B T** Limited diet and sunlight exposure
- **C T** And tendency to infection
- **D T** 'Rickety rosary'
- **E T** Especially severe if there is coexistent respiratory disease

16.
- **A T** With 'saucer deformity'
- **B T** Triggered by hypocalcaemia
- **C T** Due to high PTH and low vitamin D respectively
- **D T** Also kyphosis and cranial 'bossing'
- **E T** Principal form of vitamin D in the circulation

17.
- **A F** Bone osteoid is increased
- **B T** And occasionally tetany
- **C T** Due to proximal myopathy
- **D T** Pathognomonic radiological features (Looser's zones)
- **E T** Also occurs increased in old age and malabsorption syndromes

18.
- **A F** No chronic pain; fractures occur easily but heal
- **B T** Also inactivity and cigarette smoking
- **C F** Most apparent in vertebral bodies
- **D T** In contrast to osteomalacia
- **E F** Biochemistry is normal in absence of fracture

19.
- **A T** And also found in liver
- **B F** Absorbed as vitamin K_1
- **C T** All contain gamma-carboxyglutamic acid
- **D T** Breast milk contains little vitamin K and placental transfer is poor
- **E F** Warfarin blocks synthesis of vitamin K-dependent carboxylation of factors 2, 7, 9, 10

20.
- **A T** Ascorbic acid deficiency prevents the conversion of proline to hydroxyproline
- **B T** Recommended intake 30–75 mg
- **C F** Gingivitis only occurs in presence of teeth
- **D T** Then petechial haemorrhage and ecchymoses
- **E T** With subperiosteal haemorrhage

21.
A F Aerobic metabolism of glucose is impaired
B F Wheat, yeast and legumes are rich in vitamin B$_1$
C F Arrhythmia and high output failure
D T A mixed sensori-motor neuropathy
E T And confusion

22.
A T Dermatitis, diarrhoea and dementia
B T Add to anti-TB regimens using isoniazid
C F Sideroblastic anaemia may respond
D T Also seen in niacin deficiency
E T Also seen in niacin deficiency

23.
A T But deficiency may take years to manifest
B T Vital to tetrahydrofolate metabolism
C T Mainly in animal foodstuffs
D F Recommended intake 100 μg daily
E T And megaloblastic anaemia

24.
A T If colonic flora are reduced
B F Use monomeric feeds
C T 1 g glucose = 40 kcal
D F Use of > 10% dextrose solutions causes local phlebitis
E T Due to elevated insulin levels

25.
A T Due to hemi-cellulose
B T But stimulate flatus production
C T And hence lower the glycaemic index
D F Only small quantities of fatty acids are absorbed after digestion
E T Typical UK adult consumption

26.
A T Poor intake
B T Increased metabolic rate and enhanced losses
C T Drug-induced vomiting, hypercatabolism
D T Or body weight below 80% standard for height
E T Anti-anabolic effect

27.
A F Nutritional deficiency should be suspected in all ill patients
B T Less if mainly protein loss
C T But not specific
D T And macrocytosis
E F Lymphopenia

28.
A T Gross obesity > 40
B T Hyperinsulinaemia is common
C T But no single gene defect identified
D T But precise endocrine mechanisms unclear
E T After correction for total body mass

29.
A T And clinical gout
B T And psychosexual and anxiety disorders
C T Usually asymptomatic
D T With insulin resistance
E T And coronary artery disease

30.
A F 800–1600 kcal daily
B F 0.5–1 kg per week (1000 kcal deficit /day = 7000 kcal /week = 1 kg human tissue)
C F Reserve for refractory obesity
D F 40 g minimum recommended protein intake
E F Fat restriction < 50 g/day (calorific values fat = 9 kcal/g, CHO = 4 kcal/g)

31.
A T Adverse effects are worrying and the long-term results are disappointing
B T Walking expends 5 kcal/min (includes BMR = 1 kcal/min)
C F Even a small intake of carbohydrate prevents significant ketosis
D T Calorific value of alcohol = 7 kcal per gram
E T Effect of anti-obesity drugs plateaus at about 12 weeks

32.
- **A** T   Flat feet
- **B** T   Load-bearing joints
- **C** T   Obese subjects may be less nimble
- **D** F   Not associated with body mass index
- **E** F   Suggests rheumatoid arthritis

33.
- **A** T
- **B** T
- **C** T
- **D** F   Stimulates satiety and can help some patients lose weight
- **E** T   Increases insulin secretion

10 DISTURBANCES IN WATER, ELECTROLYTE AND ACID-BASE BALANCE

1.
- **A T** Relatively constant in health
- **B T** Approx. 28 litres
- **C F** 25% is intravascular
- **D F** Extracellular
- **E F** Intracellular

2.
- **A T** Predominantly from the oxidation of glucose
- **B F** 500–1000 ml per day
- **C T** Depends on solute load
- **D F** 100 ml
- **E T** An index of normal renal medullary function

3.
- **A F** Rare in isolation
- **B T** Usually with water depletion also
- **C T** An osmotic diuresis
- **D T** Mineralocorticoid insufficiency
- **E T** Loss into the 'third space'

4.
- **A F** But may be seen in the syndrome of inappropriate ADH secretion
- **B T** Water retention exceeds sodium retention
- **C T** Increased total body water
- **D F** But seen in adrenocortical insuffuciency
- **E T** Salt loss exceeds water loss

5.
- **A T**
- **B F** Can produce hyponatraemia
- **C T** Monitor pulse, BP and CVP carefully
- **D T** Dependent on cause of deficit
- **E T** The kidneys may be unable to excrete hydrogen ions; monitor the arterial pH

6.
- **A T** Renal tubular insensitivity to ADH
- **B T** Inadequate intake
- **C T** Inadequate intake
- **D T** Renal tubular insensitivity to ADH
- **E F** Combined salt and water depletion

7.
- **A F** Urine osmolality > 500 mosm/kg
- **B F** Hypernatraemia
- **C T** Thirst stimulated by rising plasma osmolality
- **D T** Signs of volume depletion develop more rapidly in combined salt/water depletion
- **E T** Also confusion

8.
- **A T** Unless there is significant peripheral circulatory failure
- **B F** Too rapid infusions produce cerebral oedema
- **C T**
- **D T** The use of hypotonic fluids is rarely indicated
- **E T** Signs develop more rapidly in combined salt/water depletion

9.
- **A T**
- **B T** Compared with extracellular concentrations of about 4 mmol/L
- **C T**
- **D F** Increased by bicarbonate and decreased by acidaemia
- **E T**

10.
Ⓐ T Renal tubular cell K concentration increased: excretion increased
Ⓑ T Secondary hyperaldosteronism
Ⓒ T Mineralocorticoid-like effect
Ⓓ T Primary or secondary tubular defect; also occurs with activation of renin and angiotensin
Ⓔ F Causes hyperkalaemia by an effect on the distal convoluted tubules

11.
Ⓐ T Tubular response to ADH is impaired
Ⓑ T Lethargy and immobility in the elderly
Ⓒ T QT interval is prolonged
Ⓓ T Painless distension with scanty bowel sounds
Ⓔ F Increased sensitivity to digoxin

12.
Ⓐ T Insulin promotes movement into the cells
Ⓑ T Impairment of secretion in the distal nephron
Ⓒ T Increased tissue breakdown
Ⓓ T Especially if given with ACE inhibitor
Ⓔ T Avoid concurrent supplementation

13.
Ⓐ T Relatively early changes
Ⓑ T May be the first manifestation
Ⓒ T Such symptoms are commonly overlooked
Ⓓ T Occur in severe hyperkalaemia
Ⓔ T Muscle weakness, loss of tendon reflexes and ileus; therefore check the plasma electrolytes

14.
Ⓐ F But may be necessary to prevent recurrence
Ⓑ F Give parenteral dextrose and insulin
Ⓒ T Cardioprotective effect
Ⓓ T Also correct metabolic acidosis if present with 1.26% sodium bicarbonate i. v.
Ⓔ T The resin binds potassium in exchange for calcium

15.
Ⓐ T Also tremor and choreiform movements
Ⓑ T Also from chronic diuretic therapy
Ⓒ T Excess losses in the urine
Ⓓ T Including secondary hyperaldosteronism
Ⓔ F Very poorly absorbed orally

16.
Ⓐ T
Ⓑ T Two thirds of water absorption occurs here
Ⓒ T
Ⓓ T The absence of AVP renders the collecting ducts impermeable to water
Ⓔ T

17.
Ⓐ T Dilutional hyponatraemia
Ⓑ F Typically < 250 mosm/kg
Ⓒ T Occasionally produces generalised seizures
Ⓓ F Use small volumes of hypertonic saline very cautiously
Ⓔ F ECF volume status usually appears normal

18.
Ⓐ T Pain and other stressors can induce ADH release
Ⓑ T And many other CNS disorders
Ⓒ F Water excretion is however impaired
Ⓓ T A rare complication
Ⓔ T Also other pneumonias

19.
Ⓐ F Diuretic causing sodium and water losses
Ⓑ T Inhibition of renal prostaglandin synthesis
Ⓒ T
Ⓓ F But hypothyroidism increases ADH secretion
Ⓔ F Inhibits aldosterone production

20.

Ⓐ F Major action on thick ascending limb of loop of Henle

Ⓑ T Tubular effect inhibiting urate excretion may precipitate gout

Ⓒ F Acts on the collecting ducts

Ⓓ T Causes hyperkalaemia

Ⓔ T Due to relative water excess

21.

Ⓐ T The Henderson Hasselbach equation

Ⓑ T Note nmol/L not mmol/L

Ⓒ T Unlike plasma CO_2 which is controlled by the respiratory centre via ventilation

Ⓓ F Excretion is predominantly renal

Ⓔ F Most is converted to H_2CO_3 by red cell carbonic anhydrase

22.

Ⓐ F pH is measured directly

Ⓑ T Dissociation - equilibration formula of a weak acid

Ⓒ T Useful in distinguishing between causes of metabolic acidosis

Ⓓ T Hypoventilation causes hypercapnia

Ⓔ F Normal bicarbonate 22–28 mmol/L; normal pH = 7.35–7.45

23.

Ⓐ F Plasma bicarbonate is reduced

Ⓑ T Ketoacidosis

Ⓒ F Compensatory hyperventilation

Ⓓ F Hyperchloraemic acidosis

Ⓔ F Decreased production

DISEASES OF THE KIDNEY AND GENITO-URINARY SYSTEM

11

1.
- **A** F Total number of nephrons = I million
- **B** F Efferent arterioles
- **C** T From intralobular branches of renal artery
- **D** T And arcuate arteries
- **E** F 10 mmHg

2.
- **A** F 66% of filtered water is reabsorbed
- **B** T And collecting ducts
- **C** T But only 150 mg per day excreted in urine
- **D** F 66%
- **E** F Afferent arterioles

3.
- **A** F Almost all is passively absorbed
- **B** T And in ascending limb of loop of Henle
- **C** F Active reabsorption process
- **D** T Coupled with sodium reabsorption
- **E** F 85% of bicarbonate is reabsorbed

4.
- **A** T In part regulated by mineralocorticoid
- **B** T If K^+ is low, H^+ is secreted preferentially
- **C** T Via renin-angiotensin system
- **D** T ADH increases tubular permeability to water
- **E** T Permits urinary acidification

5.
- **A** T Probably in tubular cells
- **B** F 1,25-dihydroxycholecalciferol
- **C** T Vasodilatory actions; produced in mesangium
- **D** T As do many other tissues
- **E** F Produced in adrenal cortex

6.
- **A** F Immunoelectrophoresis required
- **B** T Often with oedema and hypoalbuminaemia
- **C** F Greater when upright —'orthostatic proteinuria'
- **D** T But no red cells on microscopy
- **E** T Microalbuminuria is a sensitive predictor

7.
- **A** F Moderate 500 mg — 2.5 g but rarely more
- **B** F Usually haematuria
- **C** T Complicating dehydration in infants
- **D** T Commonest cause in childhood
- **E** F No glomerular lesion

8.
- **A** F Proteinuria is typical
- **B** T Risk factors include diabetes mellitus, NSAID usage and alcoholism
- **C** F Typically proteinuria
- **D** T Immune complex glomerulonephritis
- **E** T May be frank haematuria

9.
- **A** T pH > 8 suggests infection
- **B** T E.g. using urinary and plasma creatinine
- **C** T Assessed by ultrasound scanning
- **D** F 33% is excreted within the first hour
- **E** F Contraindicated if kidneys are small

10.
- **A** T More marked in children
- **B** T Often with generalised oedema
- **C** T With RBC casts
- **D** F Non-selective and usually not nephrotic
- **E** F Suggests C1q esterase inhibitor deficiency

11.
Ⓐ F Typically painless
Ⓑ T Transudates
Ⓒ T Diagnostic prerequisites
Ⓓ F May occur in chronic renal failure
Ⓔ F Marked sodium retention — urinary sodium < 10 mmol/L

12.
Ⓐ F Tubulointerstitial damage only
Ⓑ T And HIV
Ⓒ T Usually detectable circulating immune complexes
Ⓓ T Presents with recurrent macroscopic haematuria
Ⓔ F Immunoglobulin light chain deposits

13.
Ⓐ T With mesangial proliferation and inflammatory infiltrate
Ⓑ F But precipitating antigen unidentifiable in most
Ⓒ T Typically in children of school age
Ⓓ T And chest X-ray infiltrates
Ⓔ F Prognosis better in children

14.
Ⓐ F Hypertension is typical
Ⓑ F Tubular function normal
Ⓒ T Classical' pathway activation
Ⓓ T Or interstitial fibrosis
Ⓔ T With RBC casts

15.
Ⓐ F But can improve renal function if severely impaired
Ⓑ F Can be of value if nephrotic
Ⓒ F Often needed in oliguric phase
Ⓓ T Sodium and water restriction
Ⓔ T But drug treatment may also be necessary

16.
Ⓐ T But can occur at any age
Ⓑ F Usually < 7 days
Ⓒ T Minor proteinuria in the remainder
Ⓓ T 20% have hypertension
Ⓔ T Or focal segmental mesangial proliferation

17.
Ⓐ T More common in females
Ⓑ T Or nephrotic presentation
Ⓒ F No specific treatment
Ⓓ F 75% progress to renal failure
Ⓔ F Hypocomplementaemia

18.
Ⓐ F Acute nephritic or renal failure
Ⓑ T Early dialysis is typically required
Ⓒ F Occasional association
Ⓓ T Epithelial crescent formation occurs
Ⓔ F Only in the minority

19.
Ⓐ T Removable by plasmapheresis
Ⓑ T With linear IgG deposition
Ⓒ T Usually with acute renal failure
Ⓓ T Antibodies have pulmonary basement membrane cross-reactivity
Ⓔ F Limited response given prompt therapy

20.
Ⓐ T Uniform basement membrane thickening
Ⓑ T Or asymptomatic proteinuria
Ⓒ T Hypertension in 30%
Ⓓ F Poor prognosis
Ⓔ F No specific treatment

21.
Ⓐ F Children aged 3–15 years
Ⓑ F Minor or absent
Ⓒ F Selective proteinuria
Ⓓ F Suggests an alternative cause
Ⓔ T And atopy

22.
Ⓐ F Diagnosis in children rarely requires histological confirmation
Ⓑ F Useful in management of oedema
Ⓒ T Longer term steroids may be helpful
Ⓓ T E.g. cyclophosphamide
Ⓔ F Rarely, even in relapsing disease

23.
Ⓐ T Increases in frequency with time
Ⓑ T An immune complex nephritis
Ⓒ T 20% focal, 15% membranous
Ⓓ F Better prognosis
Ⓔ F Rare as is CNS involvement .

24.
Ⓐ F Rheumatoid arthritis and bronchiectasis
Ⓑ T Tubular insensitivity to ADH
Ⓒ T Proximal or distal
Ⓓ T Treatment does not retard progression
Ⓔ T 50% die in renal failure

25.
Ⓐ F Suggests acute pyelonephritis
Ⓑ T And urinary frequency
Ⓒ F Suggests an abnormality of the urinary tract
Ⓓ T *E. coli* in 75% of UTIs in the community
Ⓔ F Trimethoprim or co-amoxyclav

26.
Ⓐ T But ureteric obstruction may be a predisposing factor
Ⓑ T With loin or epigastric pain
Ⓒ F Typically unilateral but can be bilateral
Ⓓ F Commonly found in chilren but not adults
Ⓔ F Suggests perinephric abscess

27.
Ⓐ F 5% cf. 40% in elderly females
Ⓑ T And ureteric dilatation
Ⓒ T 40% develop symptoms if untreated
Ⓓ F Contraindicated in early pregnancy
Ⓔ F Teratogenic risk (a folate antagonist)

28.
Ⓐ T Chronic infection predisposes to phosphate stone formation
Ⓑ F Usually asymptomatic and presents with uraemia or hypertension
Ⓒ T Recurrent infections can be difficult to prevent
Ⓓ F Usually presents well before the age of 40 years
Ⓔ T 'Salt-losing nephropathy'

29.
Ⓐ F 20% of chronic dialysis patients
Ⓑ T Other aetiological factors may also be important
Ⓒ F Similar to ischaemic or tubulo-interstitial nephritis
Ⓓ F Reflux is often no longer demonstrable in adulthood
Ⓔ T As a result of a 'salt-losing' nephropathy

30.
Ⓐ F Typically normocytic or microcytic
Ⓑ T Can improve with dialysis
Ⓒ T Renal osteodystrophy with osteomalacia
Ⓓ T Even haemorrhagic pericarditis with tamponade
Ⓔ F Metabolic acidosis

31.
Ⓐ T Hence polyuria; urinary diluting ability also impaired
Ⓑ F Hyperphosphataemia
Ⓒ F Hypocalcaemia
Ⓓ T Resulting in hyperpnoea
Ⓔ F Severe proteinuria diminishes as renal failure progresses

32.
Ⓐ T Suggests severe hypertension
Ⓑ F May indicate aetiology
Ⓒ T Occurs in severe renal failure
Ⓓ T Particularly secondary hyperparathyroidism
Ⓔ T Typically progresses from this level on

33.
Ⓐ T And in elderly and diabetic patients
Ⓑ F 2 L instilled four times daily
Ⓒ F May also be preferable in patients with cardiac disease
Ⓓ T ABO compatibility is essential
Ⓔ F About 75% graft survival and 90% patient survival

34.
Ⓐ F Remember 20% of acute renal failure is non-oliguric
Ⓑ F Blood pressure is often decreased in pre-renal ARF
Ⓒ F Suggests pre-renal uraemia
Ⓓ F Suggests pre-renal uraemia
Ⓔ F Haemoglobin is typically near-normal

35.
Ⓐ T Unless severe associated illness and hypercatabolic state
Ⓑ T And calcium gluconate if severe
Ⓒ T Including estimated insensible loss
Ⓓ F Contraindicated in renal impairment
Ⓔ F An indication for urgent renal dialysis

36.
Ⓐ T Removes and replaces one litre of filtrate per hour and facilitates TPN
Ⓑ F Causes less haemodynamic disturbance
Ⓒ F Peritoneal dialysis is technically easier and less traumatic
Ⓓ T But also undertaken intermittently over 3–4 hours per day
Ⓔ F May be more effective than PD

37.
Ⓐ F Creatinine falls even more slowly
Ⓑ F Restriction should be relaxed to improve nutrition
Ⓒ T And often potassium supplementation is also necessary
Ⓓ F Increase fluid intake in parallel with renal losses
Ⓔ F Usually resolves in about 4 weeks

38.
Ⓐ T E.g. renal calculus
Ⓑ F Anuria typically suggests obstruction
Ⓒ F Intervention may avoid dialysis
Ⓓ T Demonstrates obstruction of the renal pelvis or ureter
Ⓔ F Post-obstructive diuresis occurs

39.
Ⓐ T And fever
Ⓑ F Eosinophilia is typical
Ⓒ T And neutrophil or monocytic infiltrate
Ⓓ F Typically resolves
Ⓔ T E.g. penicillin or rifampicin

40.
Ⓐ T Urine stasis and infection
Ⓑ T Or radiotherapy for such cancer
Ⓒ F Haematuria is common in either
Ⓓ T ?aberrant vessel or neuromuscular defect
Ⓔ F Typically painful

41.
Ⓐ T Typically phosphate stones
Ⓑ T Produces osteoporosis and hypercalciuria
Ⓒ F Hyperparathyroidism
Ⓓ T Normocalcaemic hypercalciuria
Ⓔ T Hypercalciuria with or without hypercalcaemia

42.
Ⓐ T Suggests total obstruction
Ⓑ F Acidification with ammonium chloride may benefit
Ⓒ F Decreases urinary calcium excretion by 30% in hypercalciuric patients
Ⓓ F Decreases urinary urate and thereby may reduce oxalate stone formation
Ⓔ F Fragmentation by lithotripsy and endoscopic removal is possible

43.
Ⓐ F Autosomal dominant
Ⓑ T But liver function tests normal
Ⓒ T And hypertension and UTI
Ⓓ F Typically bilateral
Ⓔ T 10% will have a subarachnoid haemorrhage

44.
Ⓐ T Anion gap = plasma $Na^+ - (Cl^- + HCO_3^-)$
Ⓑ T Increased chloride preserves anion gap
Ⓒ T Even in presence of systemic acidosis
Ⓓ F GFR is normal
Ⓔ F No features of uraemia

45.

Ⓐ T And amphotericin
Ⓑ T And vitamin D intoxication
Ⓒ T And SLE
Ⓓ T Also causes proximal type 2 RTA
Ⓔ T And hydronephrosis

46.

Ⓐ T Reduce dose in renal failure
Ⓑ F Contraindicated due to catabolic effect on protein metabolism
Ⓒ T Digoxin toxicity is common given the half-life of 35 hours in health
Ⓓ T Hepatic metabolism but renal excretion of active metabolites
Ⓔ T Check plasma levels daily

47.

Ⓐ T Occurs in 20% and due to increased interleukin release
Ⓑ T Typically osteolytic metastases
Ⓒ T Due to blood clot or direct tumour obstruction of ureter
Ⓓ T Erythropoietin secretion
Ⓔ F Suggests hepatoma

48.

Ⓐ T An atonic bladder
Ⓑ F Suggests spinal cord damage above conus medullaris
Ⓒ F Suggests colovesical fistula or instrumentation
Ⓓ F Suggests pelvic floor muscle weakness
Ⓔ T An anticholinergic effect

49.

Ⓐ F Typically transitional cell
Ⓑ F Painless haematuria is typical
Ⓒ F Radiotherapy is of palliative benefit
Ⓓ F Local spread occurs early and metastases late
Ⓔ T And schistosomiasis

50.

Ⓐ T As may benign prostatic disease
Ⓑ T Or haematuria
Ⓒ F Hard with obliteration of median furrow
Ⓓ T And may involve ureters
Ⓔ F Osteosclerotic metastases

51.

Ⓐ F Aged over 60 years
Ⓑ T Sometimes precipitated by UTI
Ⓒ F Associated with diminished androgen secretion
Ⓓ T Elevation suggests prostatic carcinoma
Ⓔ F Typically symmetrical

52.

Ⓐ F Typically painless
Ⓑ T Helps in the assessment of treatment response
Ⓒ F Haematogenous spread may occur
Ⓓ F Peak incidence aged 25–34 years
Ⓔ T Chemotherapy if widespread disease

12 ENDOCRINE AND METABOLIC DISEASES

1.
- **A F** Dopamine inhibits prolactin release
- **B F** Somatostatin inhibits growth hormone release
- **C T** In vivo significance of effect on prolactin is uncertain
- **D T** Gonadal steroids and inhibin modify GnRH effects
- **E T** Arginine vasopressin also effects ACTH release

2.
- **A T** Prolactin-secreting tumours are the most common
- **B T** May be visualised on CT scanning
- **C F** Usually basophil microadenoma
- **D F** Usually acidophil macroadenoma
- **E T** Other visual field losses may occur

3.
- **A T** Perhaps with prognathism and skull growth
- **B T** Or impaired glucose tolerance
- **C T** And perhaps hepatomegaly
- **D F** Growth hormone levels fail to suppress
- **E T** The skin is thickened with increased sebum production

4.
- **A F** Not usually apparent on plain films
- **B T** Impotence in men
- **C T** Impaired glucose tolerance
- **D F** Plasma cortisol is not suppressed
- **E F** Hypertension and hypokalaemia

5.
- **A T** Physiological pregnancy
- **B T** And metoclopramide, methyldopa
- **C T** TRH is elevated
- **D T**
- **E T**

6.
- **A F** Usually isolated GHRH secretory failure
- **B F** Affects the minority
- **C T** As an isolated abnormality
- **D T** With consequent short stature
- **E F** Puberty not affected

7.
- **A F** May cause gigantism
- **B T** And other chromosomal abnormalities
- **C T** And malnutrition
- **D T** Usually with obesity
- **E F** Primary hypothyroidism

8.
- **A T** Pituitary necrosis (Sheehan's syndrome)
- **B F** Usually microadenoma
- **C T** Usually macroadenoma
- **D T** Rare
- **E T** Acquired hypothalamic damage

9.
- **A F** Aldosterone secretion is maintained
- **B F** There is secondary adrenal insufficiency
- **C T** Impaired LH then FSH secretion
- **D T** There is increased insulin sensitivity
- **E T** With hypoglycaemia and hypothermia

10.
- **A F** Severe hypernatraemia only when water access denied
- **B T** Glucocorticoid insufficiency may mask diabetes insipidus
- **C T** Or secondary to pituitary tumours or sarcoid
- **D F** Carbamazepine stimulates ADH release
- **E T** An effect of long-term overhydration in psychogenic polydipsia

11.
Ⓐ T Used in manic depressive states
Ⓑ T Rarely encountered in clinical practice
Ⓒ T Also inherited in cystinosis
Ⓓ F Chlorpropamide increases renal sensitivity to vasopressin
Ⓔ F Hypokalaemia and hypercalcaemia

12.
Ⓐ T And encephalitis
Ⓑ T Even apparently minor injury
Ⓒ T And pulmonary tuberculosis
Ⓓ T And pancreas, ureter, bladder, prostatic and other malignancies
Ⓔ T As well as carbamazepine, chlorpropamide and others

13.
Ⓐ T Thyroglobulin is synthesized within thyroid cells
Ⓑ F T_4 should be regarded as a pro-hormone
Ⓒ F Bound to thyroxine-binding globulin and also to pre-albumin
Ⓓ T T_4 is deiodinated in liver, muscle and kidney
Ⓔ T Production of reverse T_3 may increase

14.
Ⓐ T With secondary hypothyroidism
Ⓑ F TSH would be elevated
Ⓒ T Free T_4 is normal
Ⓓ T And other acute illness
Ⓔ F Total T_4 increased

15.
Ⓐ F May occur in acute non-thyroidal illness
Ⓑ T Suggests primary hyperthyroidism
Ⓒ F Suggests secondary hypothyroidism
Ⓓ T Suggests autoimmune primary hypothyroidism
Ⓔ F May be seen in pregnancy

16.
Ⓐ T In around 75% of cases
Ⓑ T 15% multinodular, 5% single nodule
Ⓒ T May also cause hypothyroidism
Ⓓ T Goitre is therefore usually present
Ⓔ T And HLA B8 and DR2

17.
Ⓐ T Or persisting resting sinus tachycardia
Ⓑ T Appetite is maintained
Ⓒ F Muscular weakness may occur
Ⓓ T Occasionally with ophthalmoplegia
Ⓔ F Insulin requirements may increase

18.
Ⓐ F Controls ventricular response rate
Ⓑ F Inhibits the iodination of tyrosine
Ⓒ F TSH measurement alone should not guide therapy
Ⓓ F But titres correlate poorly with disease activity
Ⓔ T Especially patients with large goitres

19.
Ⓐ F Suggests treatment — induced hypothyroidism
Ⓑ T 40% in first year — long-term follow-up necessary
Ⓒ F Relapse is uncommon
Ⓓ T In 75% if given a standard dose
Ⓔ F In 25% if given a standard dose

20.
Ⓐ F Radioiodine is better avoided in patients < 40 years of age
Ⓑ F Potassium perchlorate is now avoided — high toxicity
Ⓒ T Beta blockers are useful for symptomatic treatment
Ⓓ T Particularly if a recurrent episode
Ⓔ T Steroids are used in thyroid crisis and severe eye complications

21.
Ⓐ T 15% are rendered permanently hypothyroid at 1 year
Ⓑ T producing dysphonia
Ⓒ T 5–10% develop post-operative hypocalcaemia
Ⓓ T 5% at 1 year
Ⓔ F No known association

22.
Ⓐ F Excessive lacrimation and conjunctivitis are more common
Ⓑ F Ophthalmopathy may precede hyperthyroidism or even follow treatment
Ⓒ F No such test available unfortunately
Ⓓ T Steroids or surgery may be needed in other cases
Ⓔ T Therefore avoid over-treatment of hyperthyroidism if possible

23.
Ⓐ T Both however are non-specific
Ⓑ T And infertility and impotence
Ⓒ T Perhaps due to oedema of the middle ear
Ⓓ T Rarely alopecia, vitiligo and dry hair
Ⓔ F Reflexes preserved with delayed relaxation

24.
Ⓐ F Free T_3 is an unreliable discriminant
Ⓑ T Rarely causing galactorrhoea
Ⓒ T Producing hyponatraemia
Ⓓ F Serum lactate dehydrogenase and creatine kinase may be elevated
Ⓔ T And serum triglyceride levels

25.
Ⓐ F There may be constipation
Ⓑ T But puberty is usually delayed
Ⓒ T May present with short stature
Ⓓ T Epiphyseal closure is delayed
Ⓔ T But a rare occurrence

26.
Ⓐ T Generalised organomegaly can occur
Ⓑ T Usually with hypothyroidism
Ⓒ T Often associated with hypothyroidism
Ⓓ T Usually no treatment required
Ⓔ T With nerve deafness; autosomal recessive

27.
Ⓐ F Goitre may occur at any age
Ⓑ T The most common cause of goitrous hypothyroidism
Ⓒ T Typically deficiency of intrathyroidal peroxidase
Ⓓ F Should suppress the serum TSH
Ⓔ F May be seen in Hashimoto's disease

28.
Ⓐ F The thyroid is typically painful
Ⓑ T Virus-induced thyroid inflammation
Ⓒ F But biochemical evidence of hyperthyroidism is common
Ⓓ T Antibodies in low titre transiently
Ⓔ F Transient hypothyroidism with thyroidal recovery usually

29.
Ⓐ F May cause painful thyroiditis with transient hypothyroidism
Ⓑ T Hypothyroidism if iodine deficiency is severe
Ⓒ F No association
Ⓓ T Secondary hypothyroidism
Ⓔ T E.g. cassava root

30.
Ⓐ F 'Hot' nodules are almost always benign
Ⓑ F Radiotherapy provides brief symptomatic relief only
Ⓒ F Total thyroidectomy, radioiodine and long-term thyroxine
Ⓓ T Papillary tumours are the most common cell type
Ⓔ F Rare despite high calcitonin levels; carcinoid syndrome can occur

31.
Ⓐ F 40% of calcium is protein-bound; normal after correction for serum albumin
Ⓑ F But metabolic alkalosis increases the level of ionised calcium
Ⓒ T Due to bone metastases (often microscopic)
Ⓓ F Decreases serum calcium levels
Ⓔ T Increases vitamin D level production with low PTH levels

32.
- **A** T But 50% are asymptomatic
- **B** F Solitary parathyroid adenoma in 90%
- **C** F A relatively late feature
- **D** T And peptic ulceration and myopathy
- **E** T With characteristic polyuria

33.
- **A** F Phosphate is usually low
- **B** F Increased 1,25 D levels
- **C** T Predisposing to stone formation
- **D** T Indicating osteoblastic activity
- **E** T Chloride is usually elevated

34.
- **A** F Feature of idiopathic hypoparathyroidism
- **B** T Secondary to hyperphosphataemia, hypocalcaemia and low vitamin D levels
- **C** F Diffuse hypertrophy of small glands
- **D** T Tertiary hyperparathyroidism
- **E** T Failure of vitamin D absorption

35.
- **A** F Autosomal dominant
- **B** T
- **C** F Type II
- **D** F Type II
- **E** T

36.
- **A** T Often via production of osteoclast activating factors
- **B** T Undetectable using standard PTH assays
- **C** T Increased vitamin D level production with low PTH levels
- **D** F Hyperthyroidism is a rare cause
- **E** T Increased vitamin D level production with low PTH levels

37.
- **A** T Features of tetany
- **B** T And mouth and oesophagus
- **C** F Features of hypercalcaemia
- **D** T Basal ganglia calcification is typical
- **E** T In prolonged hypocalcaemia

38.
- **A** T Adrenal, thyroid and ovary
- **B** T Presents in infancy
- **C** T Occurs in 1%
- **D** F Calcitonin elevation occasionally causes hypocalcaemia
- **E** F

39.
- **A** T Producing tissue resistance to PTH
- **B** F PTH concentrations rise cf. true hypoparathyroidism
- **C** F Serum phosphate is high
- **D** T And occasionally mental retardation
- **E** F Alfacalcidol treatment

40.
- **A** F Alkalosis reduces the ionised calcium
- **B** F Alkalosis reduces the ionised calcium
- **C** F Alkalosis reduces the ionised calcium
- **D** T Due to sequestration in areas of pancreatic and fat necrosis
- **E** T Vitamin D malabsorption

41.
- **A** T Usually 20 ml of a 10% solution
- **B** F Rendered ineffective by antibody formation
- **C** F Calcitonin may worsen hypocalcaemia
- **D** T But serum calcium must be monitored
- **E** F But indicated in tetany due to hyperventilation alkalosis

42.
- **A** F Principally under control of angiotensin II
- **B** T In the zona reticularis and zona fasciculata respectively
- **C** F Cortisol levels fall to a nadir at around midnight
- **D** F Hypoglycaemia stimulates cortisol release
- **E** T Anti-insulin effects

43.

Ⓐ T 'Pseudo-Cushing's' syndrome due to stress responses

Ⓑ F Pituitary microadenoma or hyperplasia

Ⓒ F Weight loss, pigmentation and metabolic alkalosis

Ⓓ T Non-ACTH-dependent Cushing's

Ⓔ F Mineralocorticoid effects

44.

Ⓐ T Protein catabolism in bone

Ⓑ F Hypertension may occur

Ⓒ T Impotence in men

Ⓓ T Muscle protein catabolism

Ⓔ F Impaired glucose tolerance

45.

Ⓐ F Diurnal pattern of secretion is lost

Ⓑ F Plasma cortisol fails to suppress with dexamethasone

Ⓒ T Sometimes used as a screening test

Ⓓ T Particularly in virilising tumours

Ⓔ F ACTH is undetectable at all times

46.

Ⓐ T Decreases mucosal resistance

Ⓑ T Increased renal sodium reabsorption

Ⓒ T Particularly likely to affect the femoral heads

Ⓓ F Sometimes used to treat severe pseudo-gout

Ⓔ T Typical; causes day-night reversal of biorhythms

47.

Ⓐ F Cf. oedema in patients with secondary hyperaldosteronism

Ⓑ T Rarely hypokalaemic paralysis

Ⓒ T Hypertension and hypokalaemia are characteristic

Ⓓ F NIDDM is however associated with primary hypoadrenalism

Ⓔ F Associated with renin suppression

48.

Ⓐ T Rare cause

Ⓑ T Commonest cause

Ⓒ T Rare

Ⓓ F Both may cause hypercalcaemia

Ⓔ T Now a rare cause

49.

Ⓐ T All features of glucocorticoid insufficiency

Ⓑ F Only new scars become pigmented

Ⓒ T Vitiligo is seen in 10–20%

Ⓓ F Increased insulin sensitivity with hypoglycaemia

Ⓔ T Loss of adrenal androgen

50.

Ⓐ T Especially if caused by an expanding pituitary lesion

Ⓑ T ACTH stimulation cannot distinguish primary from secondary failure

Ⓒ F ACTH levels are not elevated and no autoimmune association

Ⓓ F No mineralocorticoid deficiency

Ⓔ F Replacement therapy should mimic the diurnal rhythm

51.

Ⓐ T Cortisol acetate requires initial hepatic metabolism

Ⓑ F Mineralocorticoid is invariably required

Ⓒ F Patients must increase dose with intercurrent illness

Ⓓ T Pay attention to the underlying precipitant

Ⓔ F 30–40 mg per day usually

52.

Ⓐ T With defective cortisol production; 20% are due to 11-hydroxylase deficiency

Ⓑ T But mineralocorticoids preserved in two thirds

Ⓒ T Unlike females, appear normally virilised and recognition can be delayed

Ⓓ T High levels of androgens

Ⓔ T Increased ACTH secretion

53.

Ⓐ F Measurement of plasma ACTH and an ACTH stimulation test often suffice

Ⓑ T Or if severe hypoglycaemic symptoms develop

Ⓒ T Serious risk of hypoglycaemia-induced complications

Ⓓ T Plasma cortisol at 0800 hrs < 180 nmol/L

Ⓔ F Test of hypothalamic-pituitary-adrenal axis

54.

Ⓐ F Noradrenaline is a precursor of adrenaline

Ⓑ T Catecholamine secretion

Ⓒ F 90% are benign

Ⓓ T Occurs in MEN type II syndrome

Ⓔ F Symptoms worsen due to unopposed alpha-adrenoceptor activity

55.

Ⓐ T Hyperprolactinaemia and testicular dysfunction

Ⓑ T Psychogenic impotence

Ⓒ T Involving internal pudendal artery

Ⓓ T Vascular disease and autonomic neuropathy

Ⓔ T Spinal cord demyelination

56.

Ⓐ T E.g. following severe orchitis

Ⓑ F Maldescended testes in an adult should be removed

Ⓒ T Antisperm antibodies may subsequently destroy sperm

Ⓓ F No treatment is widely effective

Ⓔ F Suggests pituitary/hypothalamic cause

57.

Ⓐ F Serum LH is elevated

Ⓑ F Serum FSH is elevated

Ⓒ T Associated with anosmia

Ⓓ F Testicular damage — hypergonadotrophic

Ⓔ F Altered metabolism of testosterone — hypergonadotrophic

58.

Ⓐ F Adrenal androgen production is spared

Ⓑ F Height is excessive due to failure of epiphyseal fusion

Ⓒ T Testicular atrophy in particular

Ⓓ T Androgen deficiency

Ⓔ T Testosterone withdrawal

59.

Ⓐ T Usually 47,XXY chromosomal composition

Ⓑ T Usually 45,X

Ⓒ T May present with secondary amenorrhoea or premature menopause

Ⓓ T Affects 15% of males with leprosy

Ⓔ T May also be associated with reduced serum gonadotrophins

60.

Ⓐ T Chromosomal abnormalities are rare

Ⓑ T Occurs in the minority

Ⓒ F Sterility follows if bilateral

Ⓓ T Secondary sexual characteristics are preserved

Ⓔ F Testicular descent ensues in 40%

61.

Ⓐ F May cause dysmenorrhoea

Ⓑ T Elevated adrenal androgens

Ⓒ T Distinctive morphological features

Ⓓ T Or other severe systemic disease

Ⓔ T Or other hypothalamic or pituitary problem

62.

Ⓐ T Suppression of GnRH

Ⓑ T Failure of gonadotrophin secretion

Ⓒ T Impotence in men

Ⓓ T Or other severe systemic disease

Ⓔ T Polycystic ovary disease

63.

Ⓐ F Gonadotrophins elevated

Ⓑ F Features of androgen excess

Ⓒ F Osteoporosis develops prematurely

Ⓓ T Due to oestrogen deficiency

Ⓔ F Normal menopause occurs at this age

64.
- **A** T But 50% if NIDDM undetected
- **B** F Converse applies particularly if obese
- **C** F Inheritance is polygenic
- **D** T 70% aged over 50 years in UK
- **E** F 90% of islet cell mass must be destroyed

65.
- **A** T Patchy distribution in pancreas
- **B** T Cross-reactivity of antibodies to bovine serum albumin
- **C** T And anti-insulin antibodies
- **D** T Schmidt's syndrome
- **E** T Coded on the short arm of chromosome 6

66.
- **A** T Hypokalaemic alkalosis impairs insulin secretion
- **B** T Pancreatic fibrosis
- **C** T Conn's syndrome produces an hypokalaemic alkalosis
- **D** T Islet cell destruction
- **E** T Excessive counter-regulatory hormones

67.
- **A** F In contrast to IDDM
- **B** T Cf. 60% concordance in monozygotic twins with IDDM
- **C** F Variable insulin resistance
- **D** T Especially if combined with underactivity
- **E** T In contrast to IDDM

68.
- **A** T Due to osmotic diuresis
- **B** F Catabolism, including glycogenolysis, is increased
- **C** F Increased lipolysis and enhanced ketogenesis
- **D** T Primarily hepatic
- **E** T Intracellular to extracellular fluid shift

69.
- **A** T And increased plasma osmolality
- **B** T Compensatory respiratory alkalosis
- **C** T Thirst and hence intake may be impaired
- **D** T More profound ketogenesis occurs in IDDM
- **E** F Insulin deficiency increases their production only

70.
- **A** F Too insensitive to detect all cases
- **B** F Renal threshold may be high
- **C** T But it should never be assumed to be so
- **D** F 10–20% have serious vascular disease
- **E** T Red cells contain less glucose

71.
- **A** T IDDM or NIDDM may subsequently develop
- **B** T Predisposition to arterial disease remains
- **C** T Or thiazide diuretic therapy
- **D** F Risk of IDDM > 6%
- **E** F Risk of IDDM 36%

72.
- **A** T Or plasma glucose > 11.1 mmol/L
- **B** T Or plasma glucose > 7.8 mmol/L
- **C** F Prolonged restriction impairs glucose tolerance
- **D** T WHO standard test (1985)
- **E** F High levels occur within 120 minutes if gastric emptying is rapid

73.
- **A** F Plasma values are higher than whole blood
- **B** T But specific type of stick used should be checked
- **C** F Positive if > 0.5–1.0 mmol/L
- **D** T Normally distributed about this mean
- **E** F Unrelated to the later development of NIDDM

74.
Ⓐ T   Catabolism and osmotic diuresis
Ⓑ T   Predisposition to infection
Ⓒ T   Particularly in ketosis
Ⓓ T   Small vessel disease and neuropathy
Ⓔ T   Often detected on routine urine testing

75.
Ⓐ F   50% of new diabetics can be controlled on diet alone
Ⓑ T   Higher than that in average UK diet
Ⓒ F   Consume within diet guidelines
Ⓓ T   UK national diet tends to higher proportion of fat
Ⓔ F   Severe calorie restriction cannot be sustained for long

76.
Ⓐ F   Combined treatment may limit weight gain
Ⓑ F   Insulin secretion is stimulated
Ⓒ F   Such an action would produce insulin resistance
Ⓓ T   Thus limiting hyperglycaemia
Ⓔ T   Disulfiram-like reaction

77.
Ⓐ T   Onset of effect = 30 minutes after injection
Ⓑ T   Variably delayed onset of action
Ⓒ F   Often relative insulin resistance
Ⓓ T   But varies in other countries
Ⓔ F   Conversion to human insulin may cause hypoglycaemia

78.
Ⓐ T   Causes and effects of hypoglycaemia should be familiar to patients
Ⓑ T   Insulin resistance may decline
Ⓒ F   Unlikely to achieve good glycaemic control
Ⓓ F   Check every 2–3 months
Ⓔ F   Patients need to check blood glucose levels regularly

79.
Ⓐ T   But 50% of long term IDDM patients have no symptoms
Ⓑ T   Sympathetic nervous system activation
Ⓒ T   Neuroglycopenia
Ⓓ F   But plasma glucose may not parallel CSF glucose levels
Ⓔ T   Nocturnal hypoglycaemia may be difficult to recognise

80.
Ⓐ T   25 g of glucose
Ⓑ T   Because glucagon increases insulin secretion
Ⓒ T   Hypoglycaemia does not occur with biguanides
Ⓓ F   Can recur following initial treatment
Ⓔ F   Long-acting hypoglycaemics cause prolonged hypoglycaemia

81.
Ⓐ F   Volume depletion in ketoacidosis
Ⓑ T   Diminished in ketoacidosis
Ⓒ F   Suggests metabolic acidosis
Ⓓ T   Dehydration in ketoacidosis
Ⓔ F   An insensitive indicator of ketoacidosis

82.
Ⓐ T   Due to ketoacidosis
Ⓑ T   Due to dehydration
Ⓒ F   Skin is typically dry
Ⓓ T   Due to ketosis and dehydration
Ⓔ F   Suggests severe hypoglycaemia

83.
Ⓐ T   50% intracellular + 50% extracellular
Ⓑ T   Chloride deficit similar
Ⓒ F   Picture should be that of an acute metabolic not respiratory acidosis
Ⓓ F   Typically normal or high
Ⓔ T   Even in absence of infection

84.
A F Best replaced by 5–10% dextrose when blood glucose is near normal
B F Give none if K^+ > 5.5 mmol/L
C T Or in severe acidosis — pH < 7.0
D F Dextrose is used to correct ICF depletion and if blood glucose < 15 mmol/L
E T Central venous pressure monitoring may be necessary

85.
A F Photocoagulation is indicated
B F Often the first sign of retinopathy detectable by ophthalmoscopy
C F Regular examination is mandatory
D F Suggests glomerular dysfunction and is a sensitive indicator of microangiopathy
E T Due to cardiac autonomic neuropathy

86.
A T Due to intrauterine death, prematurity and congenital malformation
B F Typically larger than expected
C F Defer delivery to 38–39 weeks or later if possible
D F Insulin is necessary to achieve optimal control
E F Requirements increase in second trimester

87.
A T Minimise risk of intraoperative hypoglycaemia
B F Usual s.c. insulin should be substituted with GKI infusion
C T Observation alone in minor surgery
D F Often higher
E T With 2–4 hourly BM strip measurement

88.
A T Risk of pancreatitis, no atherogenic risk
B T Triglycerides variably abnormal in all except type IIa
C T May be slightly elevated in type V
D T And premature coronary atherosclerosis
E T Rare in comparison to type II

89.
A T And aim for weight reduction to body mass index < 25
B F Particularly in patients with coronary artery disease
C T Especially if refractory to dietary measures
D F Suggests better risk profile
E F Statins have such an effect

90.
A T By definition, blood glucose < 2.5 mmol/L
B T Often overlooked as cause of cerebral symptoms
C F An overnight or 12-hour fast is usually sufficient
D T Early dumping is due to the release of vasoactive amines/hormones
E T Symptoms then relieved by eating

91.
A T Rate-limiting step in biosynthesis of haem
B T Porphobilinogen accumulates
C F Typical of acute porphyria
D F Typical of the non-acute porphyrias
E T Both are hepatic porphyrias

92.
A F Decreased PD enzyme activity levels
B T Until precipitated by drugs or alcohol in some
C T Pain may mimic acute abdomen
D T Marked systemic upset
E F Barbiturates and oral contraceptives typically induce exacerbations

DISEASES OF THE BLOOD

13

1.

A F Bone marrow functional by 11–22 weeks gestation

B T Some migrate to the thymus

C T At birth most of the bone marrow is haemopoietically active

D T Proerythroblast is earliest identifiable red cell precursor

E F Produced by cells in tubules

2.

A F Membrane antigens

B F Reticulocytes stain in this way

C T Required to maintain biconcave morphology

D T Shorter (25–35 days) if measured by chromium labelling

E T By conversion to carbonic acid which then dissociates

3.

A F Two alpha and two gamma

B F Two alpha and two delta

C T Methaemoglobin contains a ferric ion

D T H^+ generated in dissociation buffered by deoxyhaemoglobin

E F Decreased

4.

A T Ranges from 40–70%

B T Around 8 hours in circulation before margination

C F Less nuclear segmentation — a shift to the left in the nuclear segmentation count (Arneth count)

D F Both derive from granulocyte-macrophage colony forming cells

E T Hence high serum vitamin B12 levels in chronic myeloid leukaemia

5.

A F 10 day lifespan

B T By the megakaryocytes

C F Found in red blood cells

D F May increase

E T And coagulation factors

6.

A F Seen in other disorders of haemoglobin synthesis e.g. thalassaemia

B T Residual ribosomal material is stained faintly

C T Sign of dyserythropoiesis

D T And lead poisoning

E T And haemoglobinopathies

7.

A T Average menstrual loss is 30 mg per month

B F Males lose 1 mg per day, females lose 2 mg per day

C T 60–70% resides in the haemoglobin molecule

D F Stored as ferritin

E T Normally about 15% of which is absorbed

8.

A T Microcytosis is the first sign

B T Sometimes poikilocytosis

C F Only in severe anaemia; hypochromia is due to microcytosis

D F Suggests hyposplenism

E T Thrombocytosis suggests active bleeding

9.

Ⓐ F Only if coexistent deficiency demonstrated

Ⓑ F Continue for 3 months to replenish stores

Ⓒ F Unless malabsorption, bleeding or poor compliance

Ⓓ T Rising counts also occur in response to bleeding

Ⓔ F Oral iron is usually effective

10.

Ⓐ F Macrocytic with polychromasia

Ⓑ T Typically a dimorphic red cell population

Ⓒ F Typically macrocytic

Ⓓ T And other haemoglobinopathies

Ⓔ T Or a normochromic normocytic picture

11.

Ⓐ F Typically macrocytic

Ⓑ T Erythropoietin deficiency

Ⓒ F Typically macrocytic

Ⓓ T Protein energy malnutrition

Ⓔ F Rarely may produce vitamin B_{12} deficiency and megaloblastosis

12.

Ⓐ T With megaloblastic marrow

Ⓑ T With polychromasia

Ⓒ T With or without cirrhosis

Ⓓ F Dimorphic, with microcytic population

Ⓔ T But variable red cell morphology

13.

Ⓐ T Commonly due to vitamin B_{12} deficiency

Ⓑ T Shift to the right in the Arneth count

Ⓒ T And red cell fragmentation

Ⓓ F Features of bleeding or haemolysis

Ⓔ F Bilirubinuria is not a feature of any anaemia

14.

Ⓐ F Feature of vitamin B_{12} deficiency only

Ⓑ T Glossitis less common in folate deficiency

Ⓒ T Mild haemolysis

Ⓓ F Features of vitamin B_{12} deficiency

Ⓔ T Partially dependent on underlying cause

15.

Ⓐ F Typically 45–65 years

Ⓑ T Found in 90% and < 50% respectively

Ⓒ T Mild haemolysis occurs

Ⓓ T Associated gastric atrophy

Ⓔ T Failure to correct suggests terminal ileal disease

16.

Ⓐ F Typically elderly patients

Ⓑ T Usually with hypercellular dysplastic marrow

Ⓒ T Normoblasts with interrupted perinuclear iron ring

Ⓓ T Particularly of chromosomes 5 and 7

Ⓔ T Risk is dependent on the precise type of myelodysplastic syndrome

17.

Ⓐ T Sometimes haemolytic anaemia alone

Ⓑ T Or penicillamine

Ⓒ T And other viral infections

Ⓓ T Especially due to vitamin B_{12} deficiency

Ⓔ T Sometimes with sideroblastic marrow change

18.

Ⓐ F Peaks about 30 years of age

Ⓑ F Thrombocytopenia

Ⓒ T Diagnosis cannot be made on peripheral blood film alone

Ⓓ F Splenomegaly occurs in under 10%

Ⓔ T Often with a chronic low-grade haemolysis

19.

Ⓐ F Bilirubin is unconjugated therefore not found in urine
Ⓑ T The latter always indicating intravascular haemolysis
Ⓒ F Decreased serum haptoglobin
Ⓓ T Most is bound to serum haptoglobin
Ⓔ T Often with reticulocytosis

20.

Ⓐ T Red cells are rich in LDH
Ⓑ T But no bilirubinuria
Ⓒ T Specific red cell abnormalities may be present e.g. spherocytes
Ⓓ T Reflects reticulocytosis
Ⓔ T With megaloblastic change if folate deficiency ensues

21.

Ⓐ T Mechanical intravascular haemolysis
Ⓑ T Associated with cold agglutinins
Ⓒ T Low-grade haemolysis
Ⓓ T Severe in blackwater fever
Ⓔ T In G6PD deficiency

22.

Ⓐ T For 5 years at least
Ⓑ F In children, defer as long as possible
Ⓒ F They represent an indication
Ⓓ T Pneumoccal immunisation is advised
Ⓔ F Indicated if severe or recurrent symptoms

23.

Ⓐ T Pigment gallstones
Ⓑ F RBC destruction occurs in the spleen
Ⓒ F Osmotic fragility is increased
Ⓓ T Often in association with parvovirus infection
Ⓔ F Suggests warm autoimmune haemolysis

24.

Ⓐ T Often precipitated by viral infection
Ⓑ F Not until HbF levels fall after the age of 3 months
Ⓒ T And bones and spleen with acute severe pain
Ⓓ F Splenic atrophy and functional hyposplenism
Ⓔ T Pneumococcal septicaemia also a feature

25.

Ⓐ T Decreased PaO_2
Ⓑ T May precipitate infarction crises
Ⓒ T
Ⓓ T Local tissue hypoxia in the bloodless field
Ⓔ T

26.

Ⓐ F Typically hypochromic microcytic
Ⓑ T In the 'major' (homozygous) form
Ⓒ T Due to bone marrow hyperplasia in early life
Ⓓ F Not until HbF synthesis declines
Ⓔ T Particularly in the 'minor' (heterozygous) form

27.

Ⓐ T Not features of increased erythrocyte production
Ⓑ T Suggesting intravascular haemolysis
Ⓒ T With warm or cold antibody
Ⓓ T Warm usually IgG, cold usually IgM
Ⓔ T CLL and lymphoma

28.

Ⓐ F ABO is commoner but milder
Ⓑ F Placental clearance of bilirubin occurs prenatally
Ⓒ T With a marked reticulocytosis (10–50%)
Ⓓ F Rhesus incompatibility is rare in the first pregnancy
Ⓔ T Must be given within 72 hours of delivery if there is a Rhesus incompatibility

29.
Ⓐ F Males over 40 years
Ⓑ T And elevated red cell mass
Ⓒ T But may be asymptomatic
Ⓓ F A feature of chronic myeloid leukaemia
Ⓔ T E.g. increased risk of stroke

30.
Ⓐ T And vitamin B_{12} deficiency
Ⓑ T And sulphonamide therapy
Ⓒ F Only if secondary folate deficiency develops
Ⓓ F Atypical lymphocytosis
Ⓔ T And propylthiouracil therapy

31.
Ⓐ T Often with neutropenia
Ⓑ F Polymorphonuclear leucocytosis
Ⓒ T Non-specific feature of many viral infections
Ⓓ F Non-Hodgkin's lymphoma
Ⓔ T Predominantly small lymphocytes

32.
Ⓐ T Or may be neutropenia in SLE
Ⓑ T And lithium therapy
Ⓒ T Variable, increases at delivery
Ⓓ F Typically lymphocytosis
Ⓔ T And myocardial infarction

33.
Ⓐ T Usually with demonstrable marrow infiltration
Ⓑ T An ominous finding
Ⓒ T And tear-drop poikilocytosis of the RBCs
Ⓓ F Lymphocytosis
Ⓔ T Rare after acute bleeding

34.
Ⓐ T Fever even without underlying infection
Ⓑ T Infection and infiltration contribute
Ⓒ T Particularly purpura
Ⓓ F Normocytic or macrocytic anaemia, with primitive white cells
Ⓔ F Hypercellular with leukaemic blast cells

35.
Ⓐ F Peaks in childhood
Ⓑ F Acute myeloid leukaemia
Ⓒ T About 100% respond cf. 70% with AML; but relapse can be problematic
Ⓓ F Acute myeloid leukaemia
Ⓔ F May complicate myelofibrosis

36.
Ⓐ T Splenomegaly in 90%
Ⓑ T Hyperuricaemia is often asymptomatic
Ⓒ F Atypical feature
Ⓓ T Variable platelet dysfunction
Ⓔ F Median survival 3 years

37.
Ⓐ T On blast transformation, platelet count may fall
Ⓑ T Mean total WCC is 220×10^9/L
Ⓒ T Philadelphia chromosome
Ⓓ F Usually decreased LAP score
Ⓔ T Occurs in 30% in ALL and 70% in AML

38.
Ⓐ F Peak age 65 years
Ⓑ T Typically warm antibody
Ⓒ F Mild organomegaly only
Ⓓ T Bacterial more than viral
Ⓔ F Overall median survival 6 years

39.
Ⓐ F Mild thrombocytopenia with usually normal urate
Ⓑ T Associated paraproteinaemia in 5%
Ⓒ T Total WCC typically $50-200 \times 10^9$/L
Ⓓ T May be associated with haemolysis
Ⓔ F Transformation is rare

40.
Ⓐ F Neither is characteristic
Ⓑ T Mild splenomegaly, generalised lymphadenopathy
Ⓒ F Moderate to massive splenomegaly, no lymphadenopathy
Ⓓ T Usually both mild
Ⓔ F Splenomegaly without lymphadenopathy

41.

Ⓐ F Massive splenomegaly can occur
Ⓑ T Characteristic finding
Ⓒ T In contrast to CML
Ⓓ T Increased cell turnover
Ⓔ F Excess of megakaryocytes

42.

Ⓐ T In males more than females
Ⓑ T 60% have urinary light chain
Ⓒ T Better in younger patients
Ⓓ T Reduction of normal plasma cells causes immunodeficiency
Ⓔ T All of which may be asymptomatic

43.

Ⓐ F Myeloma produces suppression of the other serum immunoglobulins
Ⓑ T A diagnostic prerequisite
Ⓒ T Amyloidosis occurs in 10%
Ⓓ T But the serum paraprotein may be undetectable
Ⓔ T Malignant plasma cell infiltration

44.

Ⓐ T Suggests renal amyloidosis
Ⓑ F High concentration suggests poor prognosis
Ⓒ T And thrombocytopenia
Ⓓ F No prognostic significance
Ⓔ T ADLs are useful indicators

45.

Ⓐ T A pathological hallmark
Ⓑ T Variable in degree
Ⓒ T Characterises 70% of cases
Ⓓ F In contrast to non-Hodgkin's lymphoma
Ⓔ F Usually involved though without palpable splenomegaly

46.

Ⓐ T Usually painless
Ⓑ F Suggests haemolysis
Ⓒ T Lymphopenia suggests poor prognosis
Ⓓ T And fever
Ⓔ T Dependent on staging at presentation

47.

Ⓐ T Also termed 'nodular'
Ⓑ T Typically extra-nodal at diagnosis
Ⓒ T Involves any organ
Ⓓ F 85% are B cell tumours
Ⓔ F The converse is true; prognosis also stage and age dependent

48.

Ⓐ F Measure the fibrinogen level if deficiency is suspected
Ⓑ T The Stuart–Prower factor
Ⓒ T First factor in extrinsic pathway
Ⓓ T Also affects the PTT
Ⓔ T Prothrombin

49.

Ⓐ T May not detect minor fibrinogen (Factor 1) deficiency
Ⓑ F Detected by prothrombin time
Ⓒ T Factor X also influences prothrombin time
Ⓓ F Specific assay to measure
Ⓔ T Initial factors in the intrinsic system

50.

Ⓐ T Initiated by thromboplastin
Ⓑ T An unusual complication
Ⓒ T Endothelial injury
Ⓓ T Exogenous endotoxins
Ⓔ T Commonly bronchial carcinoma

51.

Ⓐ T Microangiopathic platelet destruction
Ⓑ T May be absent in mild cases
Ⓒ F Increased
Ⓓ F Both are prolonged
Ⓔ T Factor 5, 7 and fibrinogen deficiency

52.

Ⓐ F BT is normal but petechial haemorrhages may occur
Ⓑ T Irrespective of its cause
Ⓒ F No vessel wall or platelet defect
Ⓓ F
Ⓔ T Secondary decrease in factor 8 level with a qualitative platelet defect

53.
Ⓐ F A primary vascular defect
Ⓑ T Factor 9 deficiency
Ⓒ F Reduced cutaneous capillary integrity
Ⓓ F Vasculitis without thrombocytopenia
Ⓔ T Factor 8 deficiency

54.
Ⓐ T Prenatal diagnosis is possible
Ⓑ T Usually at age over 6 months
Ⓒ F Only the PTT is prolonged
Ⓓ F Half-life = 12 hours
Ⓔ T DDAVP therapy is useful in some patients

55.
Ⓐ T Endothelial failure to synthesize vWF
Ⓑ T Impaired collagen synthesis impairs capillary support
Ⓒ T Endothelial damage
Ⓓ F Factor 9 deficiency
Ⓔ T Platelet dysfunction may also develop

56.
Ⓐ T E.g. myelofibrosis
Ⓑ T Even in absence of blood loss
Ⓒ F Thrombocytopenia
Ⓓ T With marrow infiltration
Ⓔ T Non-specific inflammatory response

57
Ⓐ T Often with leucopenia
Ⓑ T Primary, or secondary to superimposed infections
Ⓒ T Increased peripheral consumption of platelets
Ⓓ F The platelet count is normal
Ⓔ T Also many cytotoxic agents

58.
Ⓐ T Can therefore be transmitted transplacentally
Ⓑ F Usually young females
Ⓒ T Other clotting tests normal
Ⓓ F Suggests another cause of thrombocytopenia
Ⓔ T Particularly in children

59.
Ⓐ T May present with recurrent spontaneous abortion
Ⓑ T Suspect if resistance to anticoagulation with heparin
Ⓒ T And congestive heart failure
Ⓓ T Associated thrombocytosis
Ⓔ T And myelofibrosis

ONCOLOGY

14

1.
- **Ⓐ F** Ultraviolet light exposure
- **Ⓑ F** Linked to herpes simplex type II infection
- **Ⓒ T** In Africa and in Europe
- **Ⓓ T** And leukaemia and breast cancer
- **Ⓔ T** And lung cancer

2.
- **Ⓐ F** Testicular germ cell tumours
- **Ⓑ T** And testicular germ cell tumours
- **Ⓒ F** Colorectal carcinoma
- **Ⓓ F** As yet, no marker for cervical carcinoma
- **Ⓔ F** Ovarian carcinoma

3.
- **Ⓐ T** Expresses the value of a positive test i.e. the sensitivity
- **Ⓑ T** Expresses the value of a negative test i.e. the specificity
- **Ⓒ T** A limitation in all screening
- **Ⓓ F** Sensitivity
- **Ⓔ F** Specificity

4.
- **Ⓐ F** Small cell carcinoma
- **Ⓑ T** And renal and ovarian carcinoma
- **Ⓒ T** And ovarian and nasopharyngeal carcinoma
- **Ⓓ T** Eaton Lambert syndrome
- **Ⓔ T** And other gastrointestinal malignancy

5.
- **Ⓐ F** Also records the presence or absence of lymph node involvement
- **Ⓑ F** T0 = excised tumour
- **Ⓒ T** And permits assessment of treatment
- **Ⓓ T** Without new lesions appearing
- **Ⓔ F** Indicates disease on just one side of the diaphragm

6.
- **Ⓐ T** And stage IIIE if there was also extra-lymphatic involvement
- **Ⓑ F** Disease would be classified as stage IIE
- **Ⓒ T** Or other diffuse extra-lymphatic involvement
- **Ⓓ F** Classified as stage IISE
- **Ⓔ T** A = asymptomatic

7.
- **Ⓐ T** TX,N0,M0 = occult carcinoma
- **Ⓑ T** Or extension to visceral pleura/partial atelectasis
- **Ⓒ T** Or spread to heart, great vessels, mediastinum
- **Ⓓ F** Peribronchial or ipsilateral hilar
- **Ⓔ T** M1 = metastases present

8.
- **Ⓐ T** Impairing cell reproduction
- **Ⓑ F** 1 Joule per kilogram
- **Ⓒ F** Sealed sources implanted internally
- **Ⓓ F** Low energy radiation (50–100 kVp)
- **Ⓔ F** Hypoxia renders tissue less sensitive to irradiation

9.
- **Ⓐ T** An anti-metabolite
- **Ⓑ F** A plant alkaloid
- **Ⓒ F** An antibiotic anticancer drug (doxorubicin)
- **Ⓓ T** Also BCNU and CCNU
- **Ⓔ T** And transcription

10.
- **Ⓐ F** As different as possible
- **Ⓑ F** Differing modes of action
- **Ⓒ T** Against the treated tumour type
- **Ⓓ T** Or toxicity may limit benefit
- **Ⓔ F** Some reduction from optimal dose may be necessary

11.
- **Ⓐ F** Refractory to chemotherapy
- **Ⓑ F** But life sometimes prolonged
- **Ⓒ T** Also testicular teratoma
- **Ⓓ F** Life sometimes prolonged
- **Ⓔ T** But not non-Hodgkin's lymphoma

12.
- **Ⓐ T** Surgery/radiotherapy are both useful
- **Ⓑ T** Surgery is useful
- **Ⓒ T** Surgery is useful
- **Ⓓ F** Highly sensitive but rarely cured
- **Ⓔ T** Surgery is useful

13.
- **Ⓐ T** Usually reversible
- **Ⓑ F** Usually alkylating agents
- **Ⓒ T** Usually dilated (congestive)
- **Ⓓ F** Bleomycin and busulphan
- **Ⓔ T** Peripheral sensorimotor

14.
- **Ⓐ T** Testosterone suppression
- **Ⓑ T** Suppresses TSH
- **Ⓒ T** Particularly the well-differentiated tumours
- **Ⓓ F** Used in breast carcinoma
- **Ⓔ T** Blocks oestrogen binding

15.
- **Ⓐ F** Should be given regularly
- **Ⓑ T** Affects prostaglandin metabolism
- **Ⓒ F** Diamorphine can also be given in smaller volumes
- **Ⓓ F** Dihydrocodeine is more potent
- **Ⓔ F** Occasionally valuable preterminally

16.
- **Ⓐ T** A benzodiazepine
- **Ⓑ T** Blocks dopaminergic receptors
- **Ⓒ T** 5HT3 receptor antagonist
- **Ⓓ T** Given parenterally with chemotherapy
- **Ⓔ F** Chemotherapeutic agent which causes nausea and vomiting

17.
- **Ⓐ T** Typically with leukaemia
- **Ⓑ T** Impaired excretion of tumour products
- **Ⓒ F** Causes hyperkalaemia
- **Ⓓ T** Controls hyperuricaemia
- **Ⓔ T** And acute renal failure

DISEASES OF CONNECTIVE TISSUES, JOINTS AND BONES

15

1.

ⓐ F Suggests lumbar nerve root compression

ⓑ F Suggests an active inflammatory pathology

ⓒ T Overreaction to examination or stimulation lessened by distraction

ⓓ F Occasionally, serious pathology can occur without physical signs

ⓔ F Suggests inflammatory disease

2.

ⓐ F Typically asymptomatic

ⓑ F A non-specific finding in back pain of many causes

ⓒ F Exercise typically ameliorates pain in sacroiliitis

ⓓ T Especially oil-based contrast media

ⓔ T Most episodes settle within 4 weeks (3% persist more than 3 months)

3.

ⓐ F Flat feet are usually painless

ⓑ F

ⓒ T

ⓓ T Claw feet can be seen in a variety of neurological disorders

ⓔ F Often associated with secondary osteoarthritis of the first MTP joint

4.

ⓐ F A high ESR suggests another diagnosis

ⓑ T Typical of most psychosomatic disorders

ⓒ T

ⓓ F Often very chronic

ⓔ F Multiple tender points are characteristic

5.

ⓐ F Often better during activity

ⓑ F Continuous but aggravated by movement

ⓒ F Loss of normal function may be the only feature

ⓓ F

ⓔ F Typically relieved by rest

6.

ⓐ T Disc prolapse may also produce upper or lower limb neurological signs

ⓑ T Common in tension headache

ⓒ F Suggest cervical radiculopathy

ⓓ F RA typically involves atlanto-axial articulations

ⓔ T

7.

ⓐ T Either alone or associated with central chest pain

ⓑ T With characteristic painful arc on shoulder abduction

ⓒ T Suggests extra-pleural spread or bony metastases

ⓓ T Classically due to diaphragmatic irritation secondary to pleurisy

ⓔ T Due to cervical nerve root compression

8.

ⓐ T As for infraspinatus tendonitis

ⓑ F The bicipital groove may be tender

ⓒ F It suggests acromioclavicular joint disease

ⓓ T 'Frozen shoulder'

ⓔ F Pain worsens on resisted internal rotation

9.
Ⓐ T Significant pain suggests an alternative pathology such as flexor tendon tenosynovitis
Ⓑ T Also associated with knuckle pads, plantar fibromatosis and Peyronie's disease
Ⓒ T Male to female ratio = 4:1
Ⓓ T And in chronic pulmonary diseases
Ⓔ F Significant functional disability may be helped by fasciectomy

10.
Ⓐ F Lumbar disc prolapse predominates
Ⓑ F
Ⓒ F
Ⓓ F Becomes more kyphotic
Ⓔ T

11.
Ⓐ F Age of onset follows a normal distribution (no age group is exempt)
Ⓑ T After the age of 55, affects 5% of women and 2% of men
Ⓒ T In 75% of affected individuals
Ⓓ T
Ⓔ F Large and small joints can be affected

12.
Ⓐ T Especially in patients with nodules and positive rheumatoid factor
Ⓑ F CH50, C3 and C4 levels are low (activation of the classical pathway)
Ⓒ F Characteristic feature is central fibrinoid necrosis
Ⓓ T Nodes are typically non-tender
Ⓔ T Reflects chronic immune stimulation

13.
Ⓐ T Also occur with minimal joint symptoms making diagnosis difficult
Ⓑ F Anaemia is classically normochromic and normocytic
Ⓒ F Anterior uveitis is specifically associated with the seronegative spondyloarthritides
Ⓓ F Modest elevation in platelet count is common
Ⓔ T Most obvious in nodes draining actively inflamed joints

14.
Ⓐ F More suggestive of a seronegative spondyloarthritis such as ankylosing spondylitis
Ⓑ T Characteristic pattern of onset
Ⓒ T Involvement of the proximal interphalangeal and metatarsophalangeal joints respectively
Ⓓ F More suggestive of osteoarthrosis or psoriatic arthritis
Ⓔ T Often not obvious clinically but can produce cord compression

15.
Ⓐ T Due to vasculitis or ulceration of nodules
Ⓑ T The fluid is an exudate not a transudate
Ⓒ T Commonly becomes apparent as unexplained proteinuria
Ⓓ T Due to arteritis of the vasa nervorum, can be sensory, motor or mixed
Ⓔ T Relatively rare (Felty's syndrome)

16.
Ⓐ T Early morning stiffness is a characteristic feature of all inflammatory arthritides
Ⓑ T May be absent at disease onset and is not specific to rheumatoid arthritis
Ⓒ T The usual pattern; in palindromic arthritis flitting episodes are typical
Ⓓ F Scleromalacia is a painless wasting of the sclera unlike the rarer scleritis
Ⓔ F Both features can occur in RA

17.
Ⓐ F Bed rest is of great value and without risk of bony ankylosis
Ⓑ T Reduces joint pain and may reduce contractures
Ⓒ F Not usually iron deficient and reflects disease activity
Ⓓ F Low dose steroids may lessen disease progression with only a small risk of side-effects
Ⓔ F NSAIDs are not disease modifying drugs, unlike gold, penicillamine and immunosuppressants

18.

Ⓐ T 50% of patients respond in 3–6 months

Ⓑ F

Ⓒ T Benefit may not be apparent for 3 months

Ⓓ T Adverse effects are common e.g. proteinuria and marrow suppression

Ⓔ T Reserved for life-threatening or unresponsive disease

19.

Ⓐ T An explosive onset confers a relatively better prognosis

Ⓑ T Especially within 12 months of onset

Ⓒ T Indicates sero-positive disease

Ⓓ T

Ⓔ F The presence of periods of remission is a favourable sign

20.

Ⓐ T

Ⓑ T

Ⓒ T Demonstrable with the Shirmer test

Ⓓ F Female sex predominance

Ⓔ T Not diagnostic of primary Sjögren's syndrome

21.

Ⓐ T Axial joints are usually involved initially, only 10% present with peripheral joint disease

Ⓑ T E.g. the sacroiliac joints, and rare in seropositive arthritides

Ⓒ T Achilles tendonitis

Ⓓ F Typical ocular problem is acute anterior uveitis

Ⓔ F An aortitis usually causing aortic regurgitation

22.

Ⓐ T

Ⓑ F Nodules suggest seropositive arthritis especially RA

Ⓒ T Identical twins homozygous for HLA B27 may however be discordant for the disease

Ⓓ T Klebsiella carry an antigen similar to HLA B27 suggesting a possible aetiology

Ⓔ T Familial aggregation of overlapping seronegative spondyloarthritides

23.

Ⓐ T Producing difficulty standing from a chair or climbing stairs

Ⓑ F Pain may be generalised and severe

Ⓒ T Due to latent tetany

Ⓓ F 1 alpha hydroxycholecalciferol is more effective as renal hydroxylation is impaired

Ⓔ T 'Looser's zones' are translucent bands seen on X-ray

24.

Ⓐ T Due to sacroiliitis and sometimes mistaken for lumbar disc disease

Ⓑ T Lumbar lordosis may be lost in advanced disease

Ⓒ T Due to involvement of the costovertebral joints

Ⓓ T Leading to the 'bamboo spine' appearance

Ⓔ T Involvement of cartilaginous joints is a hallmark of the disease

25.

Ⓐ F Can be invaluable in acute iritis

Ⓑ F In contrast to RA, the patient with AS stiffens with bed rest

Ⓒ F Only to improve symptoms

Ⓓ T Education regarding appropriate back exercises is vital

Ⓔ T As does extra-articular disease

26.

Ⓐ F Conjunctivitis is the classical ocular manifestation

Ⓑ T Causes dysuria, frequency and suprapubic discomfort

Ⓒ F Arthritis is asymmetrical, involving large or small joints

Ⓓ T Similar delay following sexually acquired infections

Ⓔ T Similar to psoriatic skin and nail disease

27.

Ⓐ F Polymorphonuclear leucocytosis is typical in the acute phase

Ⓑ F Occur in only 15% of patients

Ⓒ F Organisms cause the preceding dysenteric illness

Ⓓ F Appear on X-ray as a periostitis

Ⓔ F 10% of patients have chronic active arthritis 20 years after onset

28.

Ⓐ T Occasionally there is no evidence of skin disease at onset

Ⓑ F Occurs in around 7%

Ⓒ T Such as pitting and onycholysis

Ⓓ F Except for patients with arthritis mutilans

Ⓔ F May precipitate an exfoliative reaction

29.

Ⓐ T Occurs in 70%

Ⓑ T Occurs in 15%

Ⓒ T Develops in 40% — may be indistinguishable from ankylosing spondylitis

Ⓓ T Occurs in 15%

Ⓔ T Occurs in 5%

30.

Ⓐ F Either as a primary disorder or in association with some connective tissue diseases

Ⓑ T Rare condition

Ⓒ F An association between coeliac disease and HLA B8 DR3 but not HLA B27

Ⓓ T Arthritis may precede evidence of ulcerative colitis or Crohn's disease

Ⓔ T Suggested by orogenital ulceration and iritis (more common in Japan)

31.

Ⓐ T Transient polyarthritis is commoner in adults 1–7 days after the rash appears

Ⓑ T A major diagnostic criterion (Duckett – Jones criteria)

Ⓒ T

Ⓓ T Purpura, abdominal pain and arthritis suggest H–S vasculitis

Ⓔ T Either a purulent monoarthritis or transient polyarthritis may occur

32.

Ⓐ F Systemic features predominate

Ⓑ T 10% of all juvenile chronic polyarthritis

Ⓒ T Especially if antinuclear factor is positive

Ⓓ T 75% are HLA B27 positive

Ⓔ F Pauciarticular disease (four or less joints affected) predominates

33.

Ⓐ T 50% of patients

Ⓑ T Especially presenting with erythema nodosum

Ⓒ T

Ⓓ T Lyme disease

Ⓔ T Neuropathic (Charcot) joints may be seen

34.
Ⓐ F Usually elevated
Ⓑ T Motor milestones are late and dentition delayed
Ⓒ T Due to hypocalcaemia (anticonvulsant therapy can also cause vitamin D deficiency)
Ⓓ F Potentially reversible although if chronically untreated, will produce limb deformity
Ⓔ F Serum alkaline phosphatase falls and serum calcium rises to normal

35.
Ⓐ F Usually acute, but less so in the elderly or the immunocompromised
Ⓑ T Also occurs after trauma or surgery
Ⓒ F Large joints are most frequently affected
Ⓓ F Haemophilus predominates in children, streptococci and staphylococci in adults
Ⓔ F Early joint aspiration is vital if the diagnosis is not to be delayed

36.
Ⓐ F Commoner in females
Ⓑ T Macular rash may also be seen
Ⓒ T Joint involvement is additive rather than flitting
Ⓓ F Positive in only 20%; always check blood and genital tract cultures
Ⓔ F Unusual

37.
Ⓐ F A rare complication
Ⓑ F X-ray change may be minimal in early infection
Ⓒ T Typically ensues 3–5 years post primary TB
Ⓓ F Synovial biopsy adds to diagnostic yield
Ⓔ F Systemic antituberculous therapy must be given

38.
Ⓐ F African American females are particularly susceptible
Ⓑ F Most commonly in the second and third decades
Ⓒ T Associated with polyclonal B lymphocyte activation
Ⓓ T Genetic factors seem to be of importance in aetiology
Ⓔ T Hormones appear to be important in disease expression

39.
Ⓐ T Not however specific to SLE
Ⓑ T Occurs in at least 50% of patients
Ⓒ F Facial rash is exacerbated or induced by sunlight
Ⓓ F Renal involvement is not infrequent and heralds a poor prognosis
Ⓔ T Especially depression and organic psychosis

40.
Ⓐ T Positive ANA is however found in many other conditions
Ⓑ T High anti-dsDNA titre is highly suggestive of SLE
Ⓒ T Rising titre may precede clinical deterioration
Ⓓ F Low titres are commonly found particularly in the elderly
Ⓔ F There are no autoantibodies of diagnostic value in PAN

41.
Ⓐ F Leucopenia and thrombocytopenia are typical
Ⓑ T Associated with an anti-cardiolipin antibody (antiphospholipid syndrome)
Ⓒ T Positive tests in low titre are however common and diagnostically unhelpful
Ⓓ F Depressed suggesting activation of the classical complement pathway
Ⓔ F Rarely elevated unless coincidental infection is present

42.
- **A** F Typically, cerebral and renal manifestations are absent
- **B** T In drug-induced lupus syndromes
- **C** T
- **D** T
- **E** F

43.
- **A** F NSAIDs may worsen renal function
- **B** T High doses are often used initially, then reduced as much as is possible
- **C** T Especially when combined with immunosuppressant drugs
- **D** T Beware retinal complications
- **E** F Little evidence to suggest that this improves the long-term prognosis

44.
- **A** T Associated with polymyositis
- **B** T
- **C** T Invariably present in this condition
- **D** F Rare
- **E** F Muscle enzymes may be elevated

45.
- **A** T Raynaud's may precede other features by years
- **B** T Gastrointestinal tract is involved in most patients
- **C** T Occurs in the majority
- **D** T 'Sausaging' of the fingers and sclerodactyly are also seen
- **E** F Speckled ANA is found in 50%; anti-DNA antibodies are not seen and complement is normal

46.
- **A** T
- **B** F ANA and RF are often positive
- **C** T
- **D** F Weight loss may occur in the absence of malignancy
- **E** T Cutaneous features suggest dermatomyositis

47.
- **A** T
- **B** T Due to claudication of the masseters
- **C** F Histological involvement is characteristically patchy
- **D** T Due to proximal myopathy
- **E** T

48.
- **A** F This finding would suggest an alternative diagnosis
- **B** F Biopsy is positive in < 40% of patients
- **C** T Absence of such response should prompt a review of the diagnosis
- **D** F Most require steroids for a minimum of 2 years
- **E** F Suggests acute ischaemic optic neuritis due to vasculitis and is a medical emergency

49.
- **A** T Diminished renal excretion of uric acid
- **B** T Increased purine turnover
- **C** T Diminished renal excretion of uric acid
- **D** T Increased purine turnover
- **E** T Diminished renal excretion of uric acid

50.
- **A** T Enzyme induction induces an acute attack
- **B** T Non-articular signs may predominate
- **C** T Onset may be explosively sudden
- **D** F Serum urate is usually elevated but may be normal
- **E** T Urate urolithiasis

51.
- **A** F Uricosuric drugs include probenecid, sulphinpyrazone and the NSAID azapropazone
- **B** F Aspirin may worsen an acute attack by reducing renal urate excretion
- **C** T
- **D** T
- **E** F Hypouricaemic therapy should be delayed unless concomitant colchicine therapy is given

52.
Ⓐ F Crystals are deposited in articular cartilage then shed into the joint space
Ⓑ T
Ⓒ T Hence 'pseudo-gout'
Ⓓ F Characteristic appearances of CPPD crystals under polarising light microscopy
Ⓔ F Such injections are often highly effective

53.
Ⓐ T Often symptomatic
Ⓑ F Females are more severely affected
Ⓒ F Synovial inflammation is mild; proliferation of new bone and cartilage is typical
Ⓓ T Collagen turnover is increased as total collagen declines
Ⓔ F Simple analgesics are equally effective and have fewer adverse effects than NSAIDs

54.
Ⓐ F More suggestive of an inflammatory arthritis such as rheumatoid arthritis
Ⓑ F Typically distal interphalangeal joint involvement
Ⓒ T
Ⓓ T
Ⓔ T

55.
Ⓐ T Male to female ratio = 2:1
Ⓑ T Other viruses, including HIV, have been implicated
Ⓒ F Systemic vasculitis affecting medium sized arteries
Ⓓ T Due to arteritis of the vasa nervorum
Ⓔ T Especially in association with renal involvement

56.
Ⓐ F Onset usually over the age of 60 years
Ⓑ T Increased bone turnover and osteoblast activity
Ⓒ T Skull is frequently involved
Ⓓ F Fractures occur more commonly but usually heal normally
Ⓔ T Rare complication suggested by bony expansion and local pain

57.
Ⓐ F Prostatic secondaries are typically osteosclerotic
Ⓑ F Serum calcium is usually normal
Ⓒ F Asymptomatic disease may be detected coincidentally on X-ray
Ⓓ F Serum alkaline phosphatase is frequently elevated due to osteoblast activation
Ⓔ T Androgen deprivation therapy is of proven value in prostatic cancer

58.
Ⓐ T Rare in later life
Ⓑ F Long bones are typically involved
Ⓒ F Blood-borne metastases occur early
Ⓓ T
Ⓔ F Even with amputation and radiotherapy 5 year survival is < 10%

59.
Ⓐ T Serum alkaline phosphatase may rise if fractures occur
Ⓑ T Accelerated bone loss occurs with oestrogen withdrawal
Ⓒ T Pain only occurs after fracture
Ⓓ F Occurs in states of corticosteroid excess
Ⓔ F Requires 40% of bone mineral content to be lost — hence the need for bone densitometry

60.
Ⓐ T
Ⓑ T
Ⓒ T Typical differential diagnosis
Ⓓ T
Ⓔ F Survival rates should be > 50%

61.
Ⓐ F Most frequently seen in the under 12s but can be seen at any age
Ⓑ T 'Sympathetic' effusion may occur in an adjacent joint
Ⓒ F X-ray changes are often delayed and isotope scan changes usually occur first
Ⓓ F Salmonella osteomyelitis is classically seen in patients with sickle-cell anaemia
Ⓔ F Disc spaces are often involved

62.
Ⓐ F Polymorphonuclear leucocytosis is typical, eosinophilia suggests Churg–Strauss vasculitis
Ⓑ F Raises the suspicion of a connective tissue disorder
Ⓒ T
Ⓓ F Typically normochromic and normocytic
Ⓔ T Renal involvement is common

63.
Ⓐ T Most often occurs in patients < 5 years old
Ⓑ T
Ⓒ F
Ⓓ T Also subcutaneous nodules though occur more often in adults
Ⓔ T Arthritis may be absent on presentation

64.
Ⓐ T Characteristic features
Ⓑ F Flitting arthralgia
Ⓒ F Peak incidence age 6 years — rare after age 15 years
Ⓓ F Infection predates the disorder by 2–3 weeks
Ⓔ F Both may occur but erythema marginatum is typical

65.
Ⓐ T Relapsing pauciarticular large joint involvement
Ⓑ T Small and large joint involvement with hypertrophic spondylosis
Ⓒ T Joint effusions
Ⓓ T Small joint involvement
Ⓔ T Small joint involvement like rheumatoid arthritis

66.
Ⓐ F Adult onset
Ⓑ T Also pelvis and scapula
Ⓒ T
Ⓓ F Loss of bone density with speckled calcification
Ⓔ T

67.
Ⓐ T
Ⓑ T Bone infarcts are common
Ⓒ T Severe osteoporosis
Ⓓ T Multifactorial
Ⓔ T

68.
Ⓐ F Onset usually in the age group 40–50 years
Ⓑ T Also with other connective tissue disorders
Ⓒ F Presents with pain and swelling of the pinna of the ear or nose
Ⓓ F But renal biopsy may show proliferative glomerulonephritis
Ⓔ F No known HLA association

DISEASES OF THE SKIN

16

1.
A T
B T 6% of body weight in health
C F They comprise 90% of epidermal cells
D F These are modified macrophages; keratinocytes synthesise vitamin D
E F Sweat glands are apocrine

2.
A F Papules < 5 mm in diameter
B T Larger than papules
C F Vesicles < 5 mm in diameter
D T They are not palpable
E F Macules are flat, with altered skin colour or texture

3.
A F Less greasy than ointments
B F Generally without emulsifiers
C F Contain finely powdered solids
D T Insoluble powders e.g. calamine lotion
E T Useful to cover larger skin areas

4.
A T There may also be purpura
B T The skin is thin and fragile
C F Systemic absorption can occur
D F Hirsutism may rarely occur
E T Local and systemic immune function may be compromised

5.
A T Epidermal oedema (spongiosis) and epidermal thickening (acanthosis)
B F This is a feature of allergic contact eczema
C F Serum IgE concentrations are elevated
D T The initial eruption occurs at the contact site
E F Occurs only in about one-third of subjects

6.
A F Nickel may cause problems
B T In sticking plasters
C T Due to wool alcohols
D T In clothing or shoes
E F

7.
A T Typically on the elbows, knees and lower back
B T Also a dermal T lymphocyte infiltrate
C T Including surgical wounds (Koebner's phenomenon)
D T Inheritance is probably polygenic
E T Also antimalarial drugs

8.
A F The scalp is frequently involved
B F Usually seen in children
C T Also subungual hyperkeratosis
D T Perhaps mimicking rheumatoid arthritis
E T Axillary folds may be similarly affected

9.
Ⓐ F Irritate these skin areas
Ⓑ T
Ⓒ T Reduce the risk of rapid relapse
Ⓓ F UVA are longwaves
Ⓔ T Or PUVA and methotrexate

10.
Ⓐ T Ducts may be obstructed
Ⓑ T Lesions elsewhere suggest an alternative diagnosis
Ⓒ T Antibiotics are helpful
Ⓓ T Largely hormonally mediated
Ⓔ T Seborrhoea (greasy skin) is often present also

11.
Ⓐ T Also tar, oils and oily cosmetics
Ⓑ T Also associated with late-onset 21-hydroxylase deficiency
Ⓒ T Also associated with androgen-secreting tumours
Ⓓ T
Ⓔ T

12.
Ⓐ T For a minimum of 3 months
Ⓑ T Antibacterials such as chlorhexidine may also help
Ⓒ F Unless given with cyproterone acetate
Ⓓ T Anti-androgen therapy often in combination with an oestrogen
Ⓔ T Reduces sebum secretion; highly teratogenic

13.
Ⓐ F Commonest in middle age
Ⓑ F Sebum secretion is normal
Ⓒ T Comedones are not seen
Ⓓ T
Ⓔ F Repeated courses may be necessary

14.
Ⓐ T But the nails are usually normal
Ⓑ T With hyperkeratosis and basal cell degeneration
Ⓒ T Perhaps with Wickham's striae
Ⓓ F Post-inflammatory pigmentation occurs
Ⓔ F But topical steroids may aid symptoms

15.
Ⓐ T Non-thrombocytopenic purpura
Ⓑ F Small and medium sized vessels are affected
Ⓒ T May be renal involvement
Ⓓ F An oligo-arthritis or mono-arthritis
Ⓔ F Used only for severe cases

16.
Ⓐ T
Ⓑ T Also caused by biliary obstruction
Ⓒ T
Ⓓ T Also caused by chronic renal failure
Ⓔ T

17.
Ⓐ F The rash is non-pruritic
Ⓑ T Usually intensely itchy
Ⓒ T Classically pruritic
Ⓓ F Non-pruritic
Ⓔ T Associated with coeliac disease

18.
Ⓐ T Perhaps with target lesions
Ⓑ T Typically on extensor surfaces
Ⓒ T Tense blood-filled lesions
Ⓓ T Superficial flaccid lesions
Ⓔ F Small scaly raised lesions

19.
Ⓐ T Also molluscum contagiosum
Ⓑ T Often extensive and resistant to nystatin
Ⓒ T Lesion of the tongue due to viral infection ?Epstein–Barr virus
Ⓓ T More common and more severe in AIDS patients
Ⓔ T Pathognomonic and responds to local radiotherapy

20.
Ⓐ T Disordered haem metabolism
Ⓑ T Perhaps progressing to chronic actinic dermatitis
Ⓒ T And also amiodarone and sulphonamides
Ⓓ F Associated with inflammatory bowel disease
Ⓔ F Unaffected by sunlight

21.
A T Or 'bull's eye' lesions
B F The eruption rapidly resolves
C F Classical features of the condition
D T May be severe systemic upset
E T Radiotherapy may precipitate such lesions

22.
A T Also orf and other viruses
B T Classical
C T Also penicillins and barbiturates
D T And other connective tissue disorders
E T And oral contraceptives

23.
A T Lesions are painful
B F Resolve over several weeks leaving bruises
C T Mild systemic upset is typical
D F Suggests an alternative diagnosis
E F More common in younger individuals

24.
A T Also brucellosis
B T Also mycoplasmal and chlamydial infections
C T Also leukaemias and Hodgkin's disease
D T Also leprosy
E T Iodides and sulphonamides

25.
A T Typically Hodgkin's disease or other lymphoma
B T Especially intra-abdominal carcinomas
C T Ovarian, gastric and nasopharyngeal carcinoma
D T Also caused by some chemotherapy
E F Especially common in HIV infection

26.
A F Most appear in early childhood
B F Should raise suspicion of malignancy
C F Not hairy and are macular
D F They are nodular
E F 6% in congenital melanocytic naevi

27.
A T 30–50% develop in this way
B T But smaller lesions may be malignant
C T Typically asymmetrical
D T Risk is also increased with fair skin and blonde hair
E T Characteristically painless

28.
A F Tend to occur in later life
B F Light exposure is not a factor
C T Pedunculated or sessile
D T With variable pigmentation
E F Not pre-malignant

29.
A T Rare in young adults
B F Spread by local invasion
C T Typically on the face or head
D T With a rolled, pearly edge
E F Radiosensitive but surgery is preferred

30.
A T Typically in Caucasians living in equatorial regions
B F Tumour comprises differentiated suprabasal cells
C T Or actinic keratosis on the skin
D F Haematogenous dissemination is rare
E F Radiosensitive but surgery is preferred

31.
A F A feature of iron deficiency
B T Also nail pitting and subungual hyperkeratosis
C T A non-specific sign of hypoalbuminaemia
D F May be associated with trauma
E T Fingernails grow faster than toenails

17 PSYCHIATRY

1.
- **Ⓐ F** Occurs in 15–20%
- **Ⓑ F** 30% of GP consultations
- **Ⓒ T** Predominantly alcohol
- **Ⓓ T** Ranges from 25–40%
- **Ⓔ F** Schizophrenia occurs in 1%

2.
- **Ⓐ T** Rarely, single gene disorder identified
- **Ⓑ T** Especially physical or sexual abuse
- **Ⓒ T** E.g. bereavement, redundancy, retirement.
- **Ⓓ T** Also acute severe physical illness
- **Ⓔ T** Particularly lack of a close relationship

3.
- **Ⓐ T** Including motor retardation
- **Ⓑ T** E.g. suicidal ideation
- **Ⓒ T** Paranoid, grandiose or depressive
- **Ⓓ T** Depersonalisation, illusions and hallucinations
- **Ⓔ T** Concentration, memory and orientation

4.
- **Ⓐ F** Suggests phobic disorder
- **Ⓑ F** Intellect frequently normal
- **Ⓒ F** Suggests affective disorder
- **Ⓓ T** Often with short term memory loss
- **Ⓔ T** Impaired concentration

5.
- **Ⓐ T** Suggestive of psychosis
- **Ⓑ T** Cf. hallucinations
- **Ⓒ T** Suggests psychosis
- **Ⓓ T** Often with derealisation
- **Ⓔ T** Typical pattern in neurosis

6.
- **Ⓐ F** Symptoms can be helped without achieving this
- **Ⓑ T** In treatment of phobias
- **Ⓒ T** With positive and negative reinforcement
- **Ⓓ F** Undertaken in interpretative psychotherapy
- **Ⓔ F** Feature of cognitive therapy

7.
- **Ⓐ F** Undertaken in psychotherapy
- **Ⓑ T** E.g. in depression
- **Ⓒ T** Altering thoughts may alter behaviour
- **Ⓓ T** And development of positive views
- **Ⓔ F** Features of psychotherapy

8.
- **Ⓐ T** May be fluctuant
- **Ⓑ T** May find simple mental arithmetic taxing
- **Ⓒ T** Usually with disorientation in time and place
- **Ⓓ T** Perceptual disturbances
- **Ⓔ T** Apathy in some cases

9.
- **Ⓐ T** Impaired consciousness suggests delirium
- **Ⓑ T** Logical reasoning is impaired
- **Ⓒ F** The converse occurs
- **Ⓓ T** Volition and interest decline
- **Ⓔ T** Mimics depressive illness

10.
- **Ⓐ T** First-rank symptoms
- **Ⓑ T** First-rank symptoms
- **Ⓒ F** Auditory hallucinations are typical
- **Ⓓ T** Or thought withdrawal
- **Ⓔ T** 'Negative' symptoms

11.
- **A** T With stable work record
- **B** F Prominent affective symptoms
- **C** F Normal premorbid personality
- **D** T Especially with precipitating factors
- **E** F Implies poorer outlook

12.
- **A** T But diurnal variation may occur
- **B** T Or early morning wakening
- **C** T 'Anhedonism' — loss of sense of enjoyment
- **D** T Perhaps with other somatic symptoms
- **E** T With delusions of worthlessness

13.
- **A** T With sense of elation or ecstasy
- **B** T With weight loss
- **C** T With pressure of speech
- **D** T Leading to reckless behaviour
- **E** T Conversation may be unsustainable

14.
- **A** F Suggest depression
- **B** T May be seen in affective disorders
- **C** T With irritability
- **D** T Typical somatic symptoms
- **E** F Features of phobic anxiety states

15.
- **A** T Delirium may also occur
- **B** T Exclude biochemically
- **C** T Measure blood glucose
- **D** T EEG may be necessary
- **E** T Rare — measure urinary catecholamines

16.
- **A** F Suggest affective disorder
- **B** T Without obvious precipitant
- **C** T Sometimes with angor animi
- **D** F Suggest psychosis
- **E** T Symptomatic overlap occurs

17.
- **A** F Females
- **B** F Rarely recalled by the patient
- **C** T Agoraphobia, i.e. fear of the market place
- **D** T And other somatic symptoms
- **E** F Only useful in short term control

18.
- **A** T E.g. fear of personal contamination
- **B** T May pass unrecognised by the patient
- **C** F Typically relapsing
- **D** T But may occur in isolation
- **E** T And selective serotonin uptake inhibitors

19.
- **A** F No conscious motivation in hysteria
- **B** T E.g. chest pain, altered bowel habit
- **C** T May be present in up to 50%
- **D** T With relatively few or no physical signs
- **E** T Pseudo-seizures are commonest in epileptic patients

20.
- **A** F Either sex, rarely non-adolescent
- **B** T With avoidance of high calorie foods
- **C** T In contrast to bulimia nervosa
- **D** F Emaciation is unrecognised by the patient
- **E** T And psychosexual retardation

21.
- **A** F Typically post-pubertal
- **B** F Body weight maintained
- **C** T With recurrent bouts of bingeing
- **D** T Or dieting after binges
- **E** F Rarely necessary

22.
- **A** T Tolerance of the effects promotes risk of organ damage
- **B** T Indicating physical dependence
- **C** T At the expense of work or social interests
- **D** F Narrowing of drinking repertoire with a fixed drinking routine
- **E** T Leading to increased consumption

23.
Ⓐ T Occasionally with malabsorption
Ⓑ T Heart failure may occur
Ⓒ T Or asymptomatic hyperuricaemia
Ⓓ T Or cerebellar degeneration
Ⓔ T Or amenorrhoea

24.
Ⓐ T Provoking early morning drinking
Ⓑ T Typically persecutory if auditory
Ⓒ T With acute confusion
Ⓓ F Suggests alcohol dependence
Ⓔ F Suggests Wernicke's encephalopathy

25.
Ⓐ T Perhaps with depersonalisation
Ⓑ T And other perceptual disorders
Ⓒ T Particularly in acute withdrawal
Ⓓ F Affect not typically disturbed
Ⓔ F Agitation rather than retardation

26.
Ⓐ F Older males
Ⓑ F Self-poisoning is frequently parasuicidal
Ⓒ F Suicide note often left and usually a history of previous attempts
Ⓓ T And drug or alcohol abuse
Ⓔ T Or bereavement

27.
Ⓐ T Especially in elderly
Ⓑ T Consider first-line
Ⓒ T Pharmacological response may take weeks
Ⓓ T E.g. cardiac disease
Ⓔ F Psychotherapy or drug therapy

28.
Ⓐ T Central tenet of cognitive therapy
Ⓑ F Life events are invariably viewed negatively by depressed subjects
Ⓒ T Depressed subjects commonly undervalue themselves
Ⓓ T
Ⓔ T The combination is better than either alone

29.
Ⓐ T Hence the extra-pyramidal features of parkinsonism
Ⓑ F These side-effects are due to dopamine receptor blockade
Ⓒ T Thioridazine has even been reported as causing retinitis pigmentosa
Ⓓ F Like gynaecomastia, a typical side-effect of dopamine receptor antagonism
Ⓔ T Serotonin receptor rather than dopamine receptor blockade

30.
Ⓐ T Also have pronounced anti-cholinergic effects including dry mouth and urinary retention
Ⓑ F Effect is often delayed for 3 weeks, unlike the adverse effects
Ⓒ F But fewer side-effects; less cardiotoxic, less sedative and less anti-cholinergic effects
Ⓓ F
Ⓔ T Probably underprescribed for less severe depressive illnesses

31.
Ⓐ F Suggests organic brain disease
Ⓑ T Especially depressive illnesses
Ⓒ F Favours organic brain disorder
Ⓓ T Common precipitants of psychiatric illness
Ⓔ F Strongly suggest organic brain syndrome

32.
Ⓐ T Permits an emergency admission without right of appeal
Ⓑ T For the purpose of assessment and treatment; patient can appeal within 14 days
Ⓒ T In order to retain in hospital; patient has no right of appeal
Ⓓ T Nurse should be RMN status and patient has no right of appeal
Ⓔ F A policeman can detain a person thought to be mentally ill and in need of safety for a 72-hour period of assessment under section 136

DISEASES OF THE NERVOUS SYSTEM

1.
- **Ⓐ T** Typically intermittent
- **Ⓑ T** With dysarthria and dysphagia
- **Ⓒ T** Soft rapid indistinct speech
- **Ⓓ F** Scanning dysarthria
- **Ⓔ F** Expressive dysphasia

2.
- **Ⓐ F** Dysphonia
- **Ⓑ T** Often due to cerebrovascular disease
- **Ⓒ T** 'Scanning' dysarthria
- **Ⓓ T** In addition to dysphonia
- **Ⓔ F** Receptive dysphasia

3.
- **Ⓐ T** Flexor or absent in lower motor neurone lesion
- **Ⓑ T** Segmental level T9–T12
- **Ⓒ T** Lower motor neurone sign
- **Ⓓ T** 'Clasp knife' rigidity is typical
- **Ⓔ T** 'Rossolimo's sign'

4.
- **Ⓐ T** Increased in upper motor neurone lesions
- **Ⓑ T** Disuse atrophy may follow prolonged paralysis from any cause
- **Ⓒ T** With flexor or absent plantar response
- **Ⓓ F** Upper motor neurone sign
- **Ⓔ F** Pattern entirely dependent on site of lesion(s)

5.
- **Ⓐ F** Resting tremor
- **Ⓑ F** 'Lead pipe' or 'cog-wheel' rigidity
- **Ⓒ T** Also other involuntary movements
- **Ⓓ F** Hypothyroidism
- **Ⓔ T** Hypokinesis

6.
- **Ⓐ F** Opposite side
- **Ⓑ F** Decussate below this level
- **Ⓒ T** And temperature sensation
- **Ⓓ F** Lowest segments outermost
- **Ⓔ F** No decussation at this level

7.
- **Ⓐ F** Reflexes preserved
- **Ⓑ T** Sensory or motor
- **Ⓒ T** In upper limbs
- **Ⓓ F** Reflexes preserved
- **Ⓔ T** With sensory ataxia

8.
- **Ⓐ T**
- **Ⓑ T** Finger flexion jerk — C8–T1
- **Ⓒ T** Same as the biceps jerk
- **Ⓓ T**
- **Ⓔ T**

9.
- **Ⓐ T** Parasympathetic innervation impaired
- **Ⓑ T** And incomplete bladder emptying
- **Ⓒ T** Internal sphincter relaxation and detrusor contraction
- **Ⓓ F** Feature of spinal cord lesions
- **Ⓔ T** And internal sphincter contraction

10.
- **Ⓐ T** 'Past pointing'
- **Ⓑ T** With loss of normal rhythm
- **Ⓒ T** Absent at rest
- **Ⓓ F** Hypotonia
- **Ⓔ F** Jerking nystagmus

11.
- **A** T The optic tract runs between optic chiasma and lateral geniculate body
- **B** T Upper fibre damage causes lower field defect
- **C** F Midline lesions cause bitemporal hemianopia
- **D** F Left lateral geniculate body
- **E** F Left monocular visual loss

12.
- **A** F Suggests sixth cranial nerve palsy
- **B** F Occurs in Horner's syndrome
- **C** T Paralysis of levator palpebrae superioris
- **D** T Impaired parasympathetic flow
- **E** T And direct light response impaired

13.
- **A** F Superior oblique
- **B** F No pupillary change
- **C** T May be difficult to detect clinically
- **D** T Head may tilt towards normal side
- **E** F Suggests internuclear ophthalmoplegia

14.
- **A** F Impaired abduction
- **B** F May be a feature of Horner's syndrome
- **C** T Usually bilateral, perhaps other ocular nerves also involved
- **D** T Infarction, haemorrhage or demyelination typically
- **E** T May be 'false localising sign' in raised intracranial pressure

15.
- **A** T Partial or complete ptosis
- **B** T With pupillary dilatation
- **C** T With pupillary constriction
- **D** F Orbicularis oculi may be affected
- **E** F No ptosis occurs

16.
- **A** T Accommodation preserved
- **B** T Defect is probably in the ciliary ganglia
- **C** T An afferent defect
- **D** F Reaction in right eye may be impaired
- **E** T Both pupils may be small but response preserved

17.
- **A** T Ophthalmic and maxillary divisions of fifth nerve
- **B** F Facial pain
- **C** T In cerebello-pontine angle
- **D** T Contralateral to site of loss
- **E** T Unilateral or bilateral

18.
- **A** T Frontalis weakness
- **B** F Decreased due to involvement of nervus intermedius
- **C** T 'Bell's' sign
- **D** F Produces hyperacusis
- **E** T Involvement of the chorda tympani

19.
- **A** T With dysphonia
- **B** T Often with aspiration
- **C** T Particularly in cerebrovascular disease
- **D** F Suggest lower motor neurone lesion twelfth nerve
- **E** F Jaw jerk is typically brisk

20.
- **A** T Test at least twice
- **B** T No response to pain = 1
- **C** T No eye opening =1
- **D** T No speech =1
- **E** T Maximum score =15

21.
- **A** F Dilated and unreactive to light
- **B** T A brain stem reflex
- **C** T 20 ml ice cold water into each ear in turn
- **D** T With $PaCO_2 > 6.7$ KPa
- **E** F All brain stem reflexes absent

22.
Ⓐ T   And other 'primitive reflexes'
Ⓑ F   Suggests a parietal lobe lesion
Ⓒ F   Posterior temporo-parietal lesion (Wernicke's area)
Ⓓ F   Temporal lobe sign
Ⓔ T   Perhaps with antisocial behaviour

23.
Ⓐ T   Contralateral to lesion
Ⓑ T   Non-dominant hemisphere
Ⓒ T   Perhaps with sensory neglect
Ⓓ F   Broca's area in the inferior frontal lobe
Ⓔ T   'Gerstmann's syndrome' of the dominant angular gyral region

24.
Ⓐ F   Suggests more sinister cause for headache
Ⓑ T   Perhaps in polycythaemia rubra vera
Ⓒ T   Central retinal artery occlusion
Ⓓ T   With hypercapnia
Ⓔ F   May cause optic atrophy

25.
Ⓐ T   Maximal on gaze towards lesion if cerebellar disease is unilateral
Ⓑ T   May be more marked in the abducting eye with disruption of the MLB
Ⓒ F   Typically present only when looking away from side of lesion
Ⓓ F   Suggests vestibulocochlear disease
Ⓔ T   Demonstrable using electronystagmography

26.
Ⓐ F   Lancinating paroxysms lasting a few seconds
Ⓑ T   'Trigger areas' may exist
Ⓒ F   No abnormal signs
Ⓓ F   Occurs in elderly subjects
Ⓔ T   E.g. carbamazepine

27.
Ⓐ T   May be disabling
Ⓑ T   Usually unilateral
Ⓒ T   Typically during attacks
Ⓓ F   Suggests benign positional vertigo
Ⓔ F   May delay progression but cannot restore auditory loss

28.
Ⓐ F   Occurs in temporal lobe epilepsy
Ⓑ T   Or other pathology of the VIII nerve
Ⓒ T   Usually associated with vertebral artery ischaemia
Ⓓ T   And other ototoxic drugs
Ⓔ T   With secondary labyrinthine inflammation

29.
Ⓐ F   Bilateral supranuclear lesions cause a spastic tongue
Ⓑ F   But can cause dysarthria, dysphonia and dysphagia
Ⓒ T   Without any sensory involvement from bulbar palsy
Ⓓ T   Invasion of the base of the skull
Ⓔ T   Causes stenosis of hypoglossal canal

30.
Ⓐ T   May follow focal EEG abnormality and symptoms — partial seizures
Ⓑ F   Often absent
Ⓒ F   Usually no obvious abnormality
Ⓓ T   TV or computer games may induce fits
Ⓔ T   Often used during the recording of an EEG

31.
Ⓐ T   With vague irritability or lethargy
Ⓑ F   audible cry may occur at the onset of the tonic phase
Ⓒ T   Tonic phase
Ⓓ T   Clonic phase
Ⓔ T   Variable duration

32.
Ⓐ T   Sometimes with loss of posture
Ⓑ F   Typically in childhood
Ⓒ T   May be detected inter-ictally
Ⓓ T   May not occur until adulthood
Ⓔ F   Rapid recovery although may occur very frequently

33.
Ⓐ T   With automatic movements e.g. lip-smacking
Ⓑ T   May be detailed with graphic descriptions
Ⓒ T   Or jamais vu (unreality)
Ⓓ T   In the minority
Ⓔ F   Todd's paresis suggests focal motor seizures

34.
Ⓐ F   Indicated if rapid recurrence
Ⓑ T   Or 3 years of nocturnal seizures only
Ⓒ T   Unless seizures limited to under 5 years of age
Ⓓ F   Primidone is metabolised to phenobarbitone
Ⓔ T   Monotherapy is preferable

35.
Ⓐ F   Suggests syncope
Ⓑ T   Not specific, especially in elderly
Ⓒ T   A good witness history is vital
Ⓓ F   Suggests vasovagal syncope
Ⓔ T   Can also feature in blackouts due to bradycardias

36.
Ⓐ F   Bradycardia and hypertension
Ⓑ T   And vomiting
Ⓒ T   And coughing
Ⓓ T   And impairment of conscious level
Ⓔ T   'False localising signs'

37.
Ⓐ T   10% of all cerebral tumours
Ⓑ F   40% of all cerebral tumours
Ⓒ T   Cerebellar tumours most frequent
Ⓓ T   Indication for CT scanning
Ⓔ F   Fourth and fifth decade

38.
Ⓐ F   Suggests an optic neuritis
Ⓑ F   Suggests chronic glaucoma
Ⓒ F   Suggests optic neuritis
Ⓓ T   Causes visual impairment
Ⓔ T   Foster–Kennedy syndrome

39.
Ⓐ T   Occurs in 50%
Ⓑ F   Typically post pubertal
Ⓒ F   May become generalised
Ⓓ T   Visual scintillations and also fortification spectra and scotomas
Ⓔ T   Focal deficits may persist > 24 hours

40.
Ⓐ F   Rare paradoxical embolism occurs if there is a right-to-left cardiac shunt
Ⓑ T   Risk dependent on other cardiac factors
Ⓒ T   With left atrial myxoma
Ⓓ T   And cerebral abscess
Ⓔ F   Occasionally if there is atrial fibrillation

41.
Ⓐ T   Usually contralateral motor, sensory, speech disturbance
Ⓑ T   Bilateral events may occur
Ⓒ T   Associated with standing
Ⓓ F   Fixed deficit stroke
Ⓔ F   Slowly progressive typically

42.
Ⓐ F   The optic pathway is only affected by larger lesions
Ⓑ F   Suggests cortical damage
Ⓒ T   Internal capsule lacunae
Ⓓ T   Internal capsule lacunae
Ⓔ T   Account for > 80% of lacunar strokes

43.
Ⓐ T   Headache is not specific to haemorrhage
Ⓑ T   In midbrain haemorrhage
Ⓒ T   With subhyaloid retinal haemorrhage
Ⓓ F   More suggestive of infarction
Ⓔ F   Suggest peripheral VIII nerve lesion

44.
- **A T** Especially pontine lesions
- **B T** With demonstrable III, IV or VI nerve lesion
- **C F** A cortical sign
- **D T** Often with vomiting
- **E T** Central type of jerking nystagmus

45.
- **A T** Worse if coma > 24 hours
- **B T** Early mortality is higher
- **C T** Suggest raised intracranial pressure or brain stem involvement
- **D T** Especially if sustained
- **E T** Functional outcome is worse with strokes of the non-dominant hemisphere

46.
- **A F** Most have no history of trauma
- **B T** Slowly progressive
- **C F** Late-onset epilepsy suggests intracerebral disease
- **D F** Suggests cerebral infarction or haemorrhage
- **E T** And impairment of consciousness

47.
- **A T** Often streptococcal in origin
- **B T** Usually staphylococcal in origin
- **C T** Typically affects the frontal lobe
- **D T** Cerebellar or temporal
- **E T** Typically staphylococcal in origin

48.
- **A F** Usually there is no suggestion of infection
- **B T** Prophylactic anticonvulsants should be considered
- **C T** Raised intracranial pressure
- **D T** With focal hemispheric signs
- **E F** Lumbar puncture may be hazardous

49.
- **A T** And general malaise
- **B T** Fever often low-grade
- **C T** Cranial nerve lesions in 25 % of cases
- **D T** Usual source of infection
- **E F** Lymphocytic meningitis

50.
- **A F** Intrathecal penicillin is both unnecessary and dangerous
- **B T** Covers meningococci, pneumococci and haemophilus
- **C F** Start therapy if the diagnosis is likely given the mortality and morbidity
- **D T** Septicaemic shock often complicates the disease
- **E F** Suggests meningococcaemia

51.
- **A T** Sometimes with encephalitis
- **B T** With subsequent anterior horn cell infection
- **C T** Lymphocytic choriomeningitis
- **D T** Common cause in UK
- **E T** Usually-self limiting

52.
- **A T** Usually no prodrome
- **B T** Occasionally a mild impairment of consciousness
- **C F** Suggests pyogenic infection
- **D F** Other viruses may cause this
- **E T** In 75% of patients

53.
- **A F** Marked post-inflammatory depigmentation may occur
- **B T** Sometimes with dysaesthesia
- **C F** Rarely anterior (motor) ganglia involved
- **D T** Rash follows in 3–4 days; initial diagnosis may be difficult
- **E F** May limit severity and duration of initial illness

54.
- **A T** Neurosyphilis can mimic many conditions
- **B T** Remember HIV infection
- **C T** Secondary syphilis
- **D T** Tabes dorsalis
- **E T** Secondary syphilis

55.
Ⓐ T 'Lightning pains'
Ⓑ T With trophic ulceration and Charcot joints
Ⓒ T And optic atrophy
Ⓓ T Plantar responses may be extensor with tabo-paresis
Ⓔ T Sensory ataxia

56.
Ⓐ F More women are affected
Ⓑ T Different haplotypes in countries outside UK
Ⓒ T Highest prevalence in the UK is in NE Scotland and Shetland
Ⓓ F The converse applies
Ⓔ F Central white matter

57.
Ⓐ F Only 25% have a chronically progressive course
Ⓑ F Rare in childhood
Ⓒ F No extrapyramidal features
Ⓓ T In spinal involvement
Ⓔ F Epilepsy and hemiplegia are unusual

58.
Ⓐ T Can detect clinically silent lesions in 75% of patients
Ⓑ T MRI most sensitive imaging technique
Ⓒ T Occurs in 70–90% of patients between attacks
Ⓓ F Non-specific abnormalities
Ⓔ F Test of lower motor neuronal disease

59.
Ⓐ T Impaired fine finger movements
Ⓑ F May coexist in the elderly
Ⓒ F Resting tremor
Ⓓ T Also 'cog-wheel' rigidity if a tremor is prominent
Ⓔ T And convergence

60.
Ⓐ F Typically arm tremor
Ⓑ T Suggests underlying cerebrovascular disease
Ⓒ T Suggests drug-induced extrapyramidal disease
Ⓓ T Suggests possible multi-system atrophy
Ⓔ F Impairment of upgaze is also common

61.
Ⓐ T Initial illness frequently unrecognised
Ⓑ T Other involuntary movement disorders
Ⓒ T And dementia
Ⓓ T 'Punch drunk' syndrome
Ⓔ T Used in some herbicides

62.
Ⓐ F Principally useful for tremor
Ⓑ F Early introduction means earlier waning of effect
Ⓒ F May be a sign of undertreatment also
Ⓓ F Neuropsychiatric problems are frequent
Ⓔ T Sustained-release preparations sometimes help

63.
Ⓐ F Autosomal dominant
Ⓑ F Onset in middle-aged subjects
Ⓒ F May help chorea
Ⓓ T But becomes generalised
Ⓔ F Suggests Friedreich's ataxia

64.
Ⓐ T Prevalence of 4 per 100 000
Ⓑ T Typically with absent reflexes
Ⓒ T Particularly tongue fasciculation
Ⓓ T Or in the upper limbs
Ⓔ T Or in the lower limbs

65.
Ⓐ T But no sensory signs in MND
Ⓑ T Look for evidence of diabetes mellitus
Ⓒ T Treatment may limit progression
Ⓓ T Protean manifestations of a number of tumours
Ⓔ T Check syphilis serology

66.
- **Ⓐ F** Changes are usually degenerative and non-specific
- **Ⓑ T** Follows the distribution of nerve root(s)
- **Ⓒ T** Only if due to disc prolapse or destructive pathology
- **Ⓓ T** Or C5–C7 involvement with appropriate reflex loss
- **Ⓔ F** Conservative management is usually adequate

67.
- **Ⓐ T** Usually extradural deposits
- **Ⓑ F** Typically elevated with xanthochromia (Froin's syndrome)
- **Ⓒ T** Pain may follow nerve root distribution
- **Ⓓ F** A late feature
- **Ⓔ T** MRI now invaluable

68.
- **Ⓐ T** Important to remember if spinal investigations are normal
- **Ⓑ T** Rare in UK in this severity
- **Ⓒ T** With vertebral collapse = Pott's disease
- **Ⓓ T** Sudden onset typically
- **Ⓔ T** Intradural pathology accounts for 20% cases of cord compression

69.
- **Ⓐ T** Spinothalamic tracts decussate after entering the spinal cord
- **Ⓑ T** Dorsal column involvement
- **Ⓒ T** Pyramidal tract involvement
- **Ⓓ F** No contralateral pyramidal signs
- **Ⓔ F** Ipsilateral dermatomal sensory changes

70.
- **Ⓐ T** Guided by sensitivities of colonising organisms
- **Ⓑ F** Immobility in itself predisposes to sore formation
- **Ⓒ F** Intermittent catheterisation is usually preferable
- **Ⓓ F** Good posturing and passive movement can minimise risk
- **Ⓔ T** Manual evacuation may be necessary

71.
- **Ⓐ T** Onset in third or fourth decade
- **Ⓑ T** Leading to trophic ulceration
- **Ⓒ T** Damage to anterior horn cells
- **Ⓓ T** A common early feature
- **Ⓔ T** Pyramidal tract damage

72.
- **Ⓐ T** Central and peripheral forms occur
- **Ⓑ T** And axillary skin freckling
- **Ⓒ T** E.g. phaeochromocytoma
- **Ⓓ T** At almost any site
- **Ⓔ T** Acoustic neuroma

73.
- **Ⓐ F** Causes peripheral neuropathy
- **Ⓑ T** Typically bilateral and associated with abnormal cyanide metabolism
- **Ⓒ T** Often reversible
- **Ⓓ T** Pyramidal tract degeneration
- **Ⓔ T** Proprioceptive loss due to dorsal column disease (SACD)

74.
- **Ⓐ F** Often develops or worsens with pregnancy
- **Ⓑ F** Supplied by the ulnar nerve
- **Ⓒ T** Radiates up the arm even to the shoulder
- **Ⓓ T** Compression of the tunnel
- **Ⓔ T** And previous wrist fracture

75.
- **Ⓐ T** Usually arthropathy apparent
- **Ⓑ T** Check chest X-ray and tuberculin test
- **Ⓒ T** Occurs in 40–50%
- **Ⓓ T** Check GTT
- **Ⓔ T** Vasculitis of the vasa nervora

76.
- **Ⓐ T** Typically sensory
- **Ⓑ T** Or mononeuritis multiplex
- **Ⓒ T** Also folate and vitamin A and E deficiency
- **Ⓓ T** And amiodarone
- **Ⓔ T** And myxoedema

77.

A T Look for haematological clues
B F Motor weakness predominates
C T Also autonomic neuropathy with local sympathetic neural dysfunction
D F The VII nerve especially is commonly involved in neurosarcoid
E T Suggests autonomic involvement

78.

A T suggests lead poisoning
B T Suggests B_{12} or folate deficiency
C T But SIADH has many causes other than small cell bronchial carcinoma
D F Wilson's disease does not cause a peripheral neuropathy
E F Not associated with a peripheral neuropathy

79.

A T 1–4 weeks, usually after viral infection
B T Paraesthesiae spread proximally
C T Muscle wasting is usually absent
D F Cranial nerves involved in 30–40%
E F CSF protein is elevated, cell count is normal

80.

A F Compression of the lateral cutaneous nerve of thigh
B F Look for an endocrine abnormality
C T A common non-metastatic syndrome
D T May be rapid in onset
E T 'Eaton–Lambert' syndrome

81.

A F Dysphonia, dysarthria and dysphagia
B T 80% have ACh receptor antibodies
C T especially occurs in females more than males
D F Only in chronic severe cases
E T Often more marked in the evenings or following exercise

82.

A T 'Cholinergic crisis'
B F Best given every 3–6 hours
C T Unless disease established for more than 7 years
D T Initiation of therapy is best undertaken in hospital
E T Even after the thymoma is removed

83.

A T As late as 10 years of age
B T With preserved tendon reflexes
C T Characteristic finding — Gower's sign
D F Serum CK is raised from birth
E T Often before the age of 20 years

84.

A T Resolves with treatment
B F Causes a variety of different peripheral nerve disorders
C T Also caused by corticosteroid treatment
D F Causes a peripheral neuropathy and spinal cord degeneration
E T Often with a peripheral neuropathy

GERIATRIC MEDICINE

19

1.
- **A** F Bone mass declines (osteoporosis) but mineralisation is normal
- **B** T Presbyacusis
- **C** F Sensitivity decreases; glucose tolerance declines
- **D** T One of many reasons for increased risk of falls
- **E** T May contribute to increase in autoimmune disease

2.
- **A** F Opiates can induce urinary retention directly and via constipating effect
- **B** T Blocks muscarinic cholinergic receptors and reduces detrusor instability
- **C** T Faecal impaction may cause overflow urinary incontinence
- **D** T Used topically to ameliorate atrophic vaginitis
- **E** T Selective alpha₁-adrenoceptor blocker useful in benign prostatic hypertrophy

3.
- **A** F Lean body mass decreases
- **B** T With decreased levels of fat-soluble drugs
- **C** T Increased activity of protein-bound drugs
- **D** T Increased initial level of some drugs
- **E** T E.g. benzodiazepine

4.
- **A** F Only 5% of subjects > 75 years have dementia
- **B** T 90% can dress
- **C** T In contrast to the hospitalised frail elderly
- **D** F 80% of subjects aged > 75 years
- **E** T

5.
- **A** F Decreased below normal of 4°C
- **B** T Young can detect 1° C change cf. the elderly who can only detect changes > 2°C
- **C** T Metabolic heat production is 50% < the young
- **D** F Shivering stops when core temperature < 32 degrees C
- **E** T Due to haemoconcentration

6.
- **A** F Increased step length variability
- **B** T A slower gait
- **C** T A broader-based gait
- **D** F Shorter steps
- **E** T Sway exhibits gender differences at all ages

7.
- **A** T With nocturia and urgency
- **B** T Due to retention and overflow
- **C** T Alzheimer's disease or multi-infarct dementia
- **D** T Sometimes improved by topical oestrogens
- **E** T With retention of urine

8.
- **A** T Reduced drug doses are frequently necessary
- **B** F But contribute to at least 10–15% of admissions
- **C** F Cardiovascular and CNS preparations
- **D** F More likely with drugs that have a low therapeutic index e.g. anticoagulants
- **E** F Poor compliance and inappropriate prescribing are major problems

20 ACUTE POISONING

1.
A F V_d = drug dose given i.v. ÷ plasma drug concentration at time zero
B F Exponential decline in drug concentration after giving the drug i.v.
C F Volume of plasma cleared of drug per unit time; Cl = dose ÷ AUC
D F Pre-systemic elimination of drugs by the liver or lungs after gut absorption
E F Amount of drug reaching the circulation when by any route other than i.v.

2.
A T Definition of drug half life
B F Half life of elimination; drug half life is measured during steady state
C T Elimination rate constant (K) = natural logarithm of 2 ÷ drug half life
D F Measured as ratio of plasma drug concentrations after i.v. and oral administration
E T Other factors oppose passive diffusion when drugs are in an ionised state

3.
A T Both sensations delay gastric emptying and hence drug absorption
B T Can be increased to 30% using a spacer device
C T Hence value in administration of nitrates in angina
D F Passes through the liver and lungs before entering systemic circulation
E F No significant quantity of any drug is absorbed through the gastric mucosa

4.
A T Drugs like propranolol also reach the plasma in chylomicrons via the thoracic duct
B F Increases bioavailability due to impaired first pass hepatic metabolism
C F Ionised drugs are less affected by the serum protein concentration
D T 'Grey baby syndrome' in neonates
E F Reduces gut flora and enterohepatic recirculation of the drug lowering drug levels

5.
A T And 6-mercaptopurine necessitating a reduction in dose of these cytotoxic drugs
B T Anti-cholinergic effect
C T Similar problem with quinidine and amiodarone
D F Increased effect due to inhibition of renal tubular secretion of methotrexate
E T Use a barrier method as well in patients on the 'Pill' and taking antibiotics

6.
A F Hepatic enzyme induction
B T Also erythromycin
C T Also fluconazole
D T Also isoniazid
E T Also rifampicin